CORE TOPICS IN CARDIAC ANAESTHESIA

For Nigel, Rebecca and Alexander Eastwood who were taken too soon

CORE TOPICS IN CARDIAC ANAESTHESIA

Edited by

Jonathan H. Mackay MRCP FRCA
Consultant Anaesthetist
Papworth Hospital
Cambridge

Joseph E. Arrowsmith MD FRCP FRCA
Consultant Anaesthetist
Papworth Hospital
Cambridge

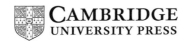
CAMBRIDGE
UNIVERSITY PRESS

CAMBRIDGE UNIVERSITY PRESS
Cambridge, New York, Melbourne, Madrid, Cape Town, Singapore, São Paulo

Cambridge University Press
The Edinburgh Building, Cambridge CB2 2RU, UK

Published in the United States of America by Cambridge University Press, New York

www.cambridge.org
Information on this title: www.cambridge.org/9780521868419

First published 2004
Reprinted by Cambridge University Press 2006

Printed in the United Kingdom at the University Press, Cambridge

A catalogue record for this publication is available from the British Library

ISBN-13 978-0-521-868419 paperback
ISBN-10 0-521-868416 hardback

CONTENTS

CONTRIBUTORS

Joseph E. Arrowsmith
Consultant Anaesthetist
Papworth Hospital
Cambridge, UK

Matthew Barnard
Consultant Anaesthetist
The Heart Hospital
London, UK

David J. Barron
Consultant Surgeon
Birmingham Children's Hospital
Birmingham, UK

John V. Booth
Assistant Professor of Anesthesiology
Duke University Medical Center
Durham, North Carolina, USA

Jonathan Byrne
Department of Cardiology
Guy's, King's and St Thomas's Hospitals
London, UK

Anne M. Campbell
Consultant Anaesthetist
The Heart Hospital
London, UK

Jim A. Chandler
Anaesthetic Specialist Registrar
Papworth Hospital
Cambridge, UK

Alan M. Cohen
Consultant Anaesthetist
Bristol Royal Infirmary
Bristol, UK

Andrew Cohen
Anaesthetic Specialist Registrar
North Thames
London, UK

Simon Colah
Cambridge Perfusion Services
Cambridge, UK

David J. Daly
Consultant Anaesthetist
The Alfred Hospital
Melbourne, Australia

Ian M. Davies
Consultant Anaesthetist
Bristol Royal Infirmary
Bristol, UK

Ravi J. De Silva
Surgical Specialist Registrar
Papworth Hospital
Cambridge, UK

David J.R. Duthie
Consultant Anaesthetist
Leeds General Infirmary
Leeds, UK

Florian Falter
Consultant Anaesthetist
Papworth Hospital
Cambridge, UK

Juliet E. Foweraker
Consultant Microbiologist
Papworth Hospital
Cambridge, UK

Andrew I. Gardner
Consultant Anaesthetist
Sir Charles Gairdner Hospital
Perth, Australia

Sunit Ghosh
Consultant Anaesthetist
Papworth Hospital
Cambridge, UK

David Gifford
Cambridge Perfusion Services
Cambridge, UK

Martin J. Goddard
Consultant Pathologist
Papworth Hospital
Cambridge, UK

Andrew A. Grace
Consultant Cardiologist
Papworth Hospital
Cambridge, UK

Jon Graham
Clinical Fellow in Anaesthesia
Austin and Repatriation Medical Centre
Melbourne, Australia

Stephen J. Gray
Consultant Anaesthetist
Papworth Hospital
Cambridge, UK

Kenneth Grixti
Consultant Anaesthetist
St Lukes Hospital
Gwardamangia, Malta

Roger M.O. Hall
Consultant Anaesthetist
Papworth Hospital
Cambridge, UK

Ian Hardy
Consultant Anaesthetist
Papworth Hospital
Cambridge, UK

David P. Jenkins
Consultant Surgeon
Papworth Hospital
Cambridge, UK

William E. Johnston
Professor and Chairman
Department of Anesthesiology
University of Texas
Southwestern Medical Center
Dallas, USA

Purna R. Joshi
Associate Professor of Anaesthesia
Tribhuvan University Hospital
Kathmandu, Nepal

John D. Kneeshaw
Consultant Anaesthetist
Papworth Hospital
Cambridge, UK

Andrew C. Knowles
Consultant Anaesthetist
Royal Victoria Hospital
Blackpool, UK

Marcella J.T. Lanzinger
Assistant Clinical Professor of Anesthesiology
Duke University Medical Center
Durham, North Carolina, USA

Trevor W.R. Lee
Assistant Professor of Anaesthesia
St Boniface Hospital
Winnipeg, Canada

A. Timothy Lovell
Consultant Anaesthetist
Bristol Royal Infirmary
Bristol, UK

Philip MacCarthy
Consultant Cardiologist
King's Hospital
London, UK

Jonathan H. Mackay
Consultant Anaesthetist
Papworth Hospital
Cambridge, UK

Jonathan B. Mark
Professor of Anesthesiology
Duke University Medical Center
Veterans Affairs Medical Center
Durham, North Carolina, USA

William T. McBride
Consultant Anaesthetist
Royal Victoria Hospital
Belfast, UK

Kenneth H. McKinlay
Fellow in Cardiothoracic Anesthesiology
Duke University Medical Center
Durham, North Carolina, USA

Sonia L. Misso
Consultant Anaesthetist
Prince Charles Hospital
Brisbane, Australia

Colin S. Moore
Anaesthetic Specialist Registrar
Edinburgh Royal Infirmary
Edinburgh, UK

Kevin P. Morris
Consultant Paediatric Intensivist
Birmingham Children's Hospital
Birmingham, UK

Bala Murali
Consultant Anaesthetist
University of North Staffordshire Hospital
Stoke on Trent, UK

Monty G. Mythen
Professor of Anaesthesia
University College Hospitals
London, UK

Samer A.M. Nashef
Consultant Surgeon
Papworth Hospital
Cambridge, UK

Mihai V. Podgoreanu
Assistant Professor of Anesthesiology
Duke University Medical Center
Durham, North Carolina, USA

Mahesh Prabhu
Consultant Anaesthetist
Freeman Hospital
Newcastle upon Tyne, UK

M. Krishna Prasad
Consultant Anaesthetist
Global Hospitals
Hyderabad, India

C. Ramaswamy Rajmohan
Anaesthetic Specialist Registrar
Papworth Hospital
Cambridge, UK

Fiona E. Reynolds
Consultant Anaesthetist
Birmingham Children's Hospital
Birmingham, UK

Maura Screaton
Critical Care Practitioner
Papworth Hospital
Cambridge, UK

Cait P. Searl
Consultant Anaesthetist
Freeman Hospital
Newcastle upon Tyne, UK

Roslyn O. Shaw
Consultant Anaesthetist
Brisbane, Australia

Julian Skoyles
Consultant Anaesthetist
City Hospital
Nottingham, UK

Jon H. Smith
Consultant Anaesthetist
Freeman Hospital
Newcastle upon Tyne, UK

Emma J.S. Taylor
Consultant Anaesthetist
Guy's and St Thomas's Hospitals
London, UK

Alain Vuylsteke
Consultant Anaesthetist
Papworth Hospital
Cambridge, UK

Isabeau A. Walker
Consultant Anaesthetist
Great Ormond Street Hospital
London, UK

Jon J. Walton
Visiting Instructor
Department of Anesthesiology
University of Michigan
Ann Arbor, Michigan, USA

Francis C. Wells
Consultant Surgeon
Papworth Hospital
Cambridge, UK

Dan W. Wheeler
Clinical Lecturer
University Department of Anaesthetics
Cambridge University
Cambridge, UK

Paul A. White
Clinical Scientist
Papworth Hospital
Cambridge, UK

PREFACE

This book is primarily aimed at anaesthetic trainees in the first 3–6 months of subspecialty training in cardiac anaesthesia and critical care. It is our response to the many trainees who have regularly asked us to recommend a small textbook on cardiac anaesthesia.

We realise that it is impossible to produce a truly comprehensive review of cardiac anaesthesia in ~120,000 words but hope that this book provides a sound grounding in all of the core topics. The content of this book has been very much guided by The Royal College of Anaesthetists' *CCST in Anaesthesia* manual, The Society of Cardiovascular Anesthesiologists' *Program Requirements for Resident Education*, and recent examination papers from the United Kingdom, North America and Australasia.

Our instructions to contributing authors and editorial aims were simple; produce a concise yet comprehensive overview of the subject emphasising pathophysiology, basic scientific principles and the key elements of practice. We hope that the use of a presentation format that relies on figures and tables in preference to text will aid comprehension and recall. We have endeavoured to avoid repetition of information, long lists of references and institutional bias. We trust that the curious trainee will turn to the larger textbooks and the Internet for more detailed discussions and exhaustive literature reviews. Finally, we hope that many sections of this book will also appeal to those preparing trainees for examinations and to clinical nurse specialists working in the field of cardiothoracic intensive care.

We would like to thank all of those who have made the publication of this volume possible; our international panel of contributors for taking the time to share their knowledge and expertise; Gill Clark and Gavin Smith of Greenwich Medical Media for their encouragement, advice and patience; and our Specialist Registrars for their advice and proof reading. Last, we wish to thank our families for their willing, and occasionally unwilling, support during this enterprise.

Jon Mackay
Joe Arrowsmith
January 2004

FOREWORD

Cardiac anaesthesia brings many divergent disciplines into one unifying practice, making it one of the most complex anaesthetic subspecialties. It requires an understanding of pathology, physiology, pharmacology, internal medicine, cardiology, cardiac surgery and intensive care. The ever-expanding nature of the specialty presents considerable challenges for both the everyday practitioner and the trainee – for whom this text is particularly targeted.

In this day and age, when a vast amount of information is already available both in print and on-line, one may be forgiven for questioning the need for yet another printed textbook. By way of an answer, the Editors (both of whom have worked in the UK and the USA) have produced a textbook (rather than a *cookbook*) that addresses a relatively unfulfilled need—a source that is specifically directed towards those who represent the future of our specialty. By incorporating contributions from authors from many countries, the Editors have largely avoided national and institutional bias.

Today's anaesthetic trainees are confronted with the seemingly impossible task of assimilating, understanding and memorizing an almost infinite body of information. Those who succeed in this task are invariably those who can confidently identify core principles without getting distracted by minute details. The Editors never intended to produce an exhaustive reference and the need to consult other sources of detailed information has, therefore, not been completely eliminated. This book does, however, provide the trainee with a very convenient framework onto which further knowledge can be added as it is acquired. The manner in which the authors have organized and presented information in this book should help the reader to more quickly see the 'bigger picture' and appreciate the subtleties of cardiac anaesthesia.

Hilary P. Grocott, MD, FRCPC
Associate Professor of Anesthesiology

Mark F. Newman, MD
Merel H. Harmel Chair and Professor of Anesthesiology

Duke University, Durham, NC, USA

ABBREVIATIONS

A

2D	Two-dimensional
AAA	Abdominal aortic aneurysm
ABG	**Arterial blood gas**
ACA	Anterior cerebral artery
ACC	American College of Cardiologists
ACE	**Angiotensin converting enzyme**
ACEI	Angiotensin converting enzyme inhibitor
ACh	Acetylcholine
ACoA	Anterior communicating (cerebral) artery
ACP	American College of Physicians
ACS	Acute coronary syndrome(s)
ACT	**Activated clotting time**
ACTH	Adrenocorticotrophic hormone
ADP	Adenosine diphosphate
AECC	American-European Consensus Conference
AED	Automatic external defibrillator
AEP	Auditory evoked potential
AF	**Atrial fibrillation**
AHA	American Heart Association
ALI	Acute lung injury
ALS	Advanced life support
AMP	Adenosine monophosphate
ANH	Acute normovolaemic haemodilution
ANP	Atrial natriuritic peptide
ANS	Autonomic nervous system
AP	Action potential
APB	Atrial premature (ectopic) beat
APC	Activated protein C
APL	Antiphospholipid
APOE	Apolipoprotein E
APTT	**Activated partial thromboplastin time**
AR	**Aortic regurgitation (incompetence)**
ARDS	**Acute respiratory distress syndrome**
ARF	**Acute renal failure**
AS	**Aortic stenosis**
ASA	**American Society of Anesthesiologists**
ASD	**Atrial septal defect**
AT	Antithrombin / Atrial tachycardia
AT-I	Angiotensin I

AT-II	Angiotensin II
ATP	Adenosine triphosphate
AV	**Aortic valve**
A-V	Atrioventricular
AVN	Atrioventricular node
AVR	**Aortic valve replacement**
AVSD	Atrioventricular septal defect
AXC	**Aortic cross clamp**

B

BA	Basilar artery
BAER	Brainstem auditory evoked response
BBB	Bundle branch block
BCPS	Bidirection cavopulmonary shunt
BIS	Bispectral (index)
BiVAD	Biventricular assist device
BLS	Basic life support
BNF	**British National Formulary**
BP	**Blood pressure**
BPEG	British Pacing and Electrophysiology Group
BSAC	British Society for Antimicrobial Chemotherapy
βTG	β-thromboglobulin
B-T	Blalock-Taussig (shunt)

C

CABG	**Coronary artery bypass graft**
CAD	Coronary artery disease
cAMP	Cyclic adenosine monophosphate
CASS	Coronary Artery Surgery Study
cAVSD	Complete atrioventricular septal defect
CBF	Cerebral blood flow
CBFV	Cerebral blood flow velocity
CCS	**Canadian Cardiovascular Society**
CCU	Critical/coronary care unit
CFAM	Cerebral function analysing monitor
CFD	Colour-flow Doppler
CFM	Cerebral function monitor
cGMP	Cyclic guanosine monophosphate
CHB	Complete (third degree) heart block
CHD	Congenital heart disease
CI	**Cardiac index**

CK–MB	Creatinine kinase MB (isoenzyme)
$CMRO_2$	Cerebral metabolic rate (for oxygen)
CNS	**Central nervous system**
CO	**Cardiac output**
CoA	Coarctation of the aorta
COPD	Chronic obstructive pulmonary disease
CPAP	Continuous positive airway pressure
CPB	**Cardiopulmonary bypass**
CP	Cavo pulmonary
CPP	Cerebral perfusion pressure
CPR	**Cardiopulmonary resuscitation**
CRI	Cardiac risk index
CSF	**Cerebrospinal fluid**
CT	**Computed tomogram/ tomography**
CVA	**Cerebrovascular accident**
CVD	Cerebrovascular disease
CVP	**Central venous pressure**
CVVHF	Continuous veno-venous haemofiltration
CWD	**Continuous-wave Doppler**
CXR	**Chest X-ray/radiograph**

D

DASI	Duke Activity Status Index
$DavO_2$	Arteriovenous oxygen difference
DC	Direct current
DDAVP	Desmopressin (1-desamino-8-D-arginine vasopressin)
DHCA	Deep hypothermic circulatory arrest
DIC	**Disseminated intravascular coagulation**
DM	**Diabetes mellitus**
DNA	**Deoxyribonucleic acid**
DNAR	Do not attempt resuscitation
DPTA	Diethylenetriaminepentacetic acid

E

E$_A$	Arterial elastance
EC	Ejection click
ECC	Extracorporeal circulation
ECG	**Electrocardiograph**
ECLS	Extracorporeal life support
ECMO	Extracorporeal membrane oxygenation
EDM	Early diastolic murmur
EDPVR	End-diastolic pressure–volume relationship
EDV	End-diastolic volume
EEG	**Electroencephalograph**
E$_ES$	End-systolic elastance
EF	Ejection fraction
EMD	Electromechanical dissociation

EPIC	Evaluation & Prevention of Ischaemic Complications (study)
ESPVR	End-systolic pressure–volume relationship
ETT	**Endotracheal tube**

F

FDG	Fluorodeoxyglucose
FDPs	Fibrin(ogen) degradation products
FFA	Free fatty acid
FFP	**Fresh-frozen plasma**
FOB	Fibreoptic bronchoscopy
FRC	Functional residual capacity
FTT	Failure to thrive
FVL	Factor V Leiden

G

GABA	Gamma amino butyric acid
GCS	Glasgow coma sale
GFR	Glomerular filtration rate
GI	**Gastrointestinal**
GMP	Guanosine monophosphate
GP	Glycoprotein
GTN	**Glyceryl trinitrate**
GTP	Guanosine triphosphate
GUCH	Grown-up congenital heart

H

Hb	**Haemoglobin**
Hb–SS	Haemoglobin-SS (Homozygous sickle)
HD	Haemodialysis
HF	Haemofiltration
HFOV	High freq. oscillatory ventilation
HIT	Heparin-induced thrombocytopenia
HITS	Heparin-induced thrombocytopenia syndrome
HLHS	Hypoplastic left heart syndrome
HMWK	High-molecular-weight kininogen
HOCM	Hypertrophic obstructive cardiomyopathy
HPVC	Hypoxic pulmonary vasoconstriction
HR	**Heart rate**

I

IABP	Intra-aortic balloon pump
ICA	Internal carotid artery
ICAM	Intercellular adhesion molecule
ICD	Implantable cardiodefibrillator

ICP	Intracranial pressure
ICS	Intercostal space
ICU	**Intensive care unit**
IDDM	**Insulin-dependent diabetes mellitus**
Ig	Immunoglobulin
IHD	Ischaemic heart disease
IHSS	Idiopathic hypertrophic subaortic stenosis
IL	Interleukin
iNO	Inducible nitric oxide
INR	International normalized ratio
IPPB	Intermittent positive pressure breathing
IPPV	Intermittent positive pressure ventilation
IRI	Ischaemia–reperfusion injury
IRV	Inverse ratio ventilation
ITP	Idiopathic thrombocytopenic purpura
ITU	Intensive therapy unit
IV	**Intravenous**
IVC	**Inferior vena cava**
IVRT	Isovolumic relaxation time
IVS	Interventricular septum

J

JGA	Juxtaglomerular apparatus
JW	Jehovah's witness

K

KIU	Kallikrein inhibitory units
KK	Kallikrein

L

LA	**Left atrium/atrial**
LAA	Left atrial appendage
LAD	**Left anterior descending (coronary artery)**
LAHB	Left anterior hemiblock
LAP	Left ventricular pressure
LAST	Left anterior short thoracotomy
LAX	Long axis
LBBB	**Left bundle branch block**
LBP	Lipopolysaccharide binding protein
LCA	Left coronary artery
LCC	Left coronary cusp
LHC	Left heart catheterization
LICA	Left internal carotid artery
LIJ	Left internal jugular
LIMA	Left internal mammary artery
LLSE	Left lower sternal edge
LMWH	Low molecular weight heparin

LMS	Left main stem (coronary artery)
LPHB	Left posterior hemiblock
LPS	Lipopolysaccharide
LSC	Late systolic click
LSCA	Left subclavian artery
LSCV	Left subclavian vein
LSPV	Left superior pulmonary vein
LUSE	Left upper sternal edge
LV	**Left ventricle/ventricular**
LVAD	Left ventricular assist device
LVEDA	Left ventricular end diastolic area
LVEDP	**Left ventricular end diastolic pressure**
LVEDV	Left ventricular end diastolic volume
LVEF	Left ventricular ejection fraction
LVESPVR	Left ventricular end-systolic pressure–volume relationship
LVESV	Left ventricular end systolic volume
LVF	Left ventricular failure
LVH	**Left ventricular hypertrophy**
LVOT	**Left ventricular outflow tract**
LVOTO	Left ventricular outflow tract obstruction

M

MAC	**Minimal alveolar concentration**
	Membrane attack complex
MAP	**Mean arterial pressure**
MAPCAs	Major aorta pulmonary collateral arteries
MCA	Middle cerebral artery
McSPI	Multicenter Study of Perioperative Ischaemia
ME	Mid-oesophageal
MEP	Motor evoked potential
MET	Medical emergency team
METs	Metabolic equivalents
MI	**Myocardial Infarction**
MIBI	Methoxyisobutyl nitrile
MIDCAB	Minimally invasive direct coronary artery bypass
MOF	Multi organ (system) failure
MPAP	Mean pulmonary artery pressure
MR	**Mitral regurgitation (incompetence)**
MRI	**Magnetic resonance imaging**
MRSA	**Methicillin-resistant *Staphylococcus Aureus***
MS	**Mitral stenosis**
MSM	Midsystolic murmur
MUGA	Multiple Gated Acquisition
MV	**Mitral valve**
MVP	Mitral valve prolapse
MVR	**Mitral valve replacement**
MW	Molecular weight

N

NAD	Nicotinamide adenine dinuleotide
NASPE	North American Society of Pacing and Electrophysiology
NCC	Non-coronary cusp
NDMR	Non-depolarizing muscle relaxant
NEC	Necrotizing enterocolitis
NG	**Nasogastric**
NIBP	**Non-invasive blood pressure**
NIDDM	**Non-insulin-dependent diabetes mellitus**
NIRS	Near infrared spectroscopy
NMB	Neuromuscular blockade/blocker
NMDA	N-methyl-D-aspartate
NO	Nitric oxide
NOS	Nitric oxide synthetase
NSAID	**Non-steroidal anti-inflammatory drug**
NSR	**Normal sinus rhythm**
NTS	Nucleus tractus solitarius
NYHA	**New York Heart Association**

O

OPCAB	Off-pump coronary artery bypass
OS	Opening snap

P

PA	**Pulmonary artery**
PAD	Pulmonary artery diastolic
PAFC	**Pulmonary artery floatation catheter**
PAI	Plasminogen activator inhibitor
PAP	**Pulmonary artery pressure**
PAPVD	Partial anomalous pulmonary venous drainage
pAVSD	Partial atrioventricular septal defect
PAWP	**Pulmonary artery wedge pressure**
PBF	Pulmonary blood flow
PCA	Patient-controlled analgesia
	Posterior cerebral artery
PCoA	Posterior communicating (cerebral) artery
PCV	Pressure-controlled ventilation
PD	Peritoneal dialysis
PDA	Patent ductus arteriosus
	Posterior descending (coronary) artery
PDE	Phosphodiesterase
PDGF	Platelet-derived growth factor
PE	Pulmonary embolus/embolism
PEEP	Positive end-expirator pressure

PET	Positron emission tomography
PF_3	Platelet factor 3
PF_4	Platelet factor 4
PFO	Patent foramen ovale
PGE_2	Prostaglandin E_2
PGI_2	Prostaglandin I_2 (prostacyclin)
PH-T	Pressure half-time
PHT	Pulmonary hypertension
PLB	Phospholamban
PONV	**Postoperative nausea and vomiting**
PPM	Permanent pacemaker
PPHN	Persistent pulmonary hypertension
PPV	Prone position ventilation
PR	**Pulmonary regurgitation (incompetence)**
PS	**Pulmonary stenosis**
PSM	Pansystolic murmur
PSV	Pressure-support ventilation
PT	Prothrombin time
PTCA	Percutaneous transluminal coronary angioplasty
PV	**Pulmonary valve**
	Pulmonary vein
PVd	Pulmonary vein diastolic
PVR	**Pulmonary vascular resistance**
PVs	Pulmonary vein systolic
PWD	**Pulsed-wave Doppler**

Q

Q_P	Pulmonary flow
Q_S	Systemic flow

R

RA	**Right atrium/atrial**
RBBB	**Right bundle branch block**
RBC	**Red blood cell**
RBF	Blood flow
RCA	Right coronary artery
RCC	Right coronary cusp
RCP	Retrograde cerebral perfusion
REMATCH	Randomized evaluation of mechanical assistance for the treatment of congestive heart failure
RHC	Right heart catheterization
RICA	Right internal carotid artery
RIJ	Right internal jugular
RIND	Reversible ischaemic neurological deficit
RNA	**Ribonucleic acid**
RR	**Respiratory rate**

RRT	Renal replacement therapy
RSCA	Right subclavian artery
RSCV	Right subclavian vein
RV	**Right ventricle/ventricular**
RVAD	Right ventricular assist device
RVH	**Right ventricular hypertrophy**
RVOT	**Right ventricular outflow tract**
RWMA	Regional wall motion abnormality

S

S_1	First heart sound
S_2	Second heart sound
S_3	Third heart sound
S_4	Fourth heart sound
SA	**Sinoatrial**
SACP	Selective antegrade cerebral perfusion
SAM	Systolic anterior motion (of the anterior mitral leaflet)
SaO$_2$	**Arterial oxygen saturation**
SAX	Short axis
SCA	Society of Cardiovascular Anesthesiologists
SCS	Spinal cord stimulation
SCUBA	Self contained underwater breathing apparatus
SERCA	Sarcoplasmic reticulum calcium ATPase
SIRS	Systemic inflammatory response to sepsis
$S_{JV}O_2$	Jugular venous oxygen saturation
SLE	Systemic lupus erythematosus
SNP	**Sodium nitroprusside**
SNS	Sympathetic nervous system
SR	Sarcoplasmic reticulum
SSEP	Somatosensory evoked potential
ST	Sinus tachycardia
SV	**Stroke volume**
SVC	**Superior vena cava**
SVG	Saphenous vein graft
S$_V$O$_2$	**Mixed venous oxygen saturation**
SVR	**Systemic vascular resistance**
SVT	**Supraventricular tachycardia**

T

T_3	Triiodothyronine
T_4	Thyroxine
TAPVD	Total anomalous pulmonary venous drainage
TCD	Transcranial Doppler
TCPC	Total cavopulmonary venous connection
TEA	Thoracic epidural analgesic

TEG	Thromboelastogram/thromboelastography
TENS	Transcutaneous electrical nerve stimulation
TGA	Transposition of the great arteries
TIA	**Transient ischaemic attack**
TIVA	Total intravenous anaesthesia
TnC	Troponin C
TnI	Troponin I
TnT	Troponin T
TNF	Tumour necrosis factor
TOE	**Transoesophageal echocardiography**
TOF	Tetrology of fallot
tPA	Tissue plasminogen activator
TPG	**Transpulmonary gradient**
TR	**Tricuspid regurgitation (incompetence)**
TS	**Tricuspid stenosis**
TT	Thrombin time
TTE	Transthoracic echocardiography
TV	**Tricuspid valve**

U

u-PA	Urokinase plasminogen activator
UTI	Urinary tract infection
UV	Umbilical vein

V

VA	Vertebral artery
VAD	Ventricular assist device
VALI	Ventilator associated lung injury
V_D	Volume of distribution
VEP	Visual evoked potential
VF	**Ventricular fibrillation**
VIP	Vasoactive intestinal peptide
VLM	Ventrolateral medulla
VO_2	Oxygen consumption
VOT	Ventricular outflow tract
VPB	Ventricular premature (ectopic) beat
VRE	Vancomycin resistant enterococcus
VSD	**Ventricular septal defect**
VT	**Ventricular tachycardia**
V_T	Tidal volume
VV	Vitelline vein
vWF	Von Willebrand factor

W

WPW	Wolf–Parkinson–White (syndrome)

ANATOMY AND PHYSIOLOGY

CARDIAC EMBRYOLOGY AND ANATOMY

1

M.J. Goddard

An appreciation of the normal development of the heart and great vessels, and normal adult cardiac anatomy is essential to the understanding of congenital and acquired heart disease.

Embryology

The heart develops entirely from splanchnic mesoderm. Union of the left and right endothelial channels results in the primitive heart tube, which starts to beat in the 3rd week of gestation. The 'arterial' end of the tube lies cephalad while the 'venous' end lies caudad. A series of dilatations form the primitive heart chambers (Figure 1.1).

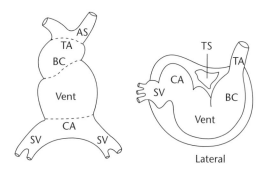

Figure 1.1 The primitive heart at around 3rd week of gestation. The sinus venosus (SV) has left and right horns, and receives blood from the vitelline and umbilical veins. The common atrium (CA) lies between the SV and single ventricle (Vent). The bulbus cordis (BC) is divided into a proximal and distal portions. The outflow tract, comprised of the distal BC and the truncus arteriosus (TA), is in continuity with the aortic sac (AS). The transverse sinus (TS) is the area of pericardial cavity lying between the arterial and venous ends of the heart tube.

Lengthening of the heart tube and differential growth cause buckling of the tube within the pericardial cavity. As a result the common atrium and sinus venosus come to lie behind the bulbus cordis and common ventricle (Figure 1.2).

Further development consists of division of the atrioventricular (A-V) canal, formation of the interatrial

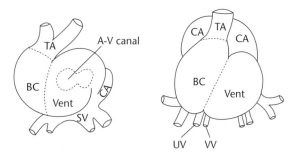

Figure 1.2 The primitive heart during the 4th and 5th weeks of gestation. The left horn of the sinus venosus (SV) receives blood from the left common cardinal vein. The right horn of the SV receives blood from the hepatocardiac canal and the right common cardinal, umbilical and vitelline veins (UV and VV, respectively). BC, bulbus cordis; CA, common atrium; TA, truncus arteriousus.

and interventricular septa and partition of the outflow tract. Development and fusion of dorsal and ventral endocardial cushions divide the A-V canal into left and right channels. During this division, enlargement of the endocardial cushions forces the channels apart while the distal bulbus cordis migrates to the left (Figure 1.3).

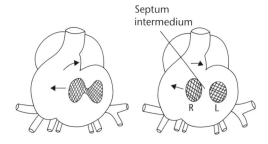

Figure 1.3 Fusion of the dorsal and ventral endocardial cushions forms the septum intermedium that divides the A-V canal into left and right channels.

Partition of the atrium begins with development of the sickle-shaped septum primum, which grows down from the dorsal wall to fuse with the septum intermedium. Before complete obliteration of the foramen primum by the septum primum, degenerative changes in the central portion of the septum result in the formation of the foramen secundum. The thicker septum secundum grows downward from the roof on the right side of the septum primum to overlie the foramen secundum. As the lower edge does not reach the septum intermedium a space between the free margin of the septum secundum and foramen secundum (known as the foramen ovale) persists (Figure 1.4). The right horn of the sinus venosus becomes incorporated into the RA (as the vena cavae) and the left horn becomes the coronary sinus.

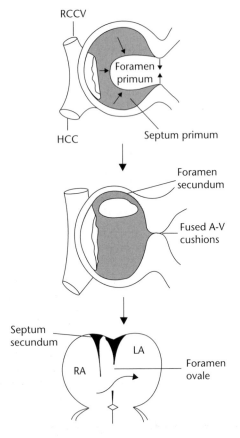

Figure 1.4 Formation of the intra-atrial septum. In the upper diagrams, the developing septum primum (shaded) is viewed from the right side of the common atrium. RCCV, right common cardinal vein (primitive SVC); HCC, hepato-cardiac channel (primitive IVC).

The interventricular septum is formed by the fusion of the inferior muscular and the membranous (bulboventricular) septa. The primary interventricular foramen, which is obliterated by formation of the septum, is bounded posteriorly by the A–V canal. The resulting separation of the bulbus cordis from the ventricle results in the formation of the RV and LV.

The truncus arteriosus, aortic sac, pharyngeal arch arteries (Figure 1.5) and dorsal aortae develop into the great vessels of the superior mediastinum.

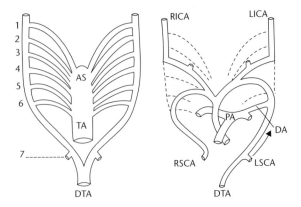

Figure 1.5 The fate of the pharyngeal arch arteries and development of the great arteries. The pharyngeal arch arteries coalesce to form the left and right dorsal aortae which join to form the primitive descending thoracic aorta (DTA). The aortic sac (AS) becomes the right half of the aortic arch, and the brachiocephalic and common carotid arteries. The left dorsal aorta forms the left half of the aortic arch. The third arch arteries form the left and right internal carotid arteries (LICA and RICA, respectively). The sixth arch arteries and truncus arteriosus (TA) form the pulmonary arteries (PA). The distal portion of the left sixth arch artery forms the ductus arteriosus (DA). The seventh intersegmental arteries form the left and right subclavian arteries (LSCA and RSCA respectively).

Partition of the outflow tract begins during formation of the interventricular septum as two pairs of ridges grow into the lumen. The left and right bulbar ridges unite to form the distal bulbar septum and the left and right aorticopulmonary ridges fuse to divide the truncus arteriosus into the aorta and main pulmonary trunk (Figure 1.6).

Differentiation of the thick myo-epicardial mantle that surrounds the primitive endocardial tube results in formation of the epicardium, myocardium and fibrous tissue of the heart. The myocardium further differentiates into a spongy, trabeculated inner layer and a compact outer layer. In the atria, the trabeculae form the pectinate muscles, whereas in the ventricles they form the chordae tendinae and papillary muscles. The myocardium of the atria remains in continuity with that of the ventricles until separated by the development of fibrous tissue in the A–V canal. The small strand of myocardium that bridges this fibrous tissue differentiates into the cardiac conducting system.

Raised folds arising from the margins of the distal ventricular outflow tracts and A–V channels become

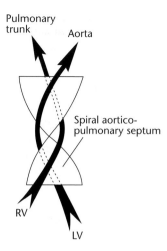

Figure 1.6 Partition of the TA by the helical aortico-pulmonary septum into the ascending aorta and main pulmonary trunk.

excavated on their downstream surfaces to form the pulmonary, aortic, tricuspid and mitral valves.

Foetal circulation

The foetal circulation (Figure 1.7) differs from the adult circulation in the following respects:

- *Umbilical vein and ductus venosus* Carries oxygenated placental blood to the IVC via the ductus venosus.
- *Foramen ovale* The opening of the IVC lies opposite the foramen ovale. Oxygenated blood is directed across the foramen by the Eustachian valve into the LA and distributed to the head and arms.
- *Pulmonary circulation* High pulmonary vascular resistance (PVR) results in minimal pulmonary blood flow and physiological RVH.
- *Ductus arteriosus* Venous blood returning from the head and arms enters the RA via the SVC. The majority of blood ejected into the main pulmonary trunk is directed into the descending thoracic aorta via the wide ductus arteriosus.
- *Umbilical arteries* These paired vessels, arising from the iliac arteries, return deoxygenated blood to the placenta.

At birth the cessation of umbilical blood flow, coupled with lung expansion and respiration yields the so-called transitional circulation. This circulation is inherently unstable and may persist for a few hours or several weeks.

- *Umbilical vessels* Close shortly after birth.
- *Ductus venosus* Becomes ligamentum venosum.

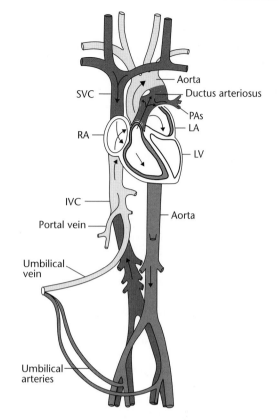

Figure 1.7 The foetal circulation.

- *Foramen ovale* When LA pressure is >RA pressure, flow across the foramen effectively ceases. May remain patent into adulthood.
- *Pulmonary circulation* Pulmonary blood flow increased with rapid decline in PVR. PVR $\cong$ SVR at 24 h. PVR continues to fall for several months.
- *Ductus arteriosus* Functional closure at birth as blood is diverted to the pulmonary circulation. Anatomical closure may take several weeks.

Normal cardiac anatomy

Pericardium

The pericardium is a cone-shaped structure composed of fibrous and serosal parts, that encloses the heart and the roots of the great vessels. The fibrous part consists of dense connective tissue that merges superiorly with the adventitia of the great arteries, and inferiorly with the central tendon of the diaphragm. The inner surface of the fibrous pericardium is lined by the parietal layer of serous pericardium, which is reflected over the surface of the heart as the visceral layer or *epicardium*. A thin film of pericardial fluid separates the two serosal layers. The pericardial reflections create the *oblique sinus*, a blind recess behind the LA bounded by the four pulmonary veins and the IVC, and the *transverse sinus* between the aorta and PA in front and the SVC and LA behind.

Heart borders

- *Right*   SVC, RA, IVC
- *Left*   Edge of LV
- *Anterior*   RA, RV, small strip of LV
- *Posterior*   LA, pulmonary veins (×4)
- *Inferior*   RV
- *Superior*   LA appendage.

Right heart chambers

The RA receives the SVC superiorly, and the coronary sinus and IVC, both guarded by rudimentary valves, inferiorly. A superior elongation, the RA appendage, overlies the root of the aorta. The *sulcus terminalis* is a groove on the surface of the RA running from the junction of the SVC and RA appendage to the IVC. The sulcus is reflected on the inner surface of the RA as a ridge of muscle; the *crista terminalis*. The character of the inner surface of the RA reflects its embryological origins. The surface posterior to the crista terminalis originates from the *sinus venosus* and is smooth, whereas that anterior to the crista originates from the primitive atrium and is trabeculated by bands of *pectinate muscle*. The *interatrial septum* forms the posteromedial wall of the RA. A shallow depression in the centre of the septum, the

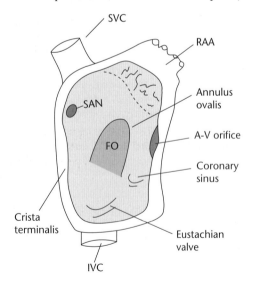

Figure 1.8 The intra-atrial septum viewed from the right side of the heart. The annulus ovalis is a sickle-shaped ridge of tissue in the septum secundum that surrounds the fossa ovalis (FO). Posterior to the crista terminalis the lining of the atrium is smooth. SAN, SA node; RAA, RA appendage.

fossa ovalis, represents that part of the *septum primum* not covered by the *septum secundum* (Figure 1.8).

The tricuspid valve (TV) separates the RA and RV. The three cusps – septal, inferior and anterior – are attached at their bases to the fibrous A-V ring. The free edges and inferior surfaces of the cusps are attached via *chordae tendinae* to papillary muscles from the trabeculae of the RV wall.

On the surface of the heart, the RA is separated from the crescent-shaped *RV* by the right A-V groove in which the right coronary artery lies. The ventricular cavity is lined by a series of ridges known as the trabeculae carnae. One of these trabeculae, the *moderator band*, lies free within the cavity and carries part of the RV conducting system. The smooth-walled outflow tract or *infundibulum* leads to the main pulmonary trunk.

The pulmonary valve (PV) consists of three semi-lunar cusps, two anterior and one posterior, attached at their bases to a fibrous ring.

Left heart chambers

The LA lies directly behind the RA from which it is separated by the interatrial septum. The small LA appendage arises from the superior aspect of the LA and overlies the RV infundibulum. The four pulmonary veins, namely – left and right, superior and inferior – drain into the posterior wall of the LA. With the exception of the LA appendage, which is trabeculated by pectinate muscles, the LA cavity is smooth walled.

The mitral valve (MV) is a complex structure composed of both valvular and subvalvular components. The valve apparatus comprises two asymmetrical leaflets attached to a flexible, saddle-shaped annulus. The subvalvular apparatus comprises chordae tendinae, papillary muscles and adjacent LV myocardium.

The LA is separated from the LV by the left A-V groove in which the *left coronary artery* lies. The ventricle is circular in cross section and has a wall thickness three to four times that of the RV. With the exception of the *aortic vestibule*, which has smooth walls, the lining of the LV cavity has prominent trabeculae carnae.

Nerve supply

The heart is innervated by afferents and efferents of both the sympathetic and parasympathetic nervous system. The parasympathetic supply comes from the vagus nerves via the cardiac plexuses. Short postganglionic fibres pass to the SA and A-V nodes and are only minimally distributed to the ventricles. The sympathetic supply arises from the cervical and upper thoracic sympathetic trunks and supplies both the atria and ventricles. Post-ganglionic fibres arise in the paired stellate ganglia. The right stellate ganglion supplies the anterior epicardial surface and the interventricular septum. The left stellate ganglion supplies the lateral and posterior surfaces of both ventricles. Although the heart has no somatic innervation, stimulation of vagal afferents may reach consciousness and be perceived as pain.

Conducting system

This is discussed in Chapter 2.

Blood supply

The *right coronary artery* arises from the anterior aortic sinus, passes between the pulmonary trunk and RA appendage and descends in the right A–V groove until it reaches the posterior interventricular groove. In 85% of patients the artery continues as the *posterior descending artery* (i.e. 'right' dominance). In its course, it gives off atrial, SA and A–V nodal, and ventricular branches before dividing into the posterior descending and RV marginal arteries.

The *left coronary artery* arises from the left posterior aortic sinus and divides into the left anterior (interventricular) descending and circumflex arteries. The LAD descends anteriorly and inferiorly to the apex of the heart. In its course it gives off one or more *diagonal* branches and a series of *septal perforating branches*, which supply the anterior interventricular septum. The *left circumflex artery* runs posteriorly in the left A–V groove until it reaches the posterior interventricular groove, where it may continue as the posterior descending artery in 15% of patients. In its course, the circumflex artery gives off one or more *obtuse marginal* branches (Figure 1.9).

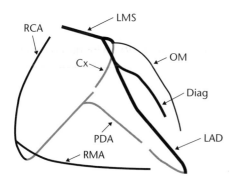

Figure 1.9 The anatomy of the coronary arteries: LMS, left main stem; RCA, right coronary artery; Cx, circumflex; OM, obtuse marginal; Diag, diagonal; LAD, left anterior descending; OM, obtuse marginal; Diag, diagonal; PDA, posterior descending artery; RMA, right marginal artery.

Venous drainage

The majority (~75%) of venous blood drains via the *coronary sinus* into the RA. The coronary sinus is 2–3 cm in length and lies adjacent to the circumflex artery in the left posterior A–V groove. Its principle tributaries are the great, small, middle and posterior LV cardiac veins (Figure 1.10).

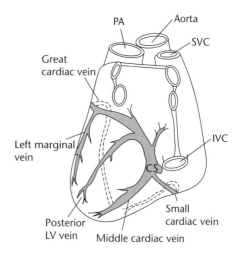

Figure 1.10 Posterior view of the heart showing the anatomy of the coronary sinus (CS) and cardiac veins.

The *anterior cardiac veins* drain the anterior part of the RV and empty directly into the RA.

The diminutive *Thebesian veins* may empty into any of the cardiac chambers and account for a small amount of venous drainage. Those draining into the left heart contribute to the 'anatomical shunt'.

Key points

- Knowledge of cardiac embryology is necessary to understand congenital heart disease.
- In the foetal circulation, oxygenated blood is directed across the foramen ovale into the LA to supply the head and arms.
- The *posterior descending artery* arises from the right coronary artery in 85% of patients.
- The venous drainage of the anterior RV does not enter the coronary sinus.

Further reading

Williams PL (Ed). *Gray's Anatomy: The Anatomical Basis of Medicine and Surgery*, 38th edition. London: Churchill Livingstone, 1995.

CARDIAC ELECTROPHYSIOLOGY

2

D.W. Wheeler & A.A. Grace

Anatomy

When in normal sinus rhythm the heart beats in an orderly sequence. Specialized cardiac muscle cells (cardiomyocytes) in the SA node generate cardiac action potentials (APs), which cause normal myocytes to contract. APs are transmitted through the heart via the conducting system (Figure 2.1).

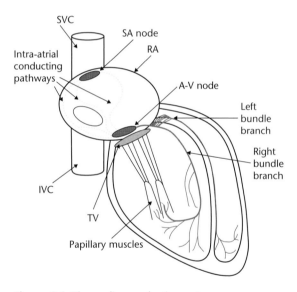

Figure 2.1 The cardiac conducting system.

The cells of the conducting system are modified general cardiomyocytes, and classified as *nodal, transitional* and *Purkinje* myocytes (Table 2.1). All myocytes in the conducting system are capable of spontaneous, rhythmic generation of cardiac APs. The anatomy and physiology of this system ensures that atrial systole precedes ventricular systole. Whichever focus produces an AP most frequently acts as the pacemaker – in sinus rhythm this is the SA node.

Sinoatrial node

The SA node lies within a groove in the wall of the RA at its junction with the SVC. Macroscopically, it is a flattened ellipse possessing a 'head', 'body' and

'tail', measuring $10 \times 3 \times 1$ mm and is often covered by a plaque of subepicardial fat.

The SA node is supplied by the right coronary artery (RCA) in 65% of hearts, and by the circumflex branch of the left coronary artery (LCA) in 35%. The largest branch of the SA nodal artery – the *ramus cristae terminalis* – runs through the centre of the SA node. It has a large lumen and thick adventitia, knitting firmly with a thick collagenous network of connective tissue within the node. It has been suggested that this structure might function as a baroreceptor for the atrial natriuretic peptide homoeostatic system. It might be expected that rhythmically discharging excitable cells have a high oxygen demand, but there are surprisingly few branches within the node. The majority of the blood flows onwards to perfuse the RA.

Pacemaker cells are nodal myocytes lying within the core of the node. Arranged in clusters, each cell has one large nucleus and pale cytoplasm containing few organelles. They are non-contractile, possessing a small number of randomly arranged myofibrils.

Intra-atrial conduction pathways

It was initially thought that the cardiac AP was conducted between the SA node and atrioventricular (A–V) node as a wave of depolarization spreading radially via gap junctions between general atrial myocytes. However, the cardiac AP reaches the A–V node more

Table 2.1 AP conduction velocities in the cardiac conducting system

Tissue	Myocyte type	Conduction rate (m s^{-1})
SA node	Nodal	0.05
Intra-atrial pathways	General and Purkinje	1
A-V node	Transitional	0.05
Bundle of His	Transitional and Purkinje	1
Purkinje system	Purkinje	4
Myocardium	General	0.6

quickly than would be expected had it been passing through ordinary myocardium. In fact there are three specialized conducting pathways consisting of Purkinje fibres in the atria: the *anterior, middle* and *posterior internodal tracts.*

Atrioventricular node

The A-V node is an oval structure measuring $8 \times 3 \times 1$ mm. It lies within the atrial septum and has a surface in the RA near the basal attachment of the septal leaflet of the TV, and a surface in the LA adjacent to the MV annulus.

Microscopically the centre of the A-V node contains a small number of nodal myocytes, surrounded by a fibrous network of long transitional myocytes – similar to that of the SA node but less dense. Transitional myocytes provide an electrical link between the nodal pacemaker cells and more distal parts of conducting system. They have a smaller diameter than general cardiac myocytes but possess similar organelles and contractile apparatus. Cardiac APs are conducted slowly in the A-V node and are therefore likely to be responsible for normal A-V conduction delay. Under normal circumstances, these cells are the only electrical link between atria and ventricles, as these chambers are electrically insulated from each other by a fibrous annulus.

The first and largest branch of the posterior septal branch of the RCA supplies the A-V node in 80% of hearts; otherwise the node derives its blood supply from the left circumflex artery.

Accessory conducting pathways

In addition to the A-V node, accessory conducting pathways may form abnormal electrical connections between the atria and ventricles. These pathways are formed as a result of disordered cardiogenesis and consist of normal cardiac myocytes or specialized conducting tissue. In these circumstances, there is incomplete formation of the mitral or tricuspid fibrous annuli that electrically insulate the atria from the ventricles. Depending on the relative refractory periods of the normal A-V nodal and the accessory conducting pathways, circumstances may arise when excitation passes retrogradely into the atria through the accessory pathway having already traversed the fibrous annulus via the A-V node. This may trigger a re-entrant tachycardia, such as that seen in the Wolff–Parkinson–White syndrome.

Bundle of His and Purkinje system

The tracts of transitional myocytes running from the A-V node narrow quickly as they pass through the fibrous annulus into the interventricular septum (IVS). The common bundle is then said to branch into the left and right bundles at the crest of the IVS. In fact, it is somewhat misleading to consider the branching as a simple bifurcation.

The right bundle runs as a discrete aggregation of fascicles until it reaches the anterior papillary muscle of the TV where it splits into a fine network of sub-endocardial Purkinje fibres, which form a network throughout the RV.

The left bundle is a flat sheet of fine fascicles, which leave the left margin of the common bundle throughout its course towards the IVS. The sheet passes over the LV aspect of the IVS and runs towards the apex of the LV. After ~3 cm it splits into anterior and posterior fascicles, maintaining the sheet-like arrangement. The anterior sheet runs towards the anterolateral papillary muscle, and posterior sheet towards the posteromedial papillary muscle. After reaching the papillary muscles, both sheets split into fine Purkinje networks penetrating the whole of the LV wall and IVS. The networks consist of Purkinje cells, which are wider and shorter than the surrounding general myocytes.

The cytoplasm of Purkinje cells is packed with mitochondria, sarcoplasmic reticulum and glycogen, but very few myofibrils. This apparatus provides the copious amounts of energy needed for the rapid conduction of APs. The Purkinje networks have large and numerous nexuses, inter-digitating with general cardiac myocytes, allowing efficient conduction of the AP to the myocardium.

Electrophysiology

The cardiac action potential

Normal cardiac function is dependent upon the generation and delivery of a wave of depolarization (the AP) from the SA node to ventricular muscle. The AP has a duration of 300–400 ms – considerably longer than APs in neuronal tissue (1–2 ms). The cardiac AP is generated in pacemaker tissue as a result of diastolic depolarization, which is the result of a complex combination of changing ionic permeabilities.

The AP is classically characterized by five distinct phases. Figures 2.2 and 2.3 describe conduction of depolarization through the heart:

- *Phase 4*   The resting membrane potential (RMP) is the period between completion of repolarization and initiation of the next AP. The RMP is primarily determined by intracellular K^+ concentration,

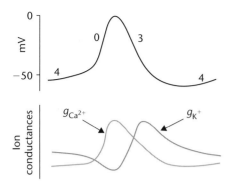

Figure 2.2 The SA node AP. Spontaneous diastolic depolarization (the pacemaker potential) is thought to occur as a result of decreasing K$^+$ conductance g_{K^+} and slightly increased Ca^{2+} $g_{Ca^{2+}}$ conductance.

and varies between -60 mV in the SA node and -90 mV in the bundle of His and Purkinje fibres. The equilibrium potential for potassium (E_K) is given by the Nernst equation:

$$E_K = -61 \log [K^+]_i / [K^+]_e$$

where $[K^+]_i$ and $[K^+]_e$ are the intracellular and extracellular potassium concentrations, respectively. For example, if $[K^+]_i = 150$ mM and $[K^+]_e = 4$ mM, then $E_K = -96$ mV. Unlike atrial and ventricular muscle, pacemaker tissue is characterized by an *unstable* RMP, secondary to a decrease in K$^+$ conductance (g_{K^+}) and a small increase Ca^{2+} conductance ($g_{Ca^{2+}}$) through transient (T-type) channels thought to underly the so-called *pacemaker potential* or *pre-potential*.

- *Phase 0* In atrial pacemaker tissue, depolarization is primarily due to Ca^{2+} influx via L-type channels, whereas beyond the A-V node depolarization is due to a 'fast' inward Na$^+$ current. For this reason, the slope of Phase 0 is flatter in SA and A-V nodal tissue (Figure 2.2) and almost vertical in non-pacemaker tissue (Figure 2.3).
- *Phase 1* Early repolarization is principally due to an increase in g_{K^+}. Complete repolarization is delayed by a simultaneous increase in $g_{Ca^{2+}}$ conductance. Phase 1 is not seen in the SA and A-V nodal AP.
- *Phase 2* The so-called *plateau phase* is due to a large increase in slow Ca^{2+} influx via L-type channels and is prominent in the distal conducting system and ventricular myocytes. Phase 2 is not seen in the SA and A-V nodal AP.
- *Phase 3* Repolarization occurs, as K$^+$ efflux increases and Ca^{2+} influx decreases (Figures 2.2 and 2.3).

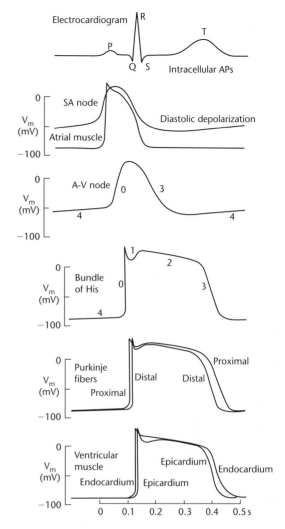

Figure 2.3 Conduction of the cardiac AP through the conducting system demonstrating the morphology and temporal relationships of the AP in different regions. From Lynch C. Cellular electrophysiology of the heart. In: Lynch III C (Ed.). *Clinical cardiac electrophysiology. Perioperative considerations* (Society of Cardiovascular Anesthesiologists Monograph). Baltimore: Lippincott, William & Wilkins ©, 1994.

Neural control of heart rate

The autonomic innervation of the heart arises from the stellate ganglion (T$_{1-4}$) and the vagus nerve.

Cholinergic stimulation of muscarinic (M$_2$) receptors in the SA node via the right vagus nerve causes membrane hyperpolarization (Phase 3 prolonged) and prolongs diastolic depolarization (reduces the slope of Phase 4 depolarization) (Figure 2.4). The net result is that the pacemaker potential takes longer to reach firing threshold and HR slows. Stimulation of

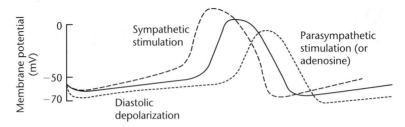

Figure 2.4 The effect of autonomic stimulation on the cardiac AP in the SA and A-V nodes. From Lynch C. Cellular electrophysiology of the heart. In: Lynch III C (Ed.). *Clinical cardiac electrophysiology. Perioperative considerations* (Society of Cardiovascular Anesthesiologists Monograph). Baltimore: Lippincott, William & Wilkins ©, 1994.

the left vagus nerve causes hyperpolarization of the transitional myocytes in the A–V node, further slowing conduction of APs between atria and ventricles.

Sympathetic stimulation increases HR and A–V nodal conduction velocity. Noradrenaline (norepinephrine) binds to β_1-adrenergic receptors on pacemaker cells in the SA node, enhancing Ca^{2+} influx. The pacemaker potential reaches firing threshold more quickly, AP conduction is more rapid, and HR increases. The left stellate ganglion has a similar effect on transitional myocytes in the A–V node, increasing the speed of transmission of cardiac APs between atria and ventricles.

Genetic influences

Advances in genetics and molecular biology are beginning to shed light on the aetiology of cardiac dysrhythmias. As well as structural defects such as accessory pathways responsible for re-entrant tachycardias, it is now clear that mutations in genes encoding ion channels that slow AP conduction in cardiac myocytes are responsible for the Brugada syndrome (a genetic condition that predisposes to sudden VF) and congenital forms of the long QT syndrome. The knowledge gained from these experiments is likely to lead to novel treatments for dysrhythmias in the future.

Key points

- All myocytes in the conducting system are capable of spontaneous, rhythmic generation of cardiac APs.

- SA nodal myocytes normally generate APs at the highest frequency and so act as the cardiac pacemaker.
- Different myocyte classes within the conducting system conduct APs at different velocities.
- The autonomic nervous system acts upon the conducting system to influence HR and rhythm.
- Knowledge of the normal anatomy, physiology and blood supply of the conducting system allows an understanding of the origins of dysrhythmias and heart block.

Further reading

Ganong WF (Ed.). *Review of Medical Physiology*, 20th edition. New York: McGraw-Hill Professional Publishing, 2001.

Lynch C. Cellular electrophysiology of the heart. In: Lynch III C (Ed.). *Clinical Cardiac Electrophysiology. Perioperative Considerations* (Society of Cardiovascular Anesthesiologists Monograph). Baltimore: William & Wilkins, 1994.

Waller BF, Gering LE, Branyas NA, Slack JD. Anatomy, histology, and pathology of the cardiac conduction system: Part I. *Clin Cardiol* 1993; **16(3):** 249–252.

Waller BF, Gering LE, Branyas NA, Slack JD. Anatomy, histology, and pathology of the cardiac conduction system: Part II. *Clin Cardiol* 1993; **16(4):** 347–352.

CARDIAC EXCITATION–CONTRACTION COUPLING

3

K.H. McKinlay & J.V. Booth

Excitation–contraction coupling is the mechanism by which membrane depolarization leads to myocardial contraction.

Anatomy

Unlike skeletal muscle, which is composed of separately innervated motor subunits, cardiac muscle cells (cardiomyocytes) interdigitate to form a syncytium. Cardiomyocytes are elliptical structures, typically $100\,\mu m$ in length and $25\,\mu m$ in diameter, which are mechanically and electrically connected to surrounding cardiomyocytes.

Cardiomyocytes comprise a bi-layer lipid membrane (the sarcolemma), cytoplasm – containing mitochondria and several cytoskeletal proteins (integrin, talin and α-actinin) and bundles of myofibrils containing contractile proteins (actin, myosin, tropomyosin and troponin) arranged in sarcomeres surrounded endoplasmic or sarcoplasmic reticulum (SR). The sarcolemma displays regular invaginations that permit the extracellular space to penetrate deep into the cardiomyocyte. These invaginations constitute the transverse tubular system. Mitochondria are prominent in cardiomyocytes, accounting for over a third of cell volume.

The boundaries of the sarcomere are demarcated by Z-lines, a band of structural protein to which the *thin filaments* are anchored (Figure 3.1).

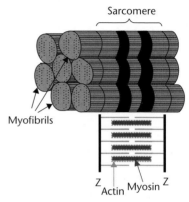

Figure 3.1 Cardiomyocytes are composed of myofibrils, each of which contains thin and thick (myo) filaments. The sarcomere lies between two Z-lines.

These filaments (7 nm in diameter) are composed of two helically arranged strands of actin polymer intertwined with a strand of tropomyosin–troponin complexes at regular intervals (Figure 3.2).

Thick filaments are composed of bundles of up to 300 molecules of myosin. Each molecule comprises two heads (which extend towards the thin filaments), a hinge and a tail, which is anchored to the M-line. Each thick filament is surrounded by a hexagonal array of thin filaments.

Individual myofibrils are connected via specialized, interdigitating areas of cell membrane known as

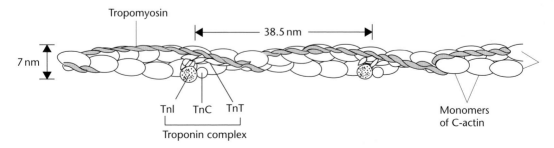

Figure 3.2 A thin filament consisting of two strands of actin polymer entwined with tropomyosin. Troponin complexes are sited at regular interval along the filament.

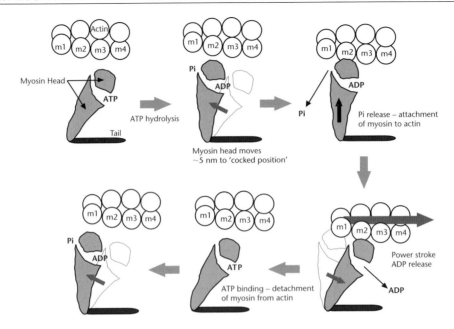

Figure 3.3 The cycle of actin–myosin interaction and force generation. From Lynch C. The biochemical and cellular basis of myocardial contractility. In: Warltier DC (Ed.). *Ventricular Function*. Baltimore: Lippincott, Williams & Wilkins ©, 1995.

intercalated discs, which coincide with the Z-line. These anchor myocytes together and allow force to be transmitted between them. Within the discs, areas of fused cell membrane called *gap junctions* provide a low-resistance pathway for propagation of electrical activity within the myocardium.

A third filament system exists, consisting mainly of the giant (30,000 kDa) protein titin, which serves to impart structural integrity and elasticity to the stretched muscle.

Force production depends upon the interaction between actin and myosin (Figure 3.3). The myosin heads contain an actin-binding site and an enzymatic site (myosin-ATPase) that hydrolyses adenosine triphosphate (ATP). During contraction, the myosin head binds to actin at a 90° angle and, with the hydrolysis of ATP, produces movement of myosin on actin by swivelling. Relaxation of this actin–myosin bond only occurs when a new ATP molecule binds to the enzymatic site. The myosin head then disconnects and reconnects at the next linkage site and the process is repeated in serial fashion. The force generated by a single sarcomere is proportional to the number of actin–myosin bonds and the significant muscle shortening depends on repetitive cycling of the above process.

The troponin–tropomyosin complex regulates actin–myosin interactions (Figure 3.4). The troponin complex

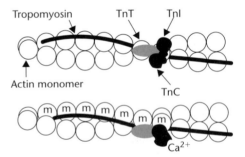

Ca^{2+} binding reveals myosin binding sites (m)

Figure 3.4 Exposure of actin–myosin-binding sites (m) by a calcium-induced conformation change in troponin-C. From Lynch C. The biochemical and cellular basis of myocardial contractility. In: Warltier DC (Ed.), *Ventricular Function*. Baltimore: Lippincott, Williams & Wilkins ©, 1995.

comprises tropomyosin-binding (TnT), calcium binding (TnC) and inhibitory (TnI) subunits. Under resting conditions TnI is tightly bound to actin and tropomyosin obscuring the actin–myosin-binding site. When Ca^{2+} binds to TnC, tropomyosin–TnI binding is weakened inducing a conformational change in tropomyosin that reveals actin–myosin-binding sites. The subsequent binding of myosin to actin is the fundamental basis of force production.

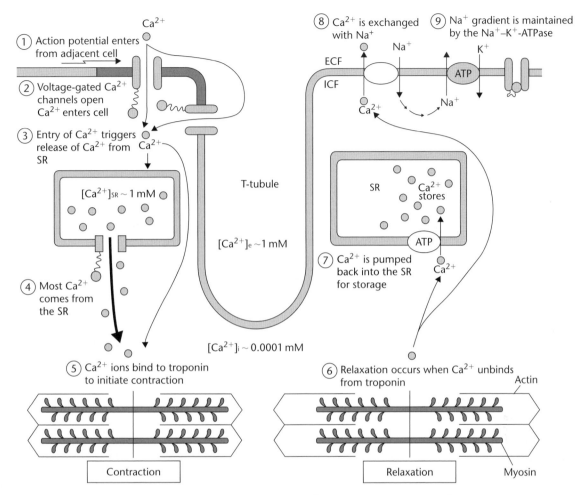

Figure 3.5 Excitation–contraction coupling and the role of Ca^{2+}. The concentration of Ca^{2+} in the extracellular space ($[Ca^{2+}]_e$) and SR ($[Ca^{2+}]_{SR}$) is around 10,000 times greater than the intracellular (cytoplasmic) Ca^{2+} concentration ($[Ca^{2+}]_i$) required to activate contraction. Modified from Figure 14.11, p 418 Human Physiology, 2nd edn. by Dee Unglaub Silverthorn. Copyright 2001 by Prentice-Hall, Inc. Reprinted by permission of Pearson Education, Inc.

The role of calcium

As fluctuations in the cytosolic concentration of Ca^{2+} modulate the actin–myosin interaction, the control of intracellular Ca^{2+} is central to excitation–contracting coupling (Figure 3.5).

Contraction

Depolarization of the sarcolemma by the cardiac AP results in activation of voltage-gated, L-type Ca^{2+} channels and a passive influx of Ca^{2+} down a huge electrochemical gradient. This in turn leads to the greater release of Ca^{2+} from the larger pool of Ca^{2+} in the SR. Although this calcium-induced calcium release is well described, its control has not been

fully elucidated. The T-tubules bring the sarcolemmal L-type channels into close proximity to the calcium-release channels – the so-called ryanodine (RyR_2) receptors – that conduct Ca^{2+} from the lumen of the SR to the cytoplasm.

Relaxation

Relaxation is dependent on the removal of Ca^{2+} from the cytosol to the SR and extracellular space. In contrast to Ca^{2+} release, which occurs down a concentration gradient, this is an active, energy consuming process. The principal mechanism of re-sequestration is SR Ca^{2+}-ATPase (SERCA); each molecule of ATP hydrolysed, returns 2 molecules of Ca^{2+} to the SR. This pump is regulated by the phosphorylation status of another SR protein, phospholamban (PLB). In the phosphorylated state, PLB facilitates calcium re-uptake by SERCA while in the dephosphorylated state it inhibits re-uptake of calcium.

Other Ca^{2+} re-uptake mechanisms include the Na^+–Ca^{2+} exchanger, sarcolemmal Ca^{2+}-ATPase and cytosolic Ca^{2+}-binding proteins, such as calmodulin and calsequestrin. Once $[Ca^{2+}]_i$ is below the $0.1\,\mu m$ threshold for activation, the interaction between actin and myosin ceases.

Key points

- Excitation–contraction coupling refers to the process by which electrical depolarization of the cardiac cell leads to myocardial contraction.
- Force production is dependent upon the interaction between actin and myosin, which is

modulated by tropomyosin and the action of Ca^{2+} on the tropinin complex.
- The concentration of Ca^{2+} in the extracellular space and the SR is around 10,000 times greater than the concentration in cardiomyocyte cytoplasm.

Further reading

Bers DM. Cardiac excitation–contraction coupling. *Nature* 2002; **415(6868)**: 198–205.

Klabunde RE. *Cardiovascular Physiology Concepts*. http://www.cvphysiology.com.

Walker C, Allyson BA, Spinale FG. The structure and function of the cardiac myocyte: a review of fundamental concepts. *J Thorac Cardiovasc Surg* 1999; **118(2)**: 375–382.

Xiao R-P, Cheng H, Zhou Y-Y, Kuschel M, Lakatta EG. Recent advances in cardiac β_2-adrenergic signal transduction. *Circ Res* 1999; **85(11)**: 1092–1100.

4

P.A. White & J.E. Arrowsmith

Ventricular performance is determined by both systolic and diastolic function – abnormalities of either may cause cardiac failure. Broadly speaking, systolic function is the ability of the ventricle to eject blood during each cardiac cycle and is dependent on three factors: preload, contractility and afterload. Normal diastolic function requires unimpeded ventricular filling and normal ventricular relaxation.

Over a wide range of physiological conditions, the outputs of the RV and LV are virtually identical. The Otto Frank and Ernest Starling Law of the Heart states, 'the energy of contraction is a function of the length of the muscle fibre'; therefore, as ventricular filling (preload) increases, stroke volume (SV) – and therefore, cardiac output (CO) – increases (Figure 4.1). Due to its dependency on preload and afterload, CO is a crude index of ventricular performance.

Preload

Preload is the passive force that stretches resting muscle fibres and determines the resting length of individual sarcomeres. The *force–length relationship* describes the relationship between the force generated upon stimulation of the muscle and preload (Figure 4.1). The magnitude of the active force generated is a function of the number of actin–myosin cross-bridges, which is itself a function of initial sarcomere length (Figure 4.2). As preload increases, there is an increase in active force up to a maximal limit – the maximum isometric force. Thus, an increase in LV preload (end-diastolic volume) leads to an increase in SV.

Afterload

The *force–length relationship* determines how alterations in preload effect force generation when the muscle length is fixed (i.e. isometric contraction). In reality, however, contracting muscle performs 'work

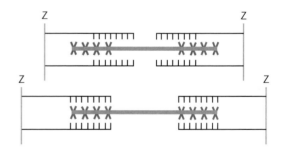

Figure 4.2 The effect on sarcomere length (distance between Z-lines) on actin–myosin overlap.

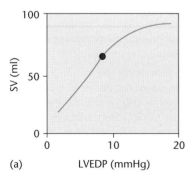

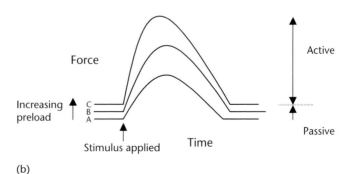

Figure 4.1 The effect of preload on force development in cardiac muscle. (a) The Frank–Starling relationship. (b) As preload increases (curves A–C) the same stimulus generates a greater force.

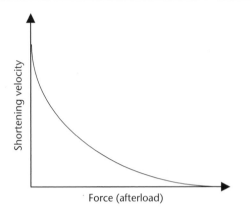

Figure 4.3 The force–velocity relationship. The greater the afterload the slower the rate of muscle shortening.

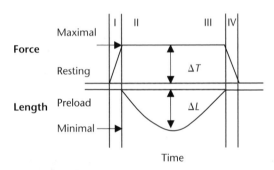

Figure 4.4 The relationship between force and length during cardiac muscle contraction.

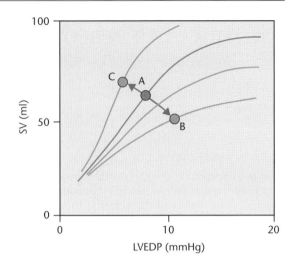

Figure 4.5 The effect of positive (C) and negative (B) inotropy on the normal (A) Frank–Starling relationship.

Inotropy

The ability to alter contractility is a property unique to cardiac muscle. For any given preload and afterload, an increase in inotropy increases the force generated during isometric contraction, and increases both the extent and velocity of muscle shortening during isotonic contraction. The net effect is an upward and leftward shift of the Frank–Starling relationship (Figure 4.5).

Pressure–volume relationship

By plotting ventricular pressure against ventricular volume throughout the cardiac cycle, a *pressure–volume loop* can be constructed. While ventricular pressure can be readily measured, measuring ventricular volume during the cardiac cycle is more problematic. Conventional techniques such as ventriculography, echocardiography, radionuclide imaging and MRI have largely been replaced by the conductance catheter, which allows beat-to-beat measurement of ventricular volume in real time.

The principle underlying the conductance catheter technique is the measurement of the electrical conductance of blood in the ventricular cavity. Blood is a good conductor of electricity whereas the ventricular wall is a relatively poor conductor. Thus when the ventricle is full, its conductance is high. The conductance catheter (Figure 4.6) has either eight or ten electrodes, typically made of platinum, mounted on a standard angiographic catheter. Typically, paired ventricular pressure and volume data are acquired at

by shortening'. The force opposing shortening can be thought of as the afterload. The *force–velocity relationship* (Figure 4.3) describes how muscles contract isotonically (i.e. shorten). As afterload increases both the rate (velocity) and extent of muscle shortening decrease. Conversely, shortening velocity increases as preload increases.

The four phases of isotonic contraction are represented in Figure 4.4.

- *Phase I* Isometric contraction – muscle length remains unchanged until the force generated overcomes preload.
- *Phase II* Isotonic contraction – when the force generated reaches the initial load, the muscle begins to shorten. The rate and extent of shortening is proportional to the preload and inversely proportional to the afterload.
- *Phase III* Isotonic relaxation – the muscle lengthens until the force reaches the preload.
- *Phase IV* Isometric relaxation – muscle length remains unchanged.

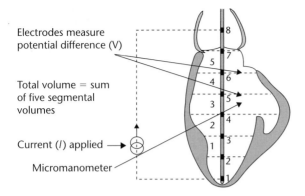

Figure 4.6 A conductance catheter. An alternating current (*I*) is applied between the two outermost electrodes by a signal conditioning and processing unit. The potential difference between pairs of consecutive electrodes is measured. The volume of blood that is measured between any two sensing electrodes can be considered to be a cylinder with boundaries defined by the endothelial surfaces of the cardiac walls and by equipotential surfaces of the electrodes. The total volume of blood within the ventricular cavity can be considered to be a column of these cylinders. Modified from van der Velde *et al*, 1992.

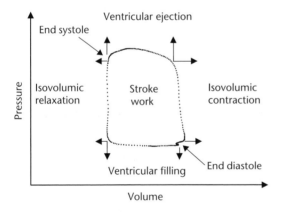

Figure 4.7 The LV pressure–volume relationship during a single cardiac cycle. Pressure (corresponding to ventricular force) is plotted on the *y*-axis, and volume (corresponding to myocardial fibre length) is plotted on the *x*-axis. The area within the pressure–volume loop is the stroke work. Note that in respiratory physiology, the axes are typically reversed.

$\geq 250\,Hz$ (i.e. at 4 ms intervals). The various phases of the pressure–volume loop can be seen in Figure 4.7.

The cycle begins at end-diastole and has four phases:

- *Isovolumic contraction*   pressure increases in the ventricle while the volume remains constant until the AV opens.

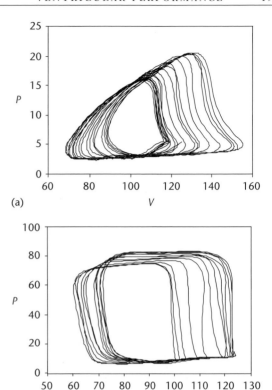

Figure 4.8 Comparison of (a) RV and (b) LV pressure–volume loops. Note that the pressure scales for the two ventricles are different (0–30 for RV and 0–150 mmHg for LV).

- *Ventricular ejection*   the AV closes when aortic pressure exceeds LV pressure (end systole).
- *Isovolumic relaxation*   the period between AV closure and MV opening.
- *Ventricular filling*   has three components: passive early filling, diastasis and active late filling during atrial systole.

The width of the loop (i.e. the difference between end-diastolic and end-systolic volumes) is the SV, and the area within the pressure–volume loop is the stroke work. Stroke work is the product of SV and mean aortic pressure during ejection. This is often simplified to the product of SV and mean aortic pressure.

Unlike the LV, ejection from the RV begins earlier in systole and, due to the high capacitance of the pulmonary vascular bed, RV pressure is not sustained throughout systole. These two factors account for the triangular RV loop morphology (Figure 4.8). For this reason and because right-heart pressures are around one-fifth of those in the left, RV stroke work is less than

LV stroke work. Although ejection during the pressure rise is mechanically efficient it is dependent on the low impedance of the pulmonary vasculature. As RV afterload increases, the RV pressure–volume relationship begins to resemble that of the LV.

Parameters derived from pressure–volume loops

By constructing pressure–volume loops under different conditions of preload and afterload, a series or family of loops can be obtained. In practice, afterload is varied using vasoactive drugs and preload by manually clamping the IVC in the operating theatre or by balloon occlusion in the catheter laboratory.

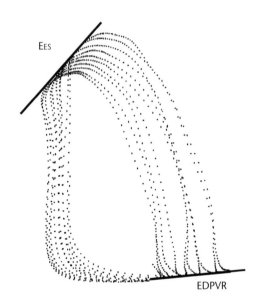

Figure 4.9 A series of LV pressure–volume loops showing the slope of the ESPVR (E$_{ES}$) and the slope of the EDPVR.

From these loops, two important relationships can be derived (Figure 4.9).

1 The slope of the end-diastolic pressure–volume relationship (EDPVR) gives information on the compliance of the ventricle. The relationship between pressure and volume at end diastole is generally curvilinear.
2 The slope of the end-systolic pressure–volume relationship (ESPVR) – also known as the end-systolic elastance (E$_{ES}$) – is a measure of ventricular contractility. Within the normal physiological range the ESPVR is linear (described by a linear regression).

The advantage of using the ESPVR as a measure of ventricular function, over more traditional methods such as ejection fraction, is that it is load independent. An increase in the contractile state of the ventricle will increase the slope of the ESPVR i.e. E$_{ES}$ (Figure 4.10).

Ventricular interdependence

As the heart is enclosed within the pericardium and both the LV and RV share superficial muscle fibres, their function is inextricably linked and interdependent. Ventricular interdependence in pathological states is dealt with in more detail elsewhere.

Overall ventricular performance is determined by preload, contractility, ventricular elastance and the manner in which the contracting ventricle interacts with the outflow tract. Whereas in the ventricle, elastance is represented by the slope of the ESPVR (i.e. E$_{ES}$), arterial elastance (E$_A$) is represented by the slope of the line joining end diastole to end systole – the relationship between SV and the pressure difference between end systole and end diastole (Figure 4.11).

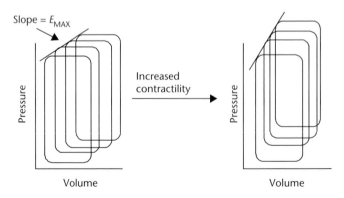

Figure 4.10 The LV ESPVR is shifted upwards and to the left demonstrating an increase in contractility.

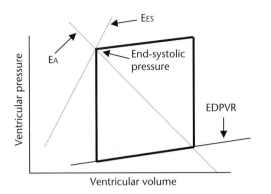

Figure 4.11 Ventriculo-arterial coupling: the relationship between E_{ES} and E_A. The E_A can be thought of as the combination of arterial resistance, impedance, capacitance and inductance. The ventricle delivers maximal (stroke) work when the E_A/E_{ES} ratio approaches 1.0.

Conclusion

The use of pressure–volume loops allows assessment of overall ventricular function, the severity of valvular incompetence and donor organ viability prior to transplantation. Later chapters will identify how the pressure–volume loop is affected in specific disease states.

Key points

- Ventricular function is dependent upon preload, contractility and afterload.
- Cardiac output is a crude, load-dependent index of ventricular function.
- The ventricular pressure–volume loop allows assessment of ventricular function and arterial elastance.
- The end-systolic pressure–volume relationship is a load-independent measure of ventricular function.

Further reading

Braunwald E, Ross J, Sonnenblick EH. *Mechanisms of Contraction of the Normal and Failing Heart*. Boston: Little, Brown & Co., 1968; pp. 31–76.

Klabunde RE. *Cardiovascular Physiology Concepts*. http://www.cvphysiology.com.

van der Velde ET, van Dijk AD, Steendijk P, Diethelm L, Chagas T, Lipton MJ. Left ventricular segmental volume by conductance catheter and Cine-CT. *Eur Heart J* 1992; **13 Suppl E**: 15-21.

Weber KT, Janicki JS. The dynamics of ventricular contraction: force, length, and shortening. *Fed Proc* 1980; **39(2)**: 188–195.

Warltier DC (Ed.). *Ventricular Function* (Society of Cardiovascular Anesthesiologists Monograph). Baltimore: Williams & Wilkins, 1995.

CORONARY PHYSIOLOGY

5

J. Byrne & P. MacCarthy

The coronary circulation is unique in that the organ supplied generates the perfusion pressure for the whole circulation. The heart relies predominantly on aerobic metabolism to meet its high-energy requirements. At rest cardiac oxygen consumption (VO_2) is 8–10 ml $100 g^{-1} min^{-1}$. The five- to six-fold increase in VO_2 caused by exercise must be met by an increase in myocardial oxygen supply. Even in the resting state oxygen extraction is near maximal, so increases in myocardial oxygen supply must be achieved by increases in coronary blood flow. There is a near-linear relationship between these two parameters (Figure 5.1).

Increased coronary flow can occur in two ways:

- by increasing coronary perfusion pressure,
- by reducing resistance to coronary blood flow.

Physiological regulation of perfusion pressure is limited and unable to meet the dramatic increase in oxygen demand when cardiac work increases. Alterations in myocardial oxygen supply under physiological conditions are therefore primarily achieved by alterations in the vascular resistance of the coronary circulation. Alteration in coronary blood flow is the critical determinant of total myocardial metabolism.

Coronary macrocirculation

Coronary blood flow is phasic and differs between right and left coronary arteries. Left coronary flow is almost exclusively diastolic as pressure in the wall of the left ventricle during systole is similar to that in the aorta. Right coronary flow also predominately occurs in diastole but lower right ventricular pressures allow some systolic flow (Figure 5.2).

Normal epicardial arteries are typically >0.3 mm in diameter, offer little measurable resistance to coronary blood flow, and play no significant role in the regulation of myocardial blood flow under physiological conditions.

Coronary microcirculation

Control of coronary flow lies entirely within the microvasculature which is composed of vessels with a diameter of <200 μm that includes small arteries, arterioles, capillaries, pericytic venules and muscular venules. Resistance to flow is inversely proportional to the fourth power of the vessel radius. While some resistance to flow occurs in small coronary arteries and large arterioles, coronary vascular resistance is largely determined by those arterioles with a diameter <150 μm. Here oxygen supply is also tightly regulated, and with a dense network of approximately 4000

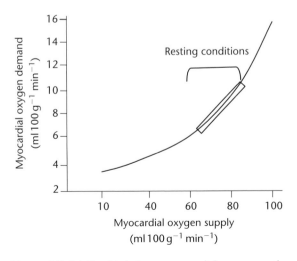

Figure 5.1 Relationship between myocardial oxygen supply and demand.

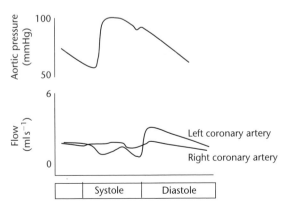

Figure 5.2 Schematic representation of flow in left and right coronary arteries.

Determinants of myocardial oxygen demand	Determinants of myocardial oxygen supply
• Wall tension	• Aortic pressure
• Myocardial contractility	• LVEDP
• HR	• Coronary vascular resistance
	• HR

Figure 5.3 Determinants of myocardial oxygen demand and supply.

capillaries per square millimetre each myocyte is in close proximity to the capillary microcirculation. Coronary arterioles themselves also appear to have particular functions dependent on their size; for example, the principle site of metabolic vasodilatation occurs in the smallest arterioles ($<100\,\mu m$) whereas larger arterioles are the site of flow-mediated vasodilatation. The number of functional arterioles depends on the myocardial oxygen requirements of the myocardium; large increases in recruitment occur as the arterial partial pressure of oxygen falls and demand increases. Regional blood flow within the myocardium is not homogenous and variations in coronary flow may be related to regional variations in myocardial metabolism.

Myocardial oxygen demand and supply

The major determinants of myocardial oxygen supply and demand are shown in Figure 5.3. Increased HR has detrimental effects on both demand and supply. An increased HR results in high ventricular wall tension and a shorter diastole. The proportional increase in the time at which wall tension is high leads to increased demand. The shorter diastole reduces the time available for coronary perfusion.

Alterations in coronary artery perfusion pressure (i.e. the difference between aortic pressure and LVEDP) play a limited role in the regulation of coronary flow. Coronary vascular resistance provides the major mechanism by which coronary flow is regulated in response to changing metabolic demand.

Coronary vascular resistance

Metabolic regulation

Metabolic control of coronary artery vasodilatation is the primary determinant of vascular tone, and can induce a five-fold reduction in vascular resistance. Adenosine plays a critical role in the modulation of resting arterial tone; although a number of other metabolites are also involved.

Adenosine

When myocardial oxygen demand exceeds supply, cardiac myocytes generate adenosine as a result of the metabolism of adenosine triphosphate (ATP). Most of the adenosine leaves the cell to reach the extracellular space where it acts to dilate vascular smooth muscle. It is chiefly the small arterioles of $25-100\,\mu m$ diameter that are the major target of adenosine-induced vasodilatation. Once in the circulation, adenosine is broken down by adenosine deaminase. Adenosine only has a role in the maintenance of coronary vascular tone when myocardial oxygen demand exceeds supply, for instance during hypoxaemia and ischaemia, or times of increased heart work. Adenosine does not help maintain coronary vascular tone under basal conditions and has a limited role during exercise.

Adenosine acts at purinergic P_1 receptors. These receptors are further subdivided into myocardial A_1 receptors and vascular A_2 receptors. Activation of vascular A_2 receptors increases the intracellular concentration of cyclic adenosine monophosphate (cAMP), leading to a reduction in intracellular calcium and the binding affinity of vascular myosin light chain kinase. This leads to relaxation of vascular smooth muscle and coronary vasodilatation (Figure 5.4). Part of the action of adenosine may also involve endothelial production of nitric oxide (NO) leading to increased intracellular cyclic guanosine monophosphate (cGMP) concentration and vasodilatation in vascular smooth muscle. Adenosine may also act via the ATP-sensitive potassium channel to cause smooth muscle hyperpolarization and vasodilatation.

Potassium

High levels of potassium lead to vasoconstriction, whereas modestly elevated levels vasodilate and may involve indirect release of NO.

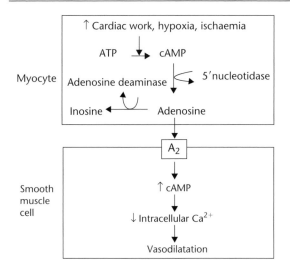

Figure 5.4 Schematic representation of the production and action of adenosine.

Hydrogen ions

Protons cause vasodilatation during anaerobic respiration.

Atrial natriuretic peptide

Atrial natriuretic peptide acts on guanylate cyclase to cause arterial vasodilatation.

Oxygen/carbon dioxide

Both hypoxaemia and hypercarbia cause vasodilatation.

Endothelial regulation

The endothelial monolayer plays a vital role in normal vascular homeostasis. Disruption or damage to these cells underlies the pathophysiology of a number of disease states.

Nitric oxide

Nitric oxide is continuously released from coronary endothelial cells under resting conditions and is the most important endothelial mediator of resting coronary artery and arteriolar tone. NO plays a crucial role in *flow-mediated* vasodilatation; the mechanism whereby increased blood flow amplifies smooth muscle relaxation and vessel dilatation. Increased blood flow leads to an increase in vascular shear stress (the force placed on the endothelium by flowing blood) and a release of NO from the endothelial layer, which in turn

leads to vasodilatation. The effects of flow-mediated vasodilatation are particularly important during exercise. As well as direct effects on arterial tone, NO also reduces platelet aggregation, and has important anti-inflammatory effects thereby reducing the risk of arteriolar occlusion. This mechanism is far more important in larger arterioles and primarily affects intermediate coronary arterioles (80–300 μm in diameter) and the larger conductance arteries. However, receptor-dependent NO release may be important at other levels of the coronary microcirculation. The production of NO is dependent on an intact endothelium and in disease states (e.g. atheromatous coronary artery disease) the endothelium may be dysfunctional or the bioavailability of NO may be reduced (e.g. by oxidative stress). When the protective effects of NO are lost, the effect of vasoconstrictors released from the endothelium may predominate. The resulting increase in coronary vascular resistance increases myocardial oxygen demand and may worsen ischaemia.

NO is generated from the conversion of the amino acid L-arginine to L-citrulline within endothelial cells, a reaction catalysed by a family of enzymes known as the NO synthases (NOS). NO increases cGMP levels within vascular smooth muscle cells, which has a number of effects, including a reduction in calcium sensitivity of the myofilaments. The net effect is smooth muscle relaxation and vasodilatation. NO diffuses across cell membranes to adjacent smooth muscle cells to exert its effects (Figure 5.5).

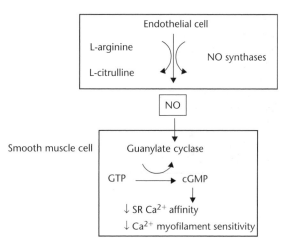

Figure 5.5 Schematic representation of the production and action of endothelial-derived NO.

Other endothelial mediators

Endothelial-dependent vasodilatation persists even after inhibition of NO suggesting the existence of alternative endothelial mediators of coronary vascular tone. The vasodilatation observed is preceded by smooth muscle hyperpolarization and is mediated by an endothelial-derived hyperpolarizing factor. Its precise nature remains uncertain, with some data suggesting that the response is mediated by endothelial-derived K^+, or dependent on cytochrome P450. A number of factors are therefore likely to be involved in this response. Other endothelial mediators have been shown to contribute to coronary vasomotor tone and may be vasodilatory (e.g. prostacyclin or bradykinin) or vasoconstrictory (e.g. endothelin-1).

Autonomic regulation

Epicardial and intramyocardial coronary arteries are densely innervated by sympathetic and parasympathetic nerve fibres. Sympathetic stimulation occurs via both vasoconstrictory (α_1 and α_2) receptors and vasodilatory (β_1, β_2 and β_3) receptors. Under *physiological* conditions both noradrenaline and adrenaline mediate coronary vasodilatation due to their β_1 effect, in contrast to their peripheral effect of vasoconstriction, which is α mediated.

α-adrenergic

The α_1-adrenergic receptors are predominantly located in vessels >100 μm in diameter, while α_2 receptors are located in the smaller arterioles. The magnitude of vasoconstriction produced by the activation of α_2 receptors is approximately double that of the α_1 receptors, and in the presence of coronary disease and a dysfunctional endothelium α_2 receptors may have a greater functional significance.

β-adrenergic

The β_1-adrenergic receptors predominate in coronary arteries and arterioles >100 μm in diamteter, whereas β_2 receptors are located in vessels <100 μm. Under normal physiological conditions, β-adrenergic stimulation causes vasodilatation of healthy coronary arteries. However, this is usually masked by increases in HR and myocardial contractility following β-receptor activation. A component of β_2-vasodilatation is thought to involve endothelial release of NO.

Cholinergic

Acetylcholine (ACh) mediates NO release from the endothelium via M_1, M_2 and M_3 receptors. While ACh is a potent coronary vasodilator when the endothelium is intact, vasoconstrictory responses may predominate in damaged endothelium due to direct effects on smooth muscle cells.

Non-adrenergic, non-cholinergic

Neuropeptides, such as vasoactive intestinal peptide (VIP) and neuropeptide Y, are also present in parasympathetic nerve fibres. Neuropeptide Y is a vasoconstrictor co-released with noradrenaline, whereas VIP causes dose-dependent relaxation of coronary arteries.

Myogenic regulation

Myogenic control refers to the intrinsic properties of vascular smooth muscle, which lead to contraction when intravascular pressure is elevated, and relaxation when pressure is reduced. The myogenic response is independent of any neural or humoral influences, although the effects may be modulated by the endothelium. The myogenic response remains incompletely understood; however the primary stimulus is the application of asymmetrical mechanical force to the vessel wall which is subsequently transduced into a signal for muscle contraction via activation of ion channels and length-dependent alterations in contractile protein function. Stretch-activated cation channels lead to increased levels of intracellular cations leading to membrane depolarization which may then lead to calcium-induced calcium release from the sarcoplasmic reticulum and smooth muscle contraction. Recent data also suggests that in conditions of increased oxidative stress, reactive oxygen species may also be involved in the myogenic response.

Autoregulation

The process whereby coronary flow is regulated by myocardial oxygen demand independently of coronary perfusion pressure is termed autoregulation and is common to a number of vascular beds. Despite quite marked alterations in coronary perfusion pressure, coronary blood flow remains relatively constant between coronary perfusion pressures from 50 to 140 mmHg. If coronary perfusion pressure falls outside these limits, flow becomes directly dependent on perfusion pressure.

Autoregulation principally occurs in vessels of diameter <150 μm. Myogenic control mechanisms play an important role, however metabolic and endothelial factors, particularly NO, are primarily involved in the control of vascular resistance during autoregulation. When NO levels are reduced or NO production is inhibited, the lower limit of autoregulation is increased and the myocardium becomes more vulnerable to hypoperfusion.

Pathophysiology

Atherosclerosis

An early pathological feature of atherosclerotic coronary artery disease is the development of endothelial dysfunction due, in part, to the reduction in bioavailability of NO. Endothelial, flow-mediated vasodilatation is significantly impaired, and vasoconstriction may occur. Furthermore, loss of NO favours platelet aggregation, the accumulation of macrophages which oxidize low-density lipoprotein and ultimately may contribute to the development of coronary atheroma. Coronary stenosis reduces the coronary perfusion pressure in the segment distal to the narrowing. The severity of the narrowing primarily determines whether any reduction in flow occurs; resistance to blood flow increases by a power of 4 as the radius decreases. However, other effects including turbulent flow, diffuse atheromatous disease and vasoconstriction due to abnormal endothelial function may further reduce blood flow.

Abnormalities of endothelial function extend to the microvasculature where loss of flow-mediated vasodilatation may reduce perfusion pressure upstream and, as perfusion pressure falls below the limits of autoregulation, the capillaries abruptly shut – at the *critical closing pressure* – and coronary flow is further reduced. The net effect will be to reduce myocardial oxygen supply and worsen ischaemia.

However, it is important to note that the net effects of atheromatous plaque formation on coronary blood flow may be attenuated by the development of collateral vessels. In some cases these may, over time, limit ischaemia even in the presence of significant arterial occlusion.

Diabetes mellitus

Abnormalities in coronary vascular function are detectable early in both type 1 and 2 DM, and occur before the development of overt vascular disease. While resting coronary blood flow is not significantly impaired, sympathetic dysfunction and dysinnervation may diminish vasodilatation and reduce coronary blood flow reserve. Furthermore, endothelial dysfunction will also reduce flow-mediated vasodilatation and lead to a blunted response when oxygen demand increases. Abnormalities of the microvasculature in DM may therefore lead to a reduction in coronary blood flow, and subsequent ischaemia even in the absence of significant angiographic coronary artery disease. However, atheromatous coronary artery disease is also more common and a reduction in the bioavailability of NO may be a major driving force for the higher plaque instability observed in diabetic patients.

Coronary spasm

Coronary spasm causes transient reductions of coronary artery blood flow and is due to focal hyperreactivity within coronary arteries. These arteries may have increased tone at rest and are sensitive to vasoconstrictory stimuli. The precise pathophysiology is unknown but may be due to a localized reduction in the bioavailability of NO or excess vasoconstrictors such as endothelin-1. Recent studies have implicated ATP-dependent K^+ channels. In the presence of a damaged endothelium, aggregated platelet thrombi may release serotonin and thromboxane which lead to vasoconstriction and worsen subsequent ischaemia.

Conclusions

Metabolic, endothelial, myogenic and neurohumoral mechanisms act in concert to regulate myocardial blood flow. Each of these processes, however, has a preferential site of action within the coronary microvasculature. Metabolic control primarily occurs in the smaller arterioles ($<100 \, \mu m$), whereas myogenic control predominates in intermediate-sized arterioles. Endothelial modulation of vascular resistance occurs in small and intermediate coronary arterioles and overlaps with, and may well modulate, myogenic microvascular control. These control mechanisms are affected by the autonomic nervous system, with β-adrenergic stimulation predominating under physiological conditions to promote vasodilatation, α-adrenergic constriction opposing metabolic vasodilatation and promoting myogenic vasoconstriction in certain areas of the coronary micro-circulation.

When myocardial oxygen demand increases, metabolic dilatation of the smallest vessels occurs first; this then leads to a reduction in myogenic tone in intermediate coronary arterioles upstream due to a reduction in pressure. The increase in flow causes endothelial-modulated, flow-mediated dilatation in larger arterioles and small arteries which further serves to increase coronary flow in response to a higher demand. Conversely, when oxygen demand is reduced, production of metabolic vasodilators is reduced and an increase in tone in the smallest arterioles occurs. This leads to a reduction in flow upstream and a downregulation of myogenic and endothelial modulation of arteriolar and small artery tone (Figure 5.6).

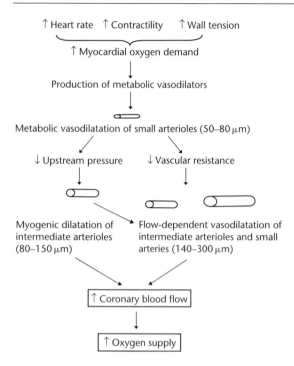

Figure 5.6 Interaction between metabolic, myogenic and endothelial control mechanisms.

The regulation of myocardial blood flow is not homogenous. Important regional variations in flow occur in response to various physiological stimuli. For instance neural and metabolic mechanisms dominate at specific sites, or microvascular domains, and biochemical and functional differences are also apparent in individual endothelial cells.

Endothelial dysfunction underlies a number of pathophysiological states and leads to loss of vasodilatory reserve in the macro- and micro-circulation. With the development of atheromatous plaque in the larger conductance arteries, and a reduction in perfusion pressure, compensatory vasodilatation is attenuated, and paradoxical vasoconstriction may occur, further reducing blood flow and worsening ischaemia.

Acknowledgement

We are grateful to Professor A.M. Shah for his review of this manuscript.

Key points

- Coronary blood flow is dependent on coronary vascular resistance and less importantly on coronary perfusion pressure (aortic pressure).
- Under physiological conditions the microcirculation controls vascular resistance and blood flow.
- Control is heterogenous between different vascular microdomains and is modulated by endothelial, metabolic, neurogenic and myogenic factors.
- In disease states, a reduction in coronary blood flow occurs due to development of atheromatous plaque, and the loss of vasodilatory reserve due to endothelial and microvascular dysfunction.

Further reading

Chilian WM. Coronary microcirculation in health and disease. Summary of an NHLBI workshop. *Circulation* 1997; **95(2)**: 522–528.

Feigl EO. Coronary physiology. *Physiol Rev* 1983; **63(1)**: 1–205.

Jones CJ, Kuo L, Davis MJ, Chilian WM. Regulation of coronary blood flow: coordination of heterogeneous control mechanisms in vascular microdomains. *Cardiovasc Res* 1995; **29(5)**: 585–596.

CARDIOVASCULAR CONTROL MECHANISMS

6

J.J. Walton & A.M. Cohen

The cardiovascular system (CVS) is a dynamic system – responding to the constantly changing demands on the circulation via a complex series of homoeostatic mechanisms. These mechanisms are either immediate or delayed, acting directly on HR, SV and vascular resistance; and indirectly via changes in circulating plasma volume. These changes are regulated via:

1 the central nervous system (CNS),
2 the endocrine system,
3 local or intrinsic mechanisms.

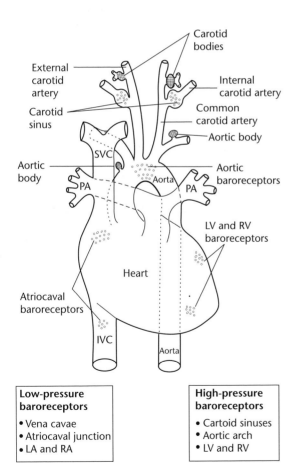

Figure 6.1 Aortic and carotid baroreceptors.

Low-pressure baroreceptors	High-pressure baroreceptors
• Vena cavae • Atriocaval junction • LA and RA	• Cartoid sinuses • Aortic arch • LV and RV

Immediate

Although considered separately for ease of explanation *in vivo*, the following components of cardiovascular homoeostasis act in concert with each other to produce a dynamic and constantly changing control system.

$$CO = SV \times HR$$

Immediate cardiac homoeostasis is primarily achieved via adjustments of HR and the three determinants of SV, namely preload, afterload and contractility.

Preload

In accordance with the Frank–Starling law, the force of myocardial muscle fibre contraction is proportional to the initial length of the fibre.

Contractility

Myocardial contractility is best described in terms of the slope of the end-systolic pressure–volume relationship (ESPVR) also known as the end-systolic elastance (E_{ES}). Extrinsic factors, such as sympathetic tone, endogenous catecholamines and exogenously administered inotropic drugs, increase contractility. *In vitro* increasing HR is associated with increased contractility – the so-called *Bowditch effect* (inochronic autoregulation). *In vivo*, the effect is less pronounced or absent in non-anaesthetized subjects.

Numerous factors, including hypoxia, anaesthetic agents and parasympathetic tone, decrease contractility.

Afterload

A sudden increase in afterload is followed by a decrease in SV that gradually increases with each successive beat. The final SV is higher than the baseline SV which persists even after aortic pressure returns to its initial value. This adaptation is known as the *Anrep effect* (homoeometric autoregulation) and is due to an initial muscle cell shortening followed by successively increasing stretch secondary to increased diastolic volumes. In the face of a sustained increase in afterload, the effect restores end-diastolic volume (EDV) by increasing contractility.

Heart rate

Although cardiac muscle possesses an intrinsic rhythmicity, its basal rate is too low to provide organ perfusion during normal metabolic activity. The autonomic nervous system (ANS) and adrenal medulla are primarily responsible for the adjustment of HR with differing metabolic needs acting via SA and atrioventricular (A-V) nodal receptors.

Increased sympathetic nervous system (SNS) activity ($C_{7/8}$–$T_{5/6}$) and circulating catecholamines decrease the time taken for the SA node to reach its firing threshold (Phase IV – slow diastolic depolarization) and increases the speed of conduction through the A-V node. This increases SA firing rate (chronotropism) and conduction velocity (dromotropism).

Increased parasympathetic (vagal) tone acts via muscarinic receptors to open K^+ channels in SA nodal cells, lowering resting membrane potential (RMP) (see Figure 2.4). Acetylcholine slows diastolic depolarization and A-V nodal conduction time, resulting in HR reduction.

Although the effects of the ANS on the heart seem well balanced, *in vivo* the SNS is dominant and capable of over-riding vagal tone.

The denervated heart

The transplanted heart lacks ANS innervation and relies on direct catecholamine stimulation of cardiac β-receptors to raise resting HR. Thyroxine increases β-receptors density. The *Bainbridge Reflex* – an autoregulatory mechanism seen in denervated hearts – describes the increase in HR seen with a rapid rise in preload.

$$V = I \times R \quad \text{(Ohm's law)}$$

$$MAP = CO \times SVR$$

$$MPAP = CO \times PVR$$

where
V   = Potential difference
I   = Current/flow
R   = Resistance
MPAP = Mean pulmonary artery pressure

SVR is the physiological term used to quantify arterial smooth muscle tone. Peripheral vascular muscle tone is under ANS control via α_1-adrenoceptors (vasoconstriction) and β_2-adrenoceptors (vasodilatation). A series of complex brainstem reflexes 'fine tunes' vascular tone.

Baroreceptor

The most important short-term regulators of MAP are the baroreceptor reflexes. The mechanoreceptors that mediate these reflexes can be subdivided into high-pressure baroreceptors (which regulate arterial pressure) and low-pressure baroreceptors (which regulate atrial filling pressures) (Figure 6.1). Afferent neural impulses travel from the baroreceptors to the CNS via the glossopharyngeal and vagus nerves.

High-pressure baroreceptors are stretch-sensitive mechanoreceptors located in the carotid sinuses and the aortic arch, which regulate MAP. Similar structures are found in the ventricles.

Low-pressure baroreceptors are located in the atria, the vena cavae and the atriocaval junctions.

Carotid sinus and aortic arch baroreceptors

A rise in MAP stimulates increased firing of the high-pressure mechanoreceptors in the carotid sinus and aortic arch. The afferent signals travel via the glossopharyngeal nerve and aortic depressor nerve (a branch of the vagus nerve) respectively to synapse in the brainstem. Within the brainstem, the *nucleus tractus solarius* (NTS) acts as a central integration site for the projection of a wide variety of inputs including CVS baroreceptors, peripheral chemoreceptors and receptors located in the airways and lungs.

Baroreceptor inputs reaching the NTS are modulated by afferents from a variety of other sites such as the hypothalamus before projecting into two further areas in the brainstem, namely the *nucleus ambiguus* and the caudal *ventrolateral medulla* (VLM). The nucleus ambiguus is the site of origin of the vagal efferent innervation of the heart and its stimulation leads to an increase in vagal tone. The caudal VLM sends inhibitory fibres to the adjacent rostral VLM. This part of the brainstem acts as the excitatory control centre of the descending sympathetic pathways to the heart. Inhibition here therefore results in a decrease in cardiac sympathetic tone.

The end result of this complex reflex arc is a decrease in HR, vasodilatation and consequent decrease in MAP (Figure 6.2). Conversely, a decrease in MAP results in increased sympathetic stimulation and reduced vagal tone leading to a rise in HR and SVR.

Autoregulation of Vascular Smooth Muscle

Although all organ systems are capable of a degree of autoregulation over a wide range of MAP (approximately 60–160 mmHg) it is particularly important in the cardiac, cerebral and renal circulations. Autoregulation is mediated by precapillary resistance

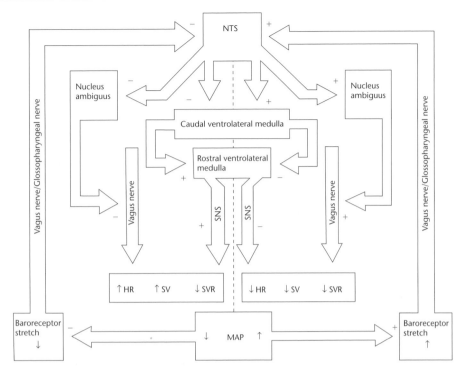

Figure 6.2 Schematic of baroreceptors reflexes.

vessels, primarily arterioles, 40–100 μm in diameter. Autoregulation has been explained as the result of two main mechanisms:

- *The myogenic mechanism* Fluctuations in perfusion pressure induce an active response in arteriolar smooth muscle tension. This damps down the change in pressure ensuring constant blood flow.
- *The metabolic mechanism* The concentration of metabolic products in the interstitial fluid has a direct effect on vascular smooth muscle. Many different substances have been investigated with regard to the metabolic mechanism of autoregulation. O_2, CO_2, nitric oxide (NO), H^+, K^+, adenosine, kinins and prostaglandins all relax vascular smooth muscles. These mechanisms are discussed in more detail in Chapter 5.

Endothelium

It is likely that vascular endothelium regulates vascular tone regardless of the source of the stimulus – neural, mechanical or metabolic. Endothelium-dependent vasodilatation is mediated by the liberation of endothelium-derived relaxing factor, which acts by increasing intracellular guanosine monophosphate levels. Thought initially to be free NO, it is now

believed that this substance is a labile NO-precursor compound, such as S-nitroso-L-cysteine. Vasoconstriction is mediated by endothelium-derived constricting factors, such as the peptide endothelin.

Chemoreceptors

Peripheral chemoreceptors situated in the carotid bodies (at the bifurcation of the carotid arteries) and in the region of the aortic arch are sensitive to changes in PaO_2, $PaCO_2$ and H^+. Although primarily concerned with respiratory regulation they have a small but important role in CVS regulation. Increased $PaCO_2$ or H^+, or decreased PaO_2 stimulates a sympathetic response leading to increased HR and SVR. This response is significantly less than that triggered by the same plasma conditions within the central chemoreceptors of the medulla.

Control of circulating volume

The above mechanisms are able to rapidly compensate for acute changes in MAP. When circulatory changes are due to changes in circulating volume, additional homoeostatic endocrine mechanisms come into play.

Antidiuretic hormone

Plasma osmolality is dependent on the quantity of total body water. Antidiuretic hormone (ADH) is secreted by the posterior pituitary gland primarily in response to an increase in plasma osmolality (sensed by osmoreceptors in the hypothalamus) but also with decreasing MAP or circulating volume (sensed by receptors in the atria, aortic arch and carotid sinuses). In addition to being a potent vasoconstrictor, ADH acts on the nephron to increase water conservation by opening ADH-sensitive water-permeable pores in the collecting ducts, stimulating active Na^+ reabsorption and increasing the collecting duct permeability to urea.

Renin–angiotensin–aldosterone system

Renin is a proteolytic enzyme synthesized, stored and released by the juxtaglomerular apparatus (JGA). The JGA is composed of modified smooth muscle cells present in every efferent and afferent glomerular arteriole. Renin is released in response to a decrease in perfusion pressure, an increase in sympathetic tone or a decrease in Na^+ at the macula densa. It acts on the hepatically synthesized protein, angiotensinogen resulting in the production of the peptide angiotensin I (AT-I).

ACE is produced by lung endothelial cells and converts AT-I to the physiologically active AT-II. AT-II has a number of important homoeostatic actions:

1 aldosterone release from the adrenal cortex,
2 ADH secretion from the posterior pituitary,
3 the sensation of thirst via the hypothalamus,
4 increased arteriolar vasoconstriction,
5 increased renal Na^+ reabsorption.

Aldosterone itself has multiple roles but primarily it reduces renal Na^+ excretion by increasing absorption in the collecting duct and loop of Henle.

Atrial natriuretic peptide

ANP is released by atrial myocytes in response to increased stretch and acts as a renin–angiotensin–aldosterone system antagonist by directly inhibiting the release of renin and aldosterone, and increasing renal Na^+ and water excretion.

Thirst response

The sensation of thirst, regulated by a thirst centre situated within the hypothalamus, is triggered by a small increase in plasma osmolality or a large decrease in blood volume or MAP.

Delayed

Chronic changes in a CVS variable (e.g. SVR in essential hypertension) may lead to a compensatory resetting of the normal homoeostatic mechanisms.

Cardiac hypertrophy

Chronic pressure overload may induce compensatory hypertrophy in the muscle of any of the cardiac chambers. Although ventricular hypertrophy initially compensates well for the increased pressure load, the increasing thickness of the ventricular wall may compromise myocardial perfusion. End-stage ventricular hypertrophy is reached when the Frank–Starling relationship no longer applies and the chamber dilates and fails.

Endocrine compensation

If volume or pressure overload persists for a period of time renin and ADH secretion is reset, resulting in Na^+ and water retention. This results in a higher resting plasma renin concentration that persists even after the CVS variables have returned to normal.

Key points

- Many factors act in concert to contribute to cardiovascular homoeostasis.
- Rapid cardiovascular changes are mediated by the autonomic and intrinsic cardiac mechanisms, augmented by changes in plasma volume under the control of the endocrine system.
- Brainstem reflexes primarily regulate the ANS control of the CVS. Efferent input is from peripheral baroreceptors and chemoreceptors.
- Local autoregulation occurs in all vascular tissue and is mediated by the vascular endothelium. It is particularly important in the cerebral, renal and coronary circulations.
- Persistent alterations in MAP and plasma volume lead to compensatory chronic changes in the cardiovascular and endocrine systems.

Further reading

Nichols CG, Hanck DA, Jewell BR. The Anrep effect: an intrinsic myocardial mechanism. *Can J Physiol Pharmacol* 1988; **66(7)**: 924–929.

Prys-Roberts C, Brown Jr BR. *International Practice of Anaesthesia*, Vol. 1. Butterworth-Heinemann International Edition, 1996; pp. 1/26/1–1/26/10.

Swanton RH. *Cardiology*, 4th edition. Blackwell Science, 1998.

ANAESTHESIA AND THE CARDIOVASCULAR SYSTEM

7

J.J. Walton & A.M. Cohen

Central nervous system (CNS) depression is the goal of general anaesthesia. In practice, however, this is accompanied by effects on other organ systems particularly the respiratory and cardiovascular systems (CVS).

Pharmacological agents

Inhalational agents

Cardiac contractility

All fluorinated agents reduce cardiomyocyte Ca^{2+} influx. A lower cytoplasmic Ca^{2+} concentration diminishes Ca^{2+}-induced Ca^{2+} release from the sarcoplasmic reticulum (SR), leaving less Ca^{2+} to bind to the myocardial muscle filaments. *In vitro*, halothane also inhibits a cell membrane Na^+–Ca^{2+} exchange pump; further diminishing Ca^{2+} flux independently of T- and L-type Ca^{2+} channels. The net effect is depressed contractility and CO.

Vascular smooth muscle

Isoflurane, sevoflurane and desflurane cause greater decreases in SVR than enflurane or halothane. In

---

PHARMACOLOGICAL

Anaesthetic agents exert their effects on the CVS in a variety of ways:

- **Direct**
  - Cardiomyocyte depression – contractility and conduction
  - Vasomotor tone in coronary and systemic circulations
- **Indirect**
  - Release of vasoactive substances (e.g. histamine)
  - Sensitization of the heart to endogenous catecholamines
  - Autonomic nervous system (ANS) depression

NON-PHARMACOLOGICAL

Effects mediated by baroreceptors, chemoreceptors and ANS.

- **Tracheal intubation/extubation**
  - Increased HR, increased contractility and vasoconstriction via the sympathetic nervous system; vagal bradycardia may occur
- **Intermittent positive-pressure ventilation (IPPV)**
  - Impaired venous return leading to decreased SV
- **Hypercarbia**
  - Increased HR, increased contractility and vasoconstriction via central chemoreceptors
- **Patient positioning**
  - Changes in venous return

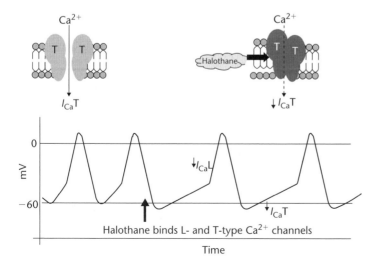

Figure 7.1 The effect of halothane on cardiomyocyte Ca^{2+} channels. Reduced Ca^{2+} influx via T- and L-type results in slowing of AP conduction and reducing the rate of pacemaker AP generation.

the coronary circulation isoflurane produces dose-dependent vasodilatation primarily in the small, high-resistance arteries (similar to SNP) while halothane exerts its vasodilatory effect on the large, low-resistance vessels (similar to glyceryl trinitrate) (Table 7.1).

Heart rate and cardiac conduction

The volatile agents have both direct and indirect effects on HR and conduction. With the exception of desflurane, which produces hyperactivity at 0.5–2.0 MAC, other volatile agents depress sympathetic activity. In addition, baroreceptor-mediated reflex tachycardia, secondary to reduced SVR and contractility, is blunted by CNS depression and slowed conduction.

Even at low concentrations, halothane directly binds to T- and L-type Ca^{2+} channels in the cell membranes of cardiomyocytes, diminishing Ca^{2+} influx. SA nodal pacemaker action potential (AP) generation is slowed or abolished (Figure 7.1), atrioventricular A-V nodal AP transmission is slowed and the refractory period is increased. Conversely, in the His–Purkinje system halothane slows AP conduction, increases AP duration and shortens the refractory period. If the SA node is inactive, other more slowly discharging foci in the atria or near the A-V junction may emerge as pacemakers, increasing the risk of dysrhythmia.

Volatile agents (particularly halothane) are more likely to cause dysrhythmias in the presence of raised circulating catecholamines. In the presence of halothane, the competing effects of α_{1A}-adrenoceptor stimulation (*reducing* His–Purkinje AP conduction velocity) and β-stimulation (*increasing* conduction velocity between Purkinje cells and myocytes), produces re-entrant circuits in the ventricular muscle with the potential to cause extrasystoles. While innocuous dysrhythmias are common, acidosis, hypokalaemia and hypocalcaemia may cause malignant dysrhythmias, such as bigeminy and multifocal ventricular extrasystoles. Sudden fluctuations in serum catecholamine levels during laryngoscopy or surgical stimulation may cause VT or VF.

The diseased heart

Most studies indicate that inhalational anaesthetics induce a degree of coronary vasodilatation. With the exception of isoflurane and desflurane, changes in coronary blood flow are in proportion to myocardial oxygen demand – autoregulation is maintained (Figure 7.2).

There is little evidence that clinically relevant doses of inhalational anaesthetics have a deleterious effect on the diseased heart. However, in the case of desflurane associated sympathetic activity has been shown to worsen myocardial ischaemia in patients undergoing coronary artery surgery.

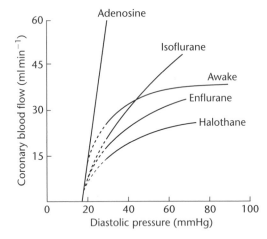

Figure 7.2 Schematic representation of the relationship between coronary blood flow and diastolic arterial pressure. Secondary to decreased myocardial O_2 demand halothane and enflurane shift the autoregulation curve to the right (coronary sinus oxygen saturation practically unchanged), whereas isoflurane (and desflurane) shift the curve to the left and straighten it. The effect of adenosine, the most potent coronary vasodilator, is shown for comparison.

Table 7.1 Effects of volatile agents on the CVS					
Properties	**HR**	**MAP**	**CO**	**SVR**	**Catecholamine sensitization**
Halothane	↓↓	↓↓	↓↓	↓	↑↑↑
Nitrous oxide	–	–	–	–	↑/↓
Enflurane	↑	↓↓	↓	↓	↑
Isoflurane	↑↑	↓↓	↓	↓↓	↑
Desflurane	↑	↓↓	↓	↓↓	↑
Sevoflurane	↑/↓	↓↓	Slight ↓	↓	↑

Coronary steal

Steal is defined as an increase in flow to a normally perfused area following coronary arteriolar vasodilatation at the expense of a decrease in perfusion to a collateral-dependent area. The prerequisite conditions for this phenomenon are (Figures 7.3 and 7.4) as follows:

- Total occlusion of the artery supplying the 'steal-prone' area.
- Perfusion of 'steal-prone' area dependent on collateral vessels.
- ≥90% stenosis in the artery supplying the collaterals.

Although isoflurane-induced coronary steal has been demonstrated in animal models there is little evidence for it in humans, indeed recent studies suggest that isoflurane improves ischaemia in some patients with ischaemic heart disease and has myocardial protective properties. It seems likely that when ischaemia has been seen in association with isoflurane, it is related to the increase in myocardial O_2 demand caused by changes in HR and SVR.

Nitrous oxide

Nitrous oxide (N_2O) produces modest dose-dependent cardiac depression. Unlike other inhalational agents this effect is offset by an increase in SVR secondary to sympathetic stimulation. The addition of N_2O to a volatile anaesthetic has been shown to result in less depression of arterial pressure than with volatile alone.

Intravenous agents

There is little evidence that any of the IV anaesthetics have a direct effect on the human cardiac conducting system. Dysrhythmias may however occur as a result of reduced myocardial blood flow and reflex tachycardia.

Barbiturates

Thiopental remains the world's most widely used IV anaesthetic agent and is the only barbiturate in common

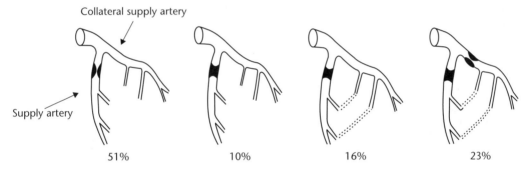

Figure 7.3 The four angiographic anatomical variants defined by the Coronary Artery Surgery Study (CASS) Registry. Total occlusion of a vessel associated with ≥50% stenosis in the collateral supply vessel was demonstrated in 23% of angiograms. However, only 12% of the 16,249 angiograms studied met the criteria for steal-prone anatomy – ≥90% stenosis of the collateral supply artery.

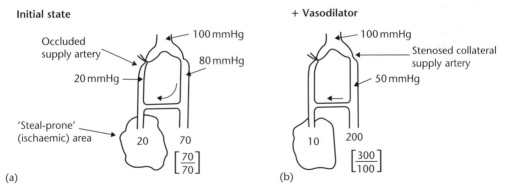

Figure 7.4 Proposed mechanism of vasodilator-induced coronary steal. In the initial state (a) a collateral supply vessel pressure of 80 mmHg (distal to the stenosis) generates a perfusion pressure of 20 mmHg in the steal-prone (ischaemic) area. Following vasodilator administration (b) increased blood flow to the non-ischaemic area reduces perfusion pressure in the steal-prone area to 10 mmHg.

use in the UK. The CVS effects include direct cardiac depression and vasodilatation. In contrast to the inhalational agents, the CVS effects are more 'patient dependent'. In young healthy subjects, CVS effects are limited to a modest fall in SVR and cardiac contractility, both compensated for by a baroreceptor-mediated increase in sympathetic tone. In the elderly and in patients with hypovolemia or decreased cardiac reserve, a profound fall in SVR and SV may occur.

Etomidate

Etomidate is the most cardiovascularly stable of the IV induction agents. Depression of the adrenocortical axis limits its clinical use.

Ketamine

The effects of ketamine on the CVS differ from those of other agents. It is the only general anaesthetic in current usage that does not produce CVS depression in patients with intact autonomic function. Modest direct myocardial depression is offset by its centrally mediated sympathomimetic actions leading to tachycardia, vasocontriction and hypertension, which in turn increase myocardial O_2 demand. In patients with impaired autonomic function however, the direct cardiac depressant effects may predominate producing cardiovascular collapse.

Propofol

Owing to its pharmacokinetic profile, propofol has become the most commonly used IV induction agent in the developed world. It has a cardiac profile very similar to that of thiopental, despite initial claims that it had minimal CVS effects. It causes direct cardiac depression and vasodilatation. Tachycardia occurs less frequently than that following thiopental administration. The deleterious CVS effects can be minimized by slow titration of the drug to observed effect.

Benzodiazepines

Diazepam, lorazepam and midazolam are often used as adjuncts to cardiac anaesthetic techniques. Although all cause hypotension secondary to myocardial depression and vasodilatation, the magnitude is less marked than that seen with barbiturates and propofol. Lorazepam has little effect on HR whereas midazolam and diazepam may be associated with either bradycardia or tachycardia. Midazolam causes a more pronounced CVS depression reflecting its faster action.

Opioids

Opioids are discussed in Chapter 13.

Neuromuscular blockers

Suxamethonium

The structural similarity to acetylcholine accounts for direct agonist action on the ANS and its effects on the CVS. Increased sympathetic tone leads to tachycardia and increased SVR, which may be exacerbated by subsequent endotracheal intubation. The resultant rise in myocardial O_2 demand is undesirable and may worsen pre-existing ischaemia. In some patients administration of the drug can lead to severe bradycardia due to a direct muscarinic effect. Bradycardia is most commonly seen in children and with repeat dosing.

Non-depolarizing drugs

Steroidal and bis-quaternary ammonium non-depolarizing muscle relaxants (NDMRs) may exert CVS side-effects by histamine release or actions on the autonomic ganglia or vagus nerve.

Histamine release is most commonly seen with atracurium. The effect is idiosyncratic.

D-tubocurarine, noted for its propensity to cause a profound autonomic ganglionic blockade, is rarely used nowadays. Clinically significant ganglionic blockade is not associated with conventional doses of commonly used NDMRs.

Pancuronium has vagolytic properties, which combined with a low propensity to cause histamine release account for its enduring popularity with cardiac anaesthetists. It can counteract some of the unwanted effects of other anaesthetic drugs – notably bradycardia. Rapid administration may cause profound tachycardia.

Regional anaesthesia

The CVS effects of regional anaesthetic techniques are the result of sympathetic blockade or inadvertent IV injection of local anaesthetic drugs.

Local anaesthetic agents

Local anaesthetics block Na^+ channels in excitable tissue, both neuronal and non-neuronal. All can be thought of as negatively inotropic and antidysrhythmic.

Lidocaine has a well-known role as a Vaughan–Williams Class 1 antidysrhythmic. It is relatively safe because of its low potency and tissue binding; consequently, a high serum concentration is necessary before cardiac toxicity is seen. Tinnitus, dizziness and perioral paraesthesia – all of which occur at lower concentrations – act as early warnings of misadministration in the conscious patient.

Bupivacaine has a narrower margin of CVS safety. Although greater tissue binding reduces the likelihood of CNS effects if used appropriately, inadvertent IV administration causes significantly greater problems. Firstly, its longer duration of action tends to cause, rather than suppress, dysrhythmias. Secondly, it has a direct toxic effect on cardiomyocyte contractile function. The overall effect of a significant IV dose of bupivacaine is refractory cardiac collapse that is only partially treatable with sympathomimetics.

Identification of D-bupivacaine as the more cardiotoxic isomer has led to the introduction of laevo (S-) bupivacaine, which has been shown to have a lower cardiac toxicity.

Sympathetic effects

All forms of regional anaesthesia have the potential for ANS blockade. Spinal anaesthesia causes a more rapid sympathetic blockade than epidural anaesthesia reflecting its faster onset. The extent of the CVS effects (primarily decreased vascular tone) is directly related to the type of block used (spinal > epidural), the dose of local anaesthetic used and the extent to which haemodynamic stability is dependent on sympathetic tone. Patients with *so-called* 'fixed CO states' such as severe aortic stenosis are particularly susceptible to sudden vasodilatation, as they are unable to increase stroke work to compensate for the drop in SVR. Spinal anaesthesia is contraindicated in these patients. In most other patients the adverse CVS effects of spinal and epidural blockade can be prevented or treated by the administration of IV fluids and direct-acting sympathomimetics such as ephedrine or α-adrenoceptor agonists like phenylephrine.

Key points

- The CNS effects of general anaesthesia are mirrored in other organ systems.
- The CVS effects of anaesthetic agents are dependent on patient age and physiological status.
- Anaesthetics have both direct and indirect actions on the CVS.
- Direct myocardial and vascular depression is often compensated for or obscured by autonomic reflexes.

Further reading

Agnew NM, Pennefather SH, Russell GN. Isoflurane and coronary heart disease. *Anaesthesia* 2002; **57(4)**: 338–347.

Ebert TJ, Muzi M. Sympathetic hyperactivity during desflurane anesthesia in healthy volunteers. A comparison with isoflurane. *Anesthesiology* 1993; **79(3)**: 444–453.

Priebe H-J. Isoflurane and coronary hemodynamics. *Anesthesiology* 1989; **71(6)**: 960–976.

Rusy BF, Komai H. Anesthetic depression of myocardial contractility: a review of possible mechanisms. *Anesthesiology* 1987; **67(5)**: 745–766.

CARDIAC PHARMACOLOGY

M.V. Podgoreanu & J.V. Booth

The homoeostatic regulation of the cardiovascular system relies on the ability of the heart to recognize and respond to many extracellular signalling molecules, including peptides, biogenic amines, steroid hormones, fatty acid derivatives and a variety of other classes of small molecules (Table 8.1). Such extracellular messengers reach their cellular targets by four different signalling routes: *endocrine* (carried in the bloodstream), *neurotransmitter* (released from nearby nerve endings), *paracrine* (diffused from an adjacent cell) and *autocrine* (released by the same cell).

The response to a given extracellular messenger (*ligand*, 'first' messenger) is mediated by *receptors*, which are proteins that recognize and bind high affinity specific ligands. After a ligand binds to receptor, a multi-step *signal transduction cascade* is set in motion that

eventually results in a response within the cell. This may be a change in intracellular ion concentration or gene expression, for example. However the biological pathways that make up the signal transduction cascade generally branch at multiple steps, loop both forward and backward, and interconnect with other pathways. This allows regulatory control to be exercised on signal transduction, which may take the form of amplification of the response, its integration with other responses, or its automatic termination to prevent runaway signalling after receptor binding. Such signal diversification explains how, during haemodynamic stress, neurohumoral-regulatory mediators (catecholamines, endothelin, angiotensin-II and vasopressin) may cause both short-term *functional responses* (positive inotropic, lusitropic, chronotropic effects, vasoconstriction and fluid retention), and also slower

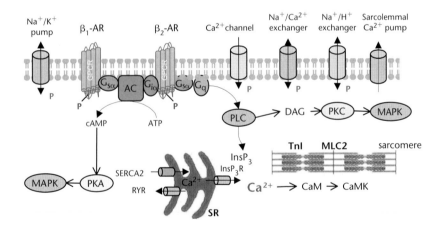

Figure 8.1 The β-adrenergic signal transduction cascade in cardiomyocytes leading to Ca^{2+}-mediated Ca^{2+} release. Agonist binding to either β1- or β2-AR stimulates $G_{s\alpha}$ protein, which binds to AC, catalysing the production of cAMP from ATP, and activation of PKA. PKA phosphorylates the voltage-dependent L-type Ca^{2+} channels, Na^+/H^+ exchange channels and Na^+/K^+ pump at the sarcolemma, the ryanodine receptor (RYR) and phospholamban (PLB) at the sarcoplasmic reticulum (SR), and troponin-I (TnI) in the sarcomeres, resulting in increased inotropic and lusitropic effects. The β2-AR is also able to bind $G_{i\alpha}$- or G_q-proteins; G_q activates phospholipase C (PLC), which causes the release of DAG and InsP3. InsP3 binds to the InsP3 receptor (InsP3R) and releases Ca^{2+} from the SR. Ca^{2+} combines with calmodulin (CaM), which activates the CaM-dependent protein kinases (CaMK) and the sarcolemmal Ca^{2+} pump, which ultimately results in the phosphorylation of PLB, myosin light chain 2 (MLC2), and Na^+/Ca^{2+} exchanger. DAG and CaM activate PKC, which in turn phosphorylates MLC2. The dephosphorylated regulatory protein PLB binds to the SR Ca^{2+} pump (SERCA2), inhibiting its activity; phosphorylation by PKA and/or CaMK causes PLB to dissociate from SERCA2, relieving the inhibitory effect. Note the activation of proliferative responses by both PKA and PKC via the MAPK pathways.

Table 8.1 Extracellular messengers involved in regulation of cardiac function

Peptides	Purines	Catecholamines	Steroids	Fatty acid derivatives	Other molecules
Growth factors	Adenosine	Epinephrine	Aldosterone	Prostaglandins	Nitric oxide (NO)
Cytokines		Norepinephrine			Acetylcholine
Angiotensin-II		Dopamine			Histamine
Endothelin					Thyroxine
Arginine vasopressin (antidiuretic hormone, ADH)					
Bradykinin					
Atrial natriuretic peptide					

Table 8.2 Plasma membrane receptors

GPCRs	Ion-channel receptors	Enzyme-linked receptors
α- and β-ARs	L-type Ca^{2+} channels	Tyrosine kinase receptors
M_2 muscarinic receptors	ACh receptors	Fibroblast growth factor (FGF) receptors
Angiotensin-II receptors	Serotonin receptors	Platelet-derived growth factor (PDGF) receptors
Adenosine receptors		Insulin-like growth factor (IGF) receptors
Arginine vasopressin (ADH) receptors		Vascular endothelial growth factor (VEGF) receptors
Bradykinin receptors		Cytokine receptors
Endothelin receptors		Tumor necrosis factor α (TNFα) receptors
Histamine receptors		Interleukin receptors
Dopaminergic receptors		Growth hormone receptors
		Transforming growth factor (TGF) receptors
		Other receptors
		Atrial natriuretic peptide (ANP) receptors

proliferative responses and programmed cell death (*apoptosis*), which play important (often maladaptive) roles in chronic heart disease.

Classification

There are three broad classes of receptors: *plasma membrane receptors* (bind ligands at the cell surface, Table 8.2), *intracellular receptors* (bind ligands that enter the cytosol) and *adhesion molecules* (involved in cell–cell and cell–matrix interactions).

The most important receptors involved in regulation of cardiac function interact with heterotrimeric guanyl nucleotide-binding proteins (*G-proteins*), and are part of one of the largest family of receptors in biology commonly called *G-protein-coupled receptors* (GPCRs). The receptors contain a conserved structure of seven hydrophobic α-helices that lie within the lipid bilayer of the cell membrane, and so are

often referred to as *seven-transmembrane-spanning* or *heptahelical* receptors. The G-protein subunits amplify and propagate the signals in the cytoplasm by modulating the activity of *effector molecules* like adenylyl cyclase (AC), phospholipases and ion channels. In turn, these effector molecules regulate the production of *second messenger molecules* (cyclic adenosine monophosphate (cAMP), cyclic guanosine monophosphate (cGMP), inositol-1,4,5-trisphosphate (InsP3), diacylglycerol and Ca^{2+}), in a highly complex pathway that ultimately activates *serine/threonine protein kinases* (protein kinase A (PKA), protein kinase C (PKC) and Ca^{2+}–calmodulin complex CAM kinase) responsible for both the *functional* and *proliferative* cellular responses (Table 8.3, Figure 8.1).

Regulation

The ligand–receptor interaction is determined by two properties of the receptor: the *binding affinity*

Table 8.3 Important GPCRs

Receptor	Tissue distribution	Ligand	Primary G-protein	Primary effector in heart tissue	Second messengers
β_1-AR	Heart	NA, A, β-agonists	G_s	AC, L-type Ca^{2+} channel	↑cAMP/PKA
β_2-AR	Heart, lung, vessels, kidney	NA, A, β-agonists	$G_s/G_i/G_q$	AC, L-type Ca^{2+} channel	↑cAMP/PKA, MAPK
β_3-AR	Adipose, heart	NA, A, β-agonists	G_s/G_i	AC	↑cAMP/PKA
$\alpha_{1A/B/D}$-AR, AT_1, ET	Heart, vessels, smooth muscle	NA, A, α-agonists; angiotensin-II; endothelin	G_q/G_{11}	PLC-β	↑DAG/InsP$_3$, PKC, MAPK
α_2-AR	Coronary vessels, CNS, pancreas, platelets	NA, A	G_i	AC	↓cAMP/PKA
M_2	Heart	Acetylcholine	G_i	AC, K^+ channels	↓cAMP/PKA, ↑outward K^+ current
A_2	Coronary vessels, heart, PA	Adenosine	G_s	AC, K_{ATP} channels, N-type Ca^{2+} channel	↑cAMP/PKA, ↑outward K^+ current

α-AR, α-adrenergic receptor subtypes (1A, 1B, 1D, 2); $\beta_{1/2/3}$-AR, subtypes 1, 2, 3; AT_1, angiotensin-II receptor subtype 1; ET, endothelin receptor; M_2, muscarinic cholinergic receptor; A_2, adenosine (purinergic) receptor subtype 2; NA, noradrenaline; A, adrenaline; PLC-β, phospholipase C-β.

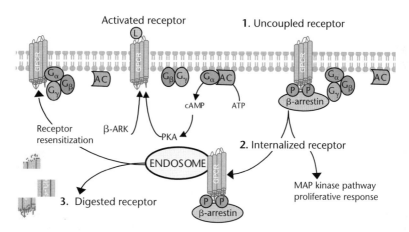

Figure 8.2 Mechanisms of β-AR desensitization: L, ligand; $G_{\alpha\beta\gamma}$, G-protein subunits.

(expressed as the dissociation constant, k_d), and the receptor *density*. Regulation of GPCR function is mediated by a process called *desensitization*, which reduces the receptor responsiveness to its extracellular messengers (Figure 8.2). Two important examples with clinical implications for the cardiac anaesthetist include the desensitization of β-adrenergic receptors (β-ARs), which can be *chronic* in the failing heart (due to chronic activation of sympathetic activity) and *acute* after CPB (due to the associated catecholamine surges). One mechanism for desensitization is receptor

downregulation, which refers to a decrease in the number of receptors expressed on the cell surface. This occurs when there is decreased transcription of the gene that encodes the receptor, destabilization of receptor messenger RNA that diminishes translation into the receptor protein, or increased receptor degradation (operates over hours). In general, receptor desensitization occurs by a sequential three-step process: *uncoupling* (phosphorylation), *internalization* (sequestration) and *digestion* (degradation). Uncoupling is a rapid process (seconds to minutes) that occurs when a protein kinase called *β-adrenergic receptor kinase* (β-ARK) phosphorylates a ligand-bound β-AR, thereby preventing it from activating a G-protein. β-ARK is one of a family of protein kinases called *G-protein receptor kinases* (GRKs). β-ARK-mediated desensitization requires a co-factor called *β-arrestin*, which binds to the phosphorylated C-terminal intracellular peptide chain. As GRKs phosphorylate only agonist-occupied GPCRs, this process is known as 'agonist-specific' or *homologous desensitization*. In contrast, second messengers can be phosphorylated by protein kinases activated by other signal transduction systems (e.g. PKA by cAMP and PKC by diacylglycerol (DAG)), in a process called 'non-agonist-specific' or *heterologous desensitization*. Uncoupling is a fully reversible step, as the receptors can be dephosphorylated by *G-protein-coupled receptor phosphatases* in process called *resensitization*. Internalization occurs when the phosphorylated β-arrestin-bound uncoupled receptors are removed from the plasma membrane and transferred inside the cell, in a process that is still reversible. Internalized β$_2$-AR–β-arrestin complexes can act as scaffolds that activate mitogen-activated protein kinase (MAPK)-mediated proliferative pathways, with significant implications in pressure-overload hypertrophy and ventricular remodelling. Manipulating myocardial β-ARK activity to improve functional responsiveness to catecholamines in cardiomyopathy and heart failure is the subject of intense research. After a prolonged exposure to an agonist, proteolytic enzymes within the cell digest the internalized receptors, which is the final, irreversible step of the desensitization process.

A reverse process, of enhanced sensitivity, can be seen after the heart is denervated or more commonly after prolonged administration of β-adrenergic blockers (*denervation sensitivity*). This appears to be the result of increased numbers of β-ARs by a process of externalization. Increased β-AR density on the cell surface makes abrupt withdrawal of β-blocker therapy dangerous and may be implicated in the aetiology of atrial dysrhythmias after cardiac surgery.

Recent studies have demonstrated a *genetic basis* for the regulation of many GPCRs. Genetic heterogeneity in the structure of both β$_1$- and β$_2$-ARs in the human population has been identified and associated with various degrees of receptor downregulation or defective coupling to G$_s$. Genetic polymorphisms in β-ARs may lead to inter-individual differences in the pathophysiology of congestive heart failure, and will allow the identification of high-risk individuals and the design of appropriate therapeutic strategies.

Receptor blockade

Classically, ligands that interact with receptors were classified as *agonists* (if binding activates the signal transduction cascade), *antagonists* (no intracellular signal) and *partial agonists* (weak activation of the signal transduction cascade, e.g. intrinsic sympathomimetic activity), all exhibiting competitive kinetics. Recent research in transgenic animals emphasizes the importance of a two-state model of receptor activation (at least for β-ARs) by competitive ligands. In the absence of a ligand, the receptor can undergo spontaneous transition from the inactivated (R) to the activated (R*) state (Figure 8.3). Ligands can be classified into *agonists*, *neutral antagonists* and *inverse agonists* according to their tendency to shift this equilibrium towards the active-state R* (agonists) or inactive-state R (inverse agonists). Although most β-adrenergic blockers act as inverse agonists, some with weak inverse agonist effects may be classified as neutral antagonists. The following β-adrenergic blockers display increasing inverse agonist effects: bucindolol < carvedilol < propranolol < metoprolol. The model explains the inability of neutral antagonists to fully block the effects of receptor overexpression, as they counteract activation by endogenous catecholamines but not by spontaneous transition into the active receptor conformation. This may be of clinical relevance with respect to the tolerability of various β-adrenergic blockers and the treatment of withdrawal syndrome.

Key points

- Regulation of cardiac performance involves three categories of mechanisms: changes in *organ physiology* (end-diastolic fibre length, Frank–Starling

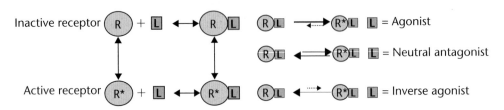

Figure 8.3 Two-state model of β-AR activation: R, inactive receptor; R*, active receptor; L, ligand.

relationship), changes in *cell biochemistry* (membrane proteins that regulate Ca^{2+} fluxes and interactions of the contractile proteins) and *proliferative responses* (long-term changes in the size and shape of the heart, cell architecture, membrane composition and expression of specific isoforms of myo-cardial proteins).

- These functional and proliferative responses are mediated by a large variety of receptors and highly complex signal transduction pathways, which allow for multiple levels of control and signal diversification.
- Understanding the mechanisms involved in receptor desensitization has important clinical application in patients with congestive heart failure and in the perioperative management of patients undergoing cardiac surgery.
- A two-state model of receptor activation has replaced classic ideas about β-receptor agonists and antagonists. The β-receptor can undergo spontaneous transition between the inactivated and activated states. These novel concepts in receptor pharmacology (e.g. inverse agonists) may facilitate the development of better therapies designed to normalize the alterations in intracellular signalling characteristic of heart disease.

- Future treatments of heart failure may be based around manipulations of receptor density as well as blocking β-receptor activation.
- Recent studies have demonstrated genetic polymorphism in the regulation of β-ARs. Different phenotypes may lead to inter-individual differences in the pathophysiology of congestive heart failure. In the future, treatments may be tailored for different groups of high-risk patients.

Further reading

Katz AM. *Physiology of the Heart*, 3rd edition. Philadelphia, PA: Lippincott Williams & Wilkins, 2001.

Rana BK, Shiina T, Insel P. Genetic variations and polymorphisms of G-protein-coupled receptors: functional and therapeutic implications. *Annu Rev Pharmacol Toxicol* 2001; **41**: 593–624.

Rockman HA, Koch WJ, Lefkowitz RJ. Seven-transmembrane-spanning receptors and heart function. *Nature* 2002; **415(6868)**: 206–212.

Zaugg M, Schaub MC, Pasch T, Spahn DR. Modulation of β-adrenergic receptor subtype activities in perioperative medicine: mechanisms and site of action. *Br J Anaesth* 2002; **88(1)**: 101–123.

ANTIHYPERTENSIVE AND VASODILATOR DRUGS 9

S.J. Gray & C.S. Moore

Control of BP can be achieved by reducing either SVR or CO. Drugs can be placed into one of three groups according to mechanism of action:

1 Vasodilatation due to activation of protein kinases.
2 Autonomically mediated antihypertensives.
3 Ion-channel mediated antihypertensives.

Clinically useful effects on both BP and CO can also be obtained by volatile anaesthetic agents and opioids (as discussed in Chapter 7).

Protein kinase activators

Both organic nitrates GTN and SNP act by increasing nitric oxide (NO) concentrations. Nitrates react with tissue thiols to produce NO_2^-, which is converted to NO whereas SNP acts as a direct NO donor. NO causes smooth muscle relaxation by increasing cyclic guanosine monophosphate (cGMP), which in turn activates protein kinases. These kinases oppose the action of vaso-constrictors such as calcium and cause vasodilatation.

Prostacyclin increases cyclic adenosine monophosphate (cAMP), which also activates protein kinases causing vasodilatation, whereas phosphodiesterase inhibitors increase cAMP concentration by inhibiting its breakdown.

Glyceryl trinitrate

GTN is a direct acting vasodilator requiring specific thiol intermediates to generate NO. It produces greater venodilatation than arteriodilatation.

Indications
- Hypertension.
- Myocardial ischaemia.
- Selective vasodilatation of more proximal larger coronary arteries has the effect of re-distributing blood via collaterals from epicardial to endocardial regions.
- Coronary spasm.
- Pulmonary hypertension (PHT).

Dose
- 0.5–$10\,\mu g\,kg^{-1}min^{-1}$; mix 25 mg in 50 ml saline.

Clinical effects
- The reduction in preload confers a number of benefits including a decrease in left ventricular wall tension, improved sub-endocardial perfusion and diminished myocardial O_2 demand. Provided filling pressures are adequate and coronary perfusion pressure is maintained.
- Superior pulmonary vasodilator in comparison to SNP.
- Reflex tachycardia.

Problems
- Methaemoglobinaemia.
- Tolerance – classically thought to be due to depletion of sulphydryl groups; currently believed to be related to the formation of peroxynitrite.

Sodium nitroprusside

Direct NO donor producing increased cGMP in vascular smooth muscle resulting in balanced arterial and venous dilatation. SNP has a short duration of action of 1–2 min.

Indications
- Hypertensive crisis.
- Perioperative hypertension.

Dose
- 0.25–$10\,\mu g\,kg^{-1}min^{-1}$; mix 50 mg in 250 ml 5% dextrose.

Clinical effects
- Potent rapidly acting arterial and venous dilator produces $\downarrow\downarrow\downarrow$ SVR, $\downarrow\downarrow\downarrow$ PVR and $\downarrow\downarrow\downarrow$ preload necessitating invasive monitoring.
- Reflex tachycardia.
- Coronary steal, arising through dilatation of more distal coronary resistance vessels, has the potential to divert blood from ischaemic regions. Reflex tachycardia and $\downarrow\downarrow$ coronary perfusion pressure add to risk of ischaemia.
- Inhibition of hypoxic pulmonary vasoconstriction promotes V/Q mismatch and hypoxia.

Problems

- Precipitous hypotension.
- Myocardial ischaemia due to decreased coronary perfusion pressure.
- Tachyphylaxis.
- Cyanide toxicity resulting from the reaction of SNP with Hb. The resulting free cyanide ions inhibit cytochrome oxidase preventing oxidative phosphorylation. Detoxification occurs by binding cyanide to thiosulphate (by rhodanase) or by binding to hydroxocobalamin. Patients at greatest risk of toxicity are as follows:
  - Cumulative dose $>1\,mg\,kg^{-1}$ over 24 h.
  - Hepatic or renal insufficiency.
  - High-dose infusion ($>8\,\mu g\,kg^{-1}min^{-1}$).
- Thiocyanate toxicity. Prolonged use with accompanying renal impairment.
- Hypoxia with inhibition of hypoxic pulmonary vasoconstriction (HPVC).
- If SNP is used in aortic dissection, additional β-blockade is necessary to counterreflex increases in HR, contractility and dP/dT.

Inhaled nitric oxide

Selective pulmonary vasodilator that acts by increasing cGMP levels in smooth muscle cells. Inhalation allows NO to be used specifically for PHT with minimal systemic effects.

Indications

- Persistent PHT of the newborn.
- Right ventricular dysfunction associated with PHT following cardiac surgery or cardiac transplantation.
- Acute respiratory distress syndrome (hypoxia relieved but long-term benefit unproven).

Dose

- Concentration used clinically 1–20 ppm.
- The concentration used should be the lowest, that is clinically effective.
- Any changes in dose should be closely monitored and the dose should be frequently re-evaluated.

Clinical effects

Inhaled NO causes preferential vasodilatation in ventilated lung units so improving V/Q matching and decreasing shunt fraction.

Problems

- Methaemoglobinaemia.
- NO_2 toxicity.
- Monitoring of NO, NO_2 and methaemoglobin along with active scavenging is mandatory.

Prostacyclin

Prostacyclin is a naturally occurring prostaglandin produced by blood vessel intima derived from arachadonic acid via cyclo–oxygenase. It is a potent vasodilator; it is also a physiologically important anticoagulant in normal blood vessels. $t_{1/2} = 2–3\,min$ with inhibition of platelet aggregation lasting up to 30 min after infusion.

Indications

- Treatment of PHT.
- Anticoagulant used for extracorporeal circuits when heparin is inadvisable.

Dose

- $2–35\,ng\,kg^{-1}min^{-1}$ IV by infusion. May be nebulized to reduce systemic effects.

Clinical effects

- Potent vasodilator decreases both SVR and PVR.
- Inhibits platelet aggregation.
- Increases renin production.

Problems

- Hypotension.
- Flushing.
- Headache.

Phosphodiesterase inhibitors

The phosphodiesterase III (PDE-III) inhibitors are classified as bipyridines (amrinone and milrinone) or an imidazolone (enoximone). As well as being inotropic agents (see Chapter 10), these agents generate substantial pulmonary and systemic vasodilatation.

Autonomic agents

Isoproterenol (isoprenaline)

Synthetic catecholamine with β-agonist ($\beta_1 > \beta_2$) and no α–activity.

Indications

- Acute bradydysrhythmias with atrioventricular node block.
- Cardiac surgery.
  - Congenital heart surgery where SV is fixed.
  - Heart and lung transplantation.
- PHT with right heart failure.
- β-blocker overdose.

Dose

- *Bolus*   20 μg (slowly).
- *Infusion*   1 mg in 250 ml 5% dextrose @ 5–20 ml/h.

Clinical effects
- Potent chronotropic effect:
  - directly by reducing refractoriness of pacemaker cells and increasing automaticity,
  - indirectly by baroreceptor activation through peripheral vasodilatation.
- Increased contractility and CO.
- Decreased aortic BP (diastolic $\gg$ systolic).
- Decreased SVR due to dilatation of all vascular beds.
- Decreased PVR (powerful pulmonary vasodilator).

Problems
- Tachycardia coupled with propensity to cause a fall in coronary perfusion pressure should caution its use in coronary artery disease.
- Dysrhythmias.
- Shortage of licensed formulation.

Esmolol

Esmolol is a rapidly acting, ultra-short duration, cardioselective β_1-blocker. Onset is <2 min, $t_{1/2} = 9$ min, reversal of effect $= 10$–20 min. It is hydrolysed by red cell esterases and is safe in bronchospastic disease.

Indications
- Emergency hypertension in the perioperative period.
- Dissecting aortic aneurysm.
- SVT and sinus tachycardias.

Dose
- *Bolus* 0.25–0.5 mg kg^{-1}.
- *Infusion* 50–$200\,\mu$g kg^{-1}min^{-1}.

Clinical effects
- May cause dramatic fall in HR, CO and BP.

Problems
- Bradycardia and hypotension.
- 10 mg ml^{-1} and 250 mg ml^{-1} similarly packaged increasing possibility of serious drug error.

Labetalol

It is a combined α- and β-blocker together with a direct vasodilatory effect. In the IV formulation the ratio of α : β-blockade is $1:7$ compared to $1:3$ when given orally. It has a relatively long $t_{1/2}$ of $\sim$6 hours and shows an eight-fold variation in bioavailability after oral administration due to extensive first-pass metabolism.

Indications
- Hypertension with accompanying tachycardia and ischaemia.

- Dissecting aortic aneurysm.
- Phaeochromocytoma.

Dose
- *Infusion* 200 mg in 200 ml 5% dextrose @ 10–50 ml/h.

Clinical effects
- Dose-related fall in HR.
- CO and SV maintained with a decrease in BP and SVR.
- No reflex tachycardia.

Problems
- Side effects of α-blockade more frequent than those of β-blockade.

Phentolamine

It is a short-acting, potent, α-adrenergic blocker. Onset is <2 min. Duration of action is 10–15 min.

Indications
- Hypertension during CPB.
- Pheochromocytoma surgery.

Dose
- *Bolus* 1–5 mg, repeat every 10 min to desired effect.

Drugs acting on ion channels

When used for BP control, calcium-channel antagonists produce generalized arteriolar vasodilatation with little effect on the venous system. Dihydropyridines, such as nicardipine and clevedipine, produce marked vasodilatation with little direct action on the heart.

Potassium-channel activators act mainly on smooth muscle to cause potassium influx into excitable tissue causing hyperpolarization of the membrane, resulting in arterial and venous vasodilatation.

Nicardipine

It is a short-acting calcium-channel blocker devoid of negative inotropic and chronotropic effects with preservation of A-V conduction. An arterial vasodilator with minimal effect on venous capacitance vessels and preload. Onset is <2 min; elimination $t_{1/2} = 40$ min.

Dose
- *Bolus* 2.5 mg over 5 min; repeat every 10 min to a maximum 12.5 mg.
- *Infusion* 2–4 mg h^{-1}; mix 50 mg in 250 ml.

Table 9.1 Antihypertensives commonly used in anaesthesia and the primary indications for their use

Antihypertensives	HR	Contractility	CO	BP	SVR/PVR	Preload
GTN	Reflex ↑	Reflex ↑	↓	↓	↓/↓	↓↓
SNP	Reflex ↑	Reflex ↑	↓	↓↓	↓↓/↓	↓↓
Isoprenaline	↑↑	↑↑	↑	↓↓	↓↓/↓↓	↓
Esmolol	↓	↓	↓↓	↓↓	↔	↔
Labetolol	↓	↓	↔	↓	↓	↔
Nicardipine	↔	↔	↔/↑	↓	↓↓	↔
Phentolamine	Reflex ↑	Reflex ↑	↑	↓↓	↓↓	↔
Hydralazine	Reflex ↑	Reflex ↑	↑	↓↓	↓↓	↔
Diazoxide	Reflex ↑	Reflex ↑	↑	↓↓	↓↓	↔
Milrinone	↔/↑	↑↑	↑↑	↓	↓↓	↓
Prostacyclin	Reflex ↑	Reflex ↑	↑	↓↓	↓↓	↔

↑, increase; ↓, decrease; ↔, no change.

Clinical effects
- No reflex tachycardia.
- No coronary steal. A potent coronary vasodilator improving blood flow to ischaemic areas.

Problems
Potential for V/Q mismatch and hypoxia – due to non-selective pulmonary vasodilator effects.

Hydralazine

It is a potassium-channel opener. A direct arterial vasodilator with little effect on venous capacitance vessels. The decrease in diastolic BP is greater than the decrease in the systolic BP. It causes reflex increased HR, contractility and CO.

Indications
- Perioperative hypertension (avoid in the presence of myocardial ischaemia).
- Pre-eclampsia.

Dose
- *Bolus* 20–40 mg slowly. Use sodium chloride 9% as diluent.

Problems
Most side effects are associated with long-term oral use.

- Fluid and water retention.
- Systemic lupus erythematosus like syndrome. Incidence of 10% – more likely in slow acetylators.
- Polyneuropathy (responsive to pyridoxine).
- Drug fever.

Diazoxide

It is a potassium-channel opener. A direct arterial vasodilator, structurally similar to thiazides but no diuretic action. Onset is <4 min. It has a relatively long duration of action (2–6 h). It causes a reflex tachycardia and increases contractility and CO.

Indications
- Perioperative hypertension without associated myocardial ischaemia.
- Hypertensive encephalopathy.
- Pre-eclampsia.

Dose
- *Bolus* 50–100 mg slowly; repeat every 10 min to desired effect.

Problems
- Salt and water retention.
- Hyperglycaemia (inhibits insulin release).
- Highly alkaline (pH = 11.0) unsuitable for intramuscular injection.
- Long duration of action.

The varying effects of the antihypertensives commonly used in anaesthesia and the primary indications for their use are outlined in Table 9.1.

Further reading

Bojar RM, Warner KG. *Manual of Perioperative Care in Cardiac Surgery*, 3rd edition. Massachusetts: Blackwell Science, Inc., 1999.

Griffin MJ, Hines RL. Management of perioperative ventricular dysfunction. *J Cardiothor Vasc Anesth* 2001; **15(1)**: 90–106.

Kaplan JA, Reich DL, Konstadt S. *Cardiac Anesthesia*, 4th edition. Philadelphia: W.B. Saunders Co., 2000.

Opie LH, Gersh BJ. *Drugs for the Heart*, 5th edition. Philadelphia: W.B. Saunders Co., 2001.

Skoyles JR, Sherry KM. Pharmacology, mechanisms of action and uses of selective phosphodiesterase inhibitors. *Br J Anaesth* 1992; **68(3)**: 293–302.

A. Cohen & S. Ghosh

A positive inotrope improves myocardial performance by increasing the force of myocardial contraction for any given preload.

Commonly used inotropic agents include:

- catecholamines (naturally occurring and synthetic),
- phosphodiesterase (PDE) inhibitors,
- digitalis glycosides.

Cellular mechanisms of myocardial contraction and the physiology of excitation–contraction coupling are covered in Chapter 3.

Cellular mechanisms

The mechanisms by which inotropes may affect alterations in intracellular Ca^{2+} homoeostasis and hence myocardial contraction can be broadly divided into those that are dependent on cyclic adenosine monophosphate (cAMP) for their activity and those that are independent of cAMP for their activity.

cAMP dependent

- Direct activation of adenyl cyclase (e.g. forskolin).
- β-adrenoceptor-mediated stimulation of adenyl cyclase (e.g. catecholamines).
- Inhibition of PDE (particularly isoenzymes types III and IV) (e.g. enoximone and milrinone).

cAMP independent

- Direct Ca^{2+} channel activation (e.g. phenylephrine).
- α_1-adrenoceptor stimulation (e.g. norepinephrine):
  - increased slow inward Ca^{2+} current;
  - increased release of Ca^{2+} from sarcoplasmic reticulum (SR);
  - increased Ca^{2+} sensitivity of contractile proteins.
- Increase in intracellular sodium:
  - inhibition of Na^+/K^+ ATPase-dependent pump by cardiac glycosides leads to increased intracellular Ca^{2+} by the effect of increased intracellular sodium on the Na^+/Ca^{2+} pump.
- Direct inhibition of Na^+/Ca^{2+} exchange pump.
- K^+-channel inhibition:
  - prolongation of cardiac action potential (AP) by inhibition of K^+ channel prolongs slow inward Ca^{2+} current and raises intracellular Ca^{2+} concentrations.

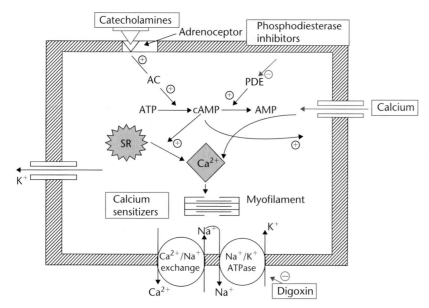

Figure 10.1 The cellular mechanisms by which inotropic drugs increase myocardial contractility. AC, adenylate cyclase; ATP, adenosine triphosphate.

- Ca^{2+} sensitizers:
  - increased Ca^{2+} sensitivity of contractile proteins (e.g. levosimendan and pimobendan).

Signal transduction

- Adrenoceptors belong to a family of receptors that span the cell membrane seven times and are coupled to guanine nucleotide-binding proteins (G-proteins) (Figure 10.2).
- G-proteins consist of three subunits: α, β and γ. Over 20 G-proteins have been identified; however, the most important being G$_s$, G$_i$, G$_q$ and G$_o$. Interaction between subunits and the receptor is dependent on the G-protein cycling from an inactive to an active state (Figure 10.3).

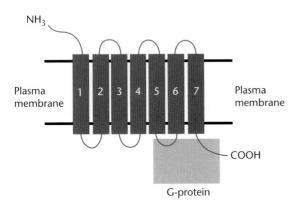

Figure 10.2 G-protein-coupled receptor spanning membrane seven times.

- The β-adrenergic receptors couple to a G$_s$-protein, activating adenylate cyclase and Ca^{2+} ion channels in some cells. G$_i$-proteins link to α$_2$-receptors and inhibit adenylate cyclase as well as inhibiting some ion channels (Figure 10.4a). α$_1$-receptors couple to a G$_q$-protein, activating phospholipases, particularly phospholipase C (Figure 10.4b).

Catecholamines

- A group of naturally occurring and synthetic compounds containing a catechol nucleus (benzene ring with hydroxyl substitution at positions 3 and 4) and an ethylamine side chain.
- All have very short plasma half lives.
- Metabolism is by oxidation by monoamine oxidase (MAO) and/or conjugation by catechol-*o*-methyl transferase (COMT).
- Catecholamines exhibit significant variability in their activity at sympathomimetic receptors (Table 10.1).

Phosphodiesterase inhibitors

- The PDE inhibitors act by inhibiting the enzyme cyclic nucleotide PDE in cardiac and vascular smooth muscle. This leads to elevated levels of cAMP and cyclic guanosine monophosphate (cGMP) by preventing their degradation.
- Molecular studies have identified seven sub-types of PDE. Selective inhibition of subtype III by bipyridines (amrinone and milrinone) or imidazolines (enoximone) allows accumulation of cAMP in the cardiac myocyte while cGMP is unaffected.

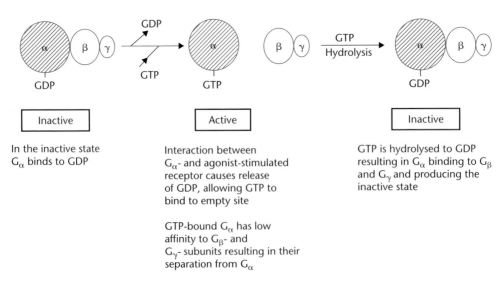

Figure 10.3 Cycling of G-protein between active and inactive states. GTP, guanosine triphosphate; GDP, guanosine diphosphate.

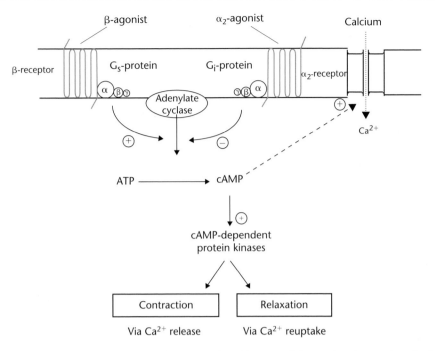

Figure 10.4(a) G-protein-mediated signal transduction mediated by G_s- and G_i-proteins. Occupation of a G_s-linked adrenoceptor activates adenylate cyclase and increases the production of cAMP while occupation of a G_i-linked adrenoceptor decreases production of cAMP.

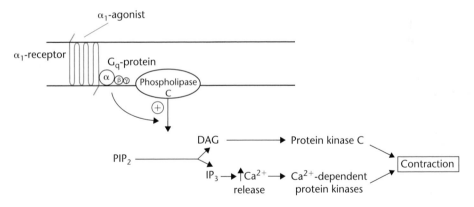

Figure 10.4(b) G-protein-mediated signal transduction mediated by G_q-protein. α_1-receptor stimulation leads to the breakdown of phosphatidyl inositol biphosphate (PIP_2) into diacylglycerol (DAG) and inositol triphosphate (IP_3) via activation of phospholipase C.

Table 10.1 Relative receptor activity of catecholamines

	α_1	α_2	β_1	β_2	DA_1	DA_2
Noradrenaline	+++	+++	+	−	−	−
Epinephrine	+++	++	+++	++	−	−
Dopamine	++	+	++	+++	+++	+++
Dobutamine	+	−	+++	+	−	−
Dopexamine	−	−	+	+++	++	++
Isoproterenol	−	−	++	++	−	−

- Accumulation of intracellular cAMP in cardiac myocytes increases phosphorylation of slow Ca^{2+} channels leading to increased contractility, while an increase in cAMP in vascular smooth muscle leads to a reduction in SVR and PVR.
- The combination of enhanced myocardial contraction and reduced afterload has led to the term inodilator in reference to these agents.

Cardiac glycosides

- Naturally occurring substances found in a number of plants including foxglove. Chemically they consist of a hydrophobic steroid nucleus and a hydrophilic lactone ring.
- Mechanism of action derives from an ability to selectively bind to the Na^+/K^+ ATPase in the cardiac myocyte. This in turn leads to an increase in intracellular Na^+, decreased activity of the Na^+/Ca^{2+} exchange mechanism and hence an increase in intracellular Ca^{2+} and enhanced myocardial contraction.
- Anti-dysrhythmic properties are discussed in Chapter 11.

Catecholamines

Dopamine

Dopamine is an endogenous precursor of norepinephrine. It is a neurotransmitter in CNS and peripheral nervous systems (PNS). It has dose-dependent activity at dopamine 1 (DA_1)-, β_1-, α_1- and 5HT-receptors (Table 10.2). It stimulates norepinephrine release from sympathetic nerves.

INDICATIONS

- Acute hypotension or shock associated with MI, endotoxic septicaemia, trauma and renal failure.

- As an adjunct after cardiac surgery where there is persistent hypotension after correction of hypovolamia.

Problem
- Dysrhythmias, commonly tachycardia.

Dobutamine

Dobutamine is a synthetic catecholamine produced by substitution of a bulky aromatic ring on the terminal amino group of dopamine. It comprises L- and D-stereoisomers:

- L-isomer stimulates α_1,
- D-isomer stimulates β_1 and β_2,
- β effects are dominant.

It shows no activity at dopaminergic receptors and does *not* cause release of norepinephrine from sympathetic nerves. Its $t_{1/2}$ is approximately 2 min and is rapidly re-distributed and metabolized by COMT to produce inactive metabolites.

Indications
- Low output cardiac failure associated with MI, cardiac surgery, cardiomyopathies, and septic/cardiogenic shock.
- Often administered by peripheral vein.
- Pharmacological stress testing.

Dose	2.5–15 µg kg^{-1}min^{-1} (β effects predominate)
CVS	↑ Myocardial contractility; ↑ HR; ↓ SVR
Renal	↑ Renal blood flow (2° to ↑ CO)
GI	↑ Splanchnic blood flow (2° to ↑ CO)

Problems
- Dose-related tachycardia.
- Hypotension.
- Tachyphylaxis (48–72 h).

Table 10.2 Dose dependent effects of dopamine

Dose	0.5–3.0 µg kg^{-1}min^{-1} (DA$_1$ effects predominate)	3.0–5.0 µg kg^{-1}min^{-1} (β$_1$ effects predominate)	>5 µg kg^{-1}min^{-1} (α$_1$ and 5HT effects predominate)
Cardiovascular system (CVS)	Modest ↑ CO	↑ Myocardial contractility; minimal change in HR/SVR	↑ HR; vasoconstriction
Renal	↑ Renal blood flow; ↓ proximal tubular sodium re-absorption	↑ Renal blood flow	↓/↑ Renal blood flow
GI	↑ Splanchnic blood flow	↑ Splanchnic blood flow	↓/↑ Splanchnic blood flow

Table 10.3 Dose dependent effects of epinephrine

Dose	0.005–$0.02\,\mu g\,kg^{-1}min^{-1}$ (β effects predominate)	$>0.02\,\mu g\,kg^{-1}min^{-1}$ (α_1 effects predominate)
CVS	↑ HR (↑ SA node activity, ↑ latent pacemakers, ↓ atrioventricular node refractory period, ↑ conduction); duration of systole shortened, diastole unaltered; ↑ myocardial contractility; peripheral arteriolar dilatation	Vasoconstriction; ↓ splanchnic; ↓ renal blood flow
Renal	↓/↑ Renal blood flow; ↑ renin secretion	↓ Renal blood flow
GI	↓/↑ Splanchnic blood flow	↓ Splanchnic blood flow
Metabolic	↑ Glucose (↓ insulin secretion, ↑ glucagon release); hypokalaemia (β_2)	Hyperglycaemia

Epinephrine

Epinephrine is a potent endogenous agonist at β_1-, β_2-, and α_1-adrenoceptors (Table 10.3).

Indications
- Cardiac arrest.
- As an adjunct after cardiac surgery where there is persistent hypotension after correction of hypovolamia.
- Anaphylactic/anaphylactoid shock.

Norepinephrine

Norepinephrine is an endogenous agonist at α_1- and α_2-receptors. It moderates β_1-agonist with little or no effect at β_2-receptors.

Indications
Main clinical use is to increase SVR in shock.

Dose	0.01–$0.1\,\mu g\,kg^{-1}min^{-1}$ (α effects predominate)
CVS	Peripheral vasoconstriction; ↑ HR and ↑ CO (β_1); modest reflex ↓ HR and ↓ CO
Renal	↓ Renal blood flow
GI	↓ Splanchnic blood flow

Problems
- Splanchnic and distal limb ischaemia.
- Metabolic acidosis.
- Increased PVR.

Dopexamine

Dopexamine is a synthetic N-substituted dopamine analogue; a potent β_2- and DA_1-receptor agonist. It has no direct β_1- or α-receptor activity. It inhibits neuronal uptake resulting in indirect sympathetic activity. The plasma $t_{1/2}$ is 6–7 min with clearance by extraneuronal uptake and the renal excretion and hepatic metabolism by COMT.

Indications
- Treatment of exacerbations of chronic heart failure, or heart failure associated with cardiac surgery when afterload reduction, combined with a mild positive inotropic effect is required.

Dose	1.0–$8\,\mu g\,kg^{-1}min^{-1}$ (β_2 and DA_1 effects predominate)
CVS	↑ Myocardial contractility; ↑ HR; ↓ SVR
Renal	↑ Renal blood flow
GI	↑ Splanchnic blood flow

Isoproterenol (isoprenaline)

Isoproterenol is a synthetic catecholamine and potent β_1- and β_2-adrenoceptor agonist.

Indications
- Refractory bradycardia (i.e. complete heart block) as a bridge to temporary or permanent pacing.
- Bradycardia in the denervated (i.e. transplanted) heart.
- Pulmonary hypertension.

Dose	0.02–$0.2\,\mu g\,kg^{-1}min^{-1}$ (β_1 effects predominate)
CVS	↑ Myocardial contractility; ↑ HR; ↓ SVR/↓ PVR
Renal	↑ Renal blood flow
GI	↑ Splanchnic blood flow

Problems
Worldwide shortage of isoprenaline hydrochloride: isoprenaline sulphate (a suitable alternative) is available, but unlicensed.

Table 10.4 PDE-III inhibitors: dose

	Inamrinone (formerly amrinone)	Milrinone	Enoximone
Structure	Bipyridine	Bipyridine	Imidazolone
Relative potency	1	15	1.5
Initial bolus	$0.75\,mg\,kg^{-1}$ in 10 min	$50\,\mu g\,kg^{-1}$ in 10 min	$0.5\,mg\,kg^{-1}$ in 20 min
Infusion	$5-20\,\mu g\,kg^{-1}\,min^{-1}$	$0.5\,\mu g\,kg^{-1}\,min^{-1}$	$20\,\mu g\,kg^{-1}\,min^{-1}$
$t_{1/2}$	3–4 h; 20% CPB tube binding	2–3 h	6–8 h
Excreted unchanged		80%	80%
Vasodilatation	++	+++	++
CVS effects	Slight ↑ HR (accelerated AV node conduction; ↑ CO (up to 45%) – minimal impact on myocardial O_2 demand; ↓ SVR/↓ PVR – ↓ CVP, ↓ PAP, ↓ PAWP, ↓ MAP; enhanced diastolic rezlaxation – improved coronary blood flow; synergism with adrenergic agonists		

Other agents

Phosphodiesterase-III inhibitors

The non-specific PDE inhibitor, aminophylline – widely used in the treatment of asthma – has long been known to improve RV function. The recent identification of isoforms of PDE has lead to the production of cardio-specific drugs.

Indications
- End-stage heart failure as a bridge to transplantation.
- Low CO syndrome after MI and cardiac surgery.
- Diastolic ventricular dysfunction (e.g. AS).
- β-adenergic receptor downregulation (e.g. prolonged CPB).
- Pulmonary hypertension.

Dose
For details see Table 10.4.

Problems
- Hypotension – concurrent norepinephrine infusion advised.
- Thrombocytopaenia (amrinone).
- Both enoximone and milrinone accumulate in renal failure. The active, sulphoxide metabolite of enoximone is wholly excreted by the kidneys.
- Enoximone requires refrigeration, cannot be mixed with glucose solutions and is best delivered through a dedicated central venous line.
- Milrinone and frusemide are incompatible.

Calcium

Half of the plasma Ca^{2+} is in the free ionized form. Plasma concentrations are increased by vitamin D and parathyroid hormone, and decreased by calcitonin.

Indications
- Treatment of hypocalcaemia (e.g. after massive blood transfusion).
- Low CO in presence of normal/elevated SVR.
- Symptomatic hyperkalaemia.
- Ca^{2+}-channel antagonist overdose.
- Symptomatic hypermagnesaemia.

Dose

Ca^{2+} dose	$2-6\,mg\,kg^{-1}$ ($0.05-0.15\,mmol\,kg^{-1}$)
Preparations	Calcium chloride 10% = 273 mg/6.8 mmol Ca^{2+} per 10 ml Calcium gluconate 10% = 89 mg/2.2 mmol Ca^{2+} per 10 ml
Clinical effects	↑ BP (↑ contractility, ↑ SVR); HR unchanged

Problems
- Life-threatening dysrhythmias in patients on digoxin.
- Inhibition of haemodynamic effects of ionotropes such as epinephrine reported.

Key point

- Catecholamines exhibit significant variability in their activity at sympathomimetic receptors.

Further reading

Bovill JG, Howie MB (Eds). *Clinical Pharmacology for Anaesthetists*. London: W.B. Saunders, 1999.

Latimer RD, Ghosh S. Inotropes, vasopressors, phosphodiesterase inhibitors. In: Prys-Roberts C, Brown BR, Nunn JF (Eds), *International Practice of Anaesthesia*. London: Butterworth-Heinemann, 1996;1/36/1-13.

ANTI-DYSRHYTHMIC DRUGS

11

S.L. Misso & R.O. Shaw

Anti-dysrhythmic drugs are traditionally classified according to their electrophysiological effects – 'The Vaughan Williams Classification' (Table 11.1).

Many drugs have more than one anti-dysrhythmic action. Several important drugs, notably digoxin, magnesium salts and adenosine, are not easily classified. Other classifications, such as 'The Sicillian Gambit', are more complex and classify drugs based on their actions (via targeted ionic currents) on dysrhythmia mechanism. Commonly used agents in the cardiac operating theatre and postoperative ICU are presented here in alphabetical order.

Adenosine

Adenosine is an endogenous purine nucleoside. It has short duration of action ($t_{1/2} < 5\,\mathrm{s}$) due to rapid metabolism by enzymatic degradation in blood and peripheral tissue.

Action

- Adenosine receptor agonist.
  - A_1 receptors are present on all cardiomyocytes.
  - A_2 receptors are present on endothelial and smooth muscle cells of the coronary and peripheral vasculature.
- *Direct effects* are mediated via A_1 receptor activation of a subset of K^+ channels. Include decreased HR, decreased conduction at SA and atrioventricular (A-V) nodes and decreased atrial contractility.
- *Indirect effects* are mediated via A_1 receptor inhibition of adenyl cyclase. Include antagonism of adrenergic effects (i.e. increased HR, conduction and contractility).
- Coronary vasodilatation is mediated by A_2 receptor enhancement of adenyl cyclase activity.

Indications

- Haemodynamically stable narrow-complex tachycardia (NCT).
- Paroxysmal SVT involving a re-entry pathway involving the A-V node.
- If the dysrhythmia is not due to the re-entry involving the A-V node or sinus node (e.g. AF, atrial flutter, atrial tachycardia (AT) or VT), then adenosine will not terminate the dysrhythmia but may produce

Table 11.1 Vaughan Williams Classification of anti-dysrhythmic drugs. Classes I and IV act on ion channels, Class II acts on receptors and Class III has mixed action

Class	Action	Drugs	APD	MRD	ERP	A-VC	Myocardial contractility
Ia	APD prolonged	Procainamide	↑	↓↓	↑	↓↓	↓
		Disopyramide	↑	↓↓	↑	↓↓	↓↓↓
		Quinidine	↑	↓↓	↑	↓↓	↓
Ib	APD shortened	Lignocaine	↓	↓	↑↑		
		Mexilitine					
Ic	APD unchanged	Flecainide	–	↓↓↓		↓↓	↓↓
II	β-blockers	Propranolol				?↓	↓↓
		Metoprolol					↓↓
III	K^+-channel blockers; APD and ERP prolonged	Amiodarone	↑↑↑		↑↑↑	↓	
		Sotalol	↑↑↑		↑↑↑	↓	↓↓
		Ibutilide	↑↑				
		Bretylium					
IV	Ca^{2+}-channel blockers	Verapamil	↓↓			↓↓	↓↓↓

APD, action potential duration; MRD, maximum rate of depolarization; ERP, effective refractory period; A-VC, atrioventricular conduction.

Table 11.2 Pharmacokinetic profiles of common anti-dysrhythmic drugs

Drug	Systemic bioavailability	Distribution	Metabolism	Excretion	Points of note
Adenosine	IV only		Metabolized in vascular endothelium and RBC	$t_{1/2} < 5$ s	No dose change with renal and hepatic disease
Amiodarone	22–86% (oral)	PPB = 96–98%; Vd = 1.3–65.8 l kg^{-1}	Extensive hepatic metabolism	Predominately excreted in the bile; 1–5% unchanged in urine; $t_{1/2}$ = 4 h to 59 days, depending on dose and route	Modify dose with hepatic disease; no dose change with renal disease; not removed by haemodialysis
Diltiazem	40–70% (oral)	PPB = 80%; Vd = 5.3 l kg^{-1}	60% hepatic metabolism; active metabolites (40% of parent drug activity)	40% unchanged in urine; $t_{1/2}$ = 3.5–6 h	Modify dose with hepatic disease; no dose change with renal disease and haemodialysis
Digoxin	60–90% (oral)	PPB = 20–30%; Vd = 5–11 l kg^{-1}	<10% hepatic metabolism	50–70% unchanged in urine	Not removed by haemodialysis
Esmolol	IV only	PPB = 50–55%; Vd = 3.43 l kg^{-1}	Hydrolysis by RBC esterases	<2% unchanged in urine; $t_{1/2}$ = 9 min	No dose change with renal and hepatic disease
Lignocaine	24–46% (oral)	PPB = 64%; Vd = 0.7–1.5 l kg^{-1}	90% hepatic metabolism; dependent on flow hepatic blood	<10% unchanged in urine; $t_{1/2} \sim$ 100 min	Modify dose with hepatic disease and heart failure; no dose change with renal disease; removed by haemodialysis
Magnesium	33% (oral)	PPB = 30%		Renal excretion proportional to GFR and plasma concentration	Removed by haemodialysis
Metoprolol	50% (oral)	PPB = 12%; Vd = 5.6 l kg^{-1}	Extensive hepatic metabolism	<5% unchanged in urine; $t_{1/2}$ = 3–5 h	Modify dose with hepatic disease; no dose change with renal disease
Verapamil	10–20% (oral)	PPB = 90%; Vd = 3.1–4.9 l kg^{-1}	65–80% hepatic metabolism; active metabolite (20% of parent drug activity)	3–4% unchanged in urine; $t_{1/2}$ = 3–7 h	Modify dose with hepatic disease; no dose change with renal disease; not removed by haemodialysis

Vd, volume of distribution; PPB, plasma protein binding; $t_{1/2}$, terminal elimination half-life; GFR, glomerular filtration rate.

transient A-V or retrograde (ventriculoatrial) block, which may clarify the diagnosis.
- Stable wide-complex tachycardia (WCT) of supraventricular origin.
- No longer recommended to discriminate between VT and SVT, in the diagnosis of stable WCT of uncertain origin, as hazardous if mediated by accessory pathways.

Dose
- Initial adult dose: 3 mg as a rapid IV bolus over 1–3 s followed by a saline flush.
- Further doses of 6 and 12 mg after 1–2 min if no response observed.

Problems
- Common transient side effects are flushing, dyspnoea, chest pain, headache and hypotension.
- Bronchospasm.
- Acceleration of accessory pathway conduction.
- Concurrent methylxanthine administration may reduce efficacy.
- Effects potentiated/prolonged by dipyridamole and carbamazepine.
- Effects prolonged in transplanted (denervated) heart.

Amiodarone

Amiodarone is a benzofuran derivative and its structure is similar to thyroxine and tri-iodothyronine. The drug is a broad spectrum anti-dysrhythmic and has a long duration of action ($t_{1/2}$: 1–2 months) with extensive tissue binding and an enormous volume of distribution.

Action
- Although considered to be a Class III anti-dysrhythmic (major action is K^+-channel antagonism) amiodarone also has Class I, II and IV actions, giving it a unique pharmacological and anti-dysrhythmic profile.
- Oral amiodarone takes days to work in ventricular tachy-dysrhythmias, but IV amiodarone has immediate effect and can be used in life-threatening ventricular dysrhythmias.

Indications
- Cardiac arrest with persistent VT or VF.
- Haemodynamically stable:
  - WCT of uncertain origin;
  - monomorphic and polymorphic VT (normal baseline QT interval);
  - narrow-complex SVT.
- Ventricular rate control of AF/atrial flutter:
  - First-line drug for patients with co-existing congestive heart failure (CHF) and pre-excited AF/atrial flutter.
- Cardioversion of AF/atrial flutter:
  - If direct current (DC) cardioversion undesirable or contraindicated.
- Narrow-complex SVT:
  - Unresponsive to adenosine, vagal stimulation and/or DC cardioversion.
- Prophylaxis against perioperative AF in cardiac surgical patients.
- Amiodarone administered IV following out-of-hospital cardiac arrest due to VF improves survival to hospital admission.

Dose
- Initially 5 mg kg^{-1} (300 mg) IV over 60 min, followed by 15 mg kg^{-1} (900 mg) over 23 h.
- Maintenance: 600 mg *per orem* (PO) daily for 1 week, 400 mg daily for 1 week, followed by 200 mg daily thereafter.
- Following cardiac arrest – 300 mg IV.
- Maximum daily dose is 2.2 g.

Problems
- Bradycardia, heart block, increased defibrillation threshold.
- Vasodilatation and negative inotropy.
- Pulmonary fibrosis.
- Haemodynamic instability with anaesthesia following chronic therapy.
- Long-term therapy is associated with corneal micro-deposits, optic neuritis, blindness, photo-sensitivity, hypo- and hyperthyroidism, proximal muscle weakness, ataxia, GI symptoms and liver dysfunction.
- Potentiated by drugs that prolong the QT interval.

β-blockers

With the exception of sotalol, which is discussed below, these are covered in Chapter 9.

Calcium-channel blockers

Calcium-channel blockers are a heterogeneous group of compounds that block the slow inward Ca^{2+} current via (L-type) channels. While verapamil and diltiazem possess Class IV anti-dysrhythmic properties, the dihydropyridines (e.g. nifedipine) have minimal myocardial effects.

Action (verapamil and diltiazem)
- Decreased conduction and increased refractoriness in A-V node.

Indications
- Narrow-complex paroxysmal SVT.
- Ventricular rate control in AF/atrial flutter and multi-focal AT.
- A-V nodal re-entrant tachydysrhythmias.

Dose

Verapamil
- Initially 2.5–5 mg IV over 2 min.
- A further 5–10 mg every 15–30 min if no response, to a maximum of 20 mg.

Diltiazem
- Initially 0.25 mg kg^{-1}, followed by a second dose of 0.35 mg kg^{-1}, although IV preparation not licensed in the UK.
- May also be given by infusion of 5–15 mg h^{-1} to control the ventricular rate in AF/atrial flutter.

Problems
- Decreased myocardial contractility (verapamil > diltiazem).

Digoxin

One of a family of cardiac glycosides derived from the foxglove.

Action
- Primary direct effect is inhibition of Na$^+$/K$^+$ ATPase.
- Increased intracellular Na$^+$ and Ca^{2+}/decreased intracellular K$^+$.
- Increased slope 4 depolarization and decreased resting membrane potential in conduction tissue.
- Delayed A-V conduction.
- Increased vagal activity (indirect effect).
- Increased inotropy.

Indications
- Rate control of AF/atrial flutter.

Dose
- Adult IV dose (undigitalized):
  - initial IV dose 10–15 μg kg^{-1}, over 30 min (usually 500 μg);
  - repeat after 6 h until desired effect is achieved (up to 20 μg kg^{-1});
  - maintenance is 5–10 μg kg^{-1} day^{-1} in divided doses.
- Child IV dose (undigitalized):
  - initial IV dose 15 μg kg^{-1} over 30 min;
  - then 5 μg kg^{-1} 6 h later;
  - maintenance 5 μg kg^{-1} for every 12 h.

Reduce dose if previously digitalized, elderly or renal impairment. Therapeutic range is 0.5–1.5 ng ml^{-1}.

Problems
- Side effects are common.
- CVS – any form of dysrhythmia, including:
  - junctional bradycardia, ventricular bigeminy and heart block.
- GI – anorexia, nausea, vomiting, diarrhoea and abdominal pain.

- CNS – headache, drowsiness, confusion, visual disturbances and muscle weakness.

Disopyramide

Class I anti-dysrhythmic with Class III properties.

Action
- Similar to quinidine and procainamide, but with more pronounced anticholinergic activity.

Indications
- A-V nodal, A-V re-entrant and ventricular dysrhythmias.
- Prevention of paroxysmal AF/atrial flutter.

Dose
- *IV*   2 mg kg^{-1} (up to 150 mg) over 5 min. Repeated up to 300 mg in the 1st hour, then 0.4 mg kg^{-1} h^{-1}.
- *Oral*   300–800 mg day^{-1} in divided doses.

Problems
- Anticholinergic effects.
- VT/torsade de pointes.
- Heart block.

Flecainide

Flecainide hydrochloride is a Class Ic anti-dysrhythmic.

Action
- Slows conduction (particularly in the His–Purkinje system) and suppresses accessory conduction pathways.
- Available for oral and IV (outside USA) administration.

Indications
- Atrial flutter and AF.
- Ectopic atrial tachycardia.
- A-V nodal re-entrant tachycardia.
- SVT associated with an accessory pathway (Wolff–Parkinson–White syndrome).
- Ventricular dysrhythmias.

Dose
- *IV*   2 mg kg^{-1} at 10 mg min^{-1}, followed by 0.2 mg kg^{-1} h^{-1} for 12 h.
- *Oral*   Initially 50 mg b.d. to a maximum of 300 mg day^{-1}.

Clinical effects
- Rapid cardioversion (within 2–4 h) of recent-onset AF.
- Suppression of ventricular ectopic foci.

Problems
- Significant negative inotropic effects. Increased mortality in patients with ventricular dysfunction and dysrhythmias limits use.

- Increased mortality has been observed in patients following acute MI, possibly due to pro-dysrhythmic effects.
- Reversible hepatotoxicity, dizziness, paraesthesia, headaches and nausea.
- Increases plasma digoxin levels by 15%.

Ibutilide

Ibutilide is a potent, short-acting, pure Class III agent, derived from sulphonamides.

Action
- Increased action potential (AP) duration and refractory period.

Indications
- Acute pharmacological conversion of atrial flutter or AF.
- Administration to patients with atrial flutter or AF prior to DC cardioversion increases the chances of conversion to sinus rhythm.
- Termination of re-entrant atrial dysrhythmias.
- Most effective agent for atrial flutter or AF of short duration.

Dose
- Only available for IV administration.
- For adults $\geq$60 kg, 1 mg over 10 min, repeated after 10 min, if unsuccessful.
- For adults <60 kg, initial dose 0.01 mg kg^{-1}.
- Should continuously monitor for dysrhythmias at time of administration and for 4–6 h after administration (longer if hepatic dysfunction as the clearance of ibutilide may be prolonged).

Clinical effects
Fewer clinically important adverse haemodynamic effects, even in patients with depressed ventricular function, than Class I agents.

Problems
- Relatively high incidence of ventricular pro-dysrhythmia (QT prolongation), including polymorphic VT and torsade de pointes.
- Pro-dysrhythmia may be increased in severe LV dysfunction.
- Short duration of action, compared to other agents, limits effectiveness for maintaining sinus rhythm.

Lidocaine (Lignocaine)

Lidocaine is a Class Ib anti-dysrhythmic used to suppress ventricular dysrhythmias associated with acute MI and cardiac surgery.

Action
- Na$^+$-channel blocker.
- Main action is depression of phase 4 diastolic depolarization.

- Decreased automaticity of pacemaker tissue in Purkinje fibres.
- Decreased automaticity in SA node only when diseased.
- Minimal effect on AP duration or conduction in normal circumstances; however, conduction may be delayed in diseased myocardium.
- Greater efficacy in the presence of a relatively high serum [K$^+$].

Indications
- Acute sustained ventricular tachy-dysrhythmias.
- Second-line treatment behind amiodarone, procainamide and sotalol.
- Control of haemodynamically compromising premature ventricular contractions (PVCs).
- No proven short- or long-term efficacy in cardiac arrest.

Dose
- For pulseless VT/VF cardiac arrest after failure of defibrillation and where amiodarone is contraindicated, initial bolus of 1.0–1.5 mg kg^{-1}.
- Infusion: 4 mg min^{-1} for 30 min, 2 mg min^{-1} for 2 h, reducing to 1 mg min^{-1}.

Problems
- *CNS toxicity* altered level of consciousness, muscle twitching and seizures.
- *CVS toxicity* bradycardia, hypotension and cardiac arrest.
- Increases defibrillation threshold.
- Can precipitate complete heart block in patients with impaired A-V conduction.

Magnesium

Magnesium may decrease the incidence of dysrhythmias in patients undergoing cardiac surgery, though empirical use in cardiac surgery remains controversial.

Action
- Direct effect on stabilizing the myocardial cell membrane.
- Direct/indirect effect on cellular [K$^+$] and [Na$^+$].
- Antagonism of Ca^{2+} entry into sarcoplasmic reticulum.
- Prevention of coronary artery spasm and coronary artery dilatatation.
- Catecholamine antagonism.

Indications
- Use in cardiac arrest if torsade de pointes or hypomagnesaemia is suspected.
- Refractory VF.
- Torsade de pointes with a pulse.

- Life-threatening ventricular dysrhythmias due to digitalis toxicity.

Dose
- Cardiac arrest (for torsade de pointes or hypo-magnesaemia): 1–2 g $MgSO_4$ IV bolus.
- Torsade de pointes (cardiostable): 1–2 g $MgSO_4$ IV over 5–60 min, followed by $0.5–1.0\,g\,h^{-1}$.

Problems
- Hypotension, bradycardia and AV block.
- Muscle weakness and sedation.
- Inhibition of platelet aggregation.
- Cardiac arrest in overdose.
- Interaction with Ca^{2+}-channel blockers, causing hypotension.

Procainamide

Procainamide is a Class Ia agent – anti-dysrhythmic agent.

Action
- Slows conduction.
- Increases effective refractory period in atria and His–Purkinje system.

Indications
- Ventricular dysrhythmias, especially those unresponsive or incompletely responsive to lignocaine.
- Conversion of AF and atrial flutter to sinus rhythm.
- Control of rapid ventricular rate due to accessory pathways in pre-excited atrial dysrhythmias.
- Chronic suppression of PVCs.

Dose
- Given as an infusion of $20\,mg\,min^{-1}$ until either:
  - the dysrhythmias is suppressed
  - hypotension ensues
  - the QRS complex is prolonged by 50% or
  - a total of $17\,mg\,kg^{-1}$ has been given (1.2 g for a 70-kg patient).
- Oral administration is also available.

Clinical effects and problems
- Precipitous hypotension following rapid administration.
- QT prolongation – torsade de pointes.
- Risk of accumulation in renal and hepatic dysfunction, and congestive cardiac failure.
- Other side effects include, GI disturbances, CNS symptoms (headaches and sleep disturbance), rash and agranulocytosis.
- Hypersensitivity reactions, a lupus-like syndrome and the need to monitor serum drug and N-acetyl metabolite levels limit use.

Sotalol

Sotalol is a nonselective β-blocker with class III anti-dysrhythmic properties.

Action
- Increases AP duration and refractory period.
- Onset of action more rapid than oral amiodarone.

Indications
- Ventricular and supraventricular dysrhythmias.
- Prevention of paroxysmal SVT – including postoperative AF (efficacy similar to amiodarone).

Dose
- *IV* $1–1.5\,mg\,kg^{-1}$ at $10\,mg\,min^{-1}$.
- *Oral* 40–160 mg b.d.

Problems
- Bradycardia and hypotension – particularly in patients with poor LV function.
- Increased risk of torsade de pointes.
- IV administration is limited by need to infuse slowly.

Key points

- For any unstable tachydysrhythmia, the first-line treatment is electrical cardioversion.
- Pro-dysrhythmic side effects are more likely when more than one drug is used.
- Class III agents cause less haemodynamic instability than Class I agents.

Further reading

Boyd WC, Thomas SJ. Pro: Magnesium should be administered to all coronary artery bypass graft surgery patients undergoing cardiopulmonary bypass. *J Cardiothorac Vasc Anesth* 2000; **14(3)**: 339–343.

Grigore AM, Mathew JP. Con: Magnesium should not be administered to all coronary artery bypass graft surgery patients undergoing cardiopulmonary bypass. *J Cardiothorac Vasc Anesth* 2000; **14(3)**: 344–346.

Kudenchuk PJ, Cobb LA, Copass MK, Cummins RO, Doherty AM, Fahrenbruch CE *et al.* Amiodarone for resuscitation after out-of-hospital cardiac arrest due to ventricular fibrillation. *N Engl J Med* 1999; **341(12)**: 871–878.

The American Heart Association in collaboration with the International Liaison Committee on Resuscitation. Guidelines 2000 for Cardiopulmonary Resuscitation and Emergency Cardiovascular Care. *Circulation* 2000; **102 (8 Suppl I)**: I1–I384.

ANTICOAGULANTS AND PROCOAGULANTS 12

J.H. Mackay & C.S. Moore

Few cardiac operations are undertaken without heparin and protamine. This chapter discusses important features of these key drugs, their alternatives, and commonly used pharmacological adjuncts to prevent bleeding.

Heparin

This polyanionic mucopolysaccharide, which was originally identified in 1916 from liver tissue, is now derived from either bovine lung or porcine intestinal mucosa. Unfractionated heparin contains molecules with molecular weight (MW) of 5–30 kDa. The molecules are highly negatively charged due to the presence of sulphhydryl groups ($CH_2OSO_3^-$) on side chains. Rapid onset and reversibility together with easy point-of-care monitoring have given heparin a virtual monopoly as anticoagulant CPB.

Action
- Requires presence of antithrombin (AT) for anticoagulant effect.
- AT–heparin complex has >1000-fold increased affinity for thrombin than AT without heparin.
- AT–heparin complex prevents thrombin-mediated fibrinogen conversion to fibrin, platelet activation and release of tissue plasminogen activator (tPA).

Dose
- Standard dose is 300 units kg^{-1} (3 mg kg^{-1}) via central vein prior to aortic cannulation.
- Dose by volume is 0.3 ml kg^{-1} of 1000 units ml^{-1} heparin.

Problems
1 Heparin resistance (2° to decreased AT levels) is defined as failure of heparin 500 units kg^{-1} to prolong ACT to ⩾480 s. Treatment is with FFP or AT concentrate:
   - *Acquired*
     - Patients given preoperative heparin at increased risk due to hepatic clearance of AT–heparin–thrombin complexes.
     - Hepatic failure.
   - *Congenital*
     - Incidence is 1 in 1000.
2 Heparin-induced thrombocytopaenia syndrome (HITS):
   - IgG mediated.
   - Thrombocytopenia, heparin tachyphylaxis and arterial thrombosis.
   - Treatment consists of stopping heparin, removal of heparin from flushes and substitution of alternative anticoagulant.
3 Transient hypotension due to histamine release and binding of negatively charged heparin with Ca^{2+}; usually clinically insignificant.

Heparin alternatives

Proven heparin allergy and HITS are absolute contraindications to heparin. All heparin substitutes have limitations in the surgical setting.

Low-molecular-weight-heparins

Low-molecular-weight heparins (LMWHs) have short chains (mean MW, 4–5 kDa), which act via factor Xa inhibition. Effect on APTT is considerably less than unfractionated heparin. Cross reaction may occur in HITS. Lack of potency, difficulty monitoring efficacy, long elimination $t_{1/2}$ and inability to reverse with protamine make LMWHs unsuitable for cardiac surgery.

Thrombin inhibitors (hirudin, lepirudin and argatroban)

These agents bind tightly to thrombin and block all thrombin-catalysed reactions. Due to short elimination $t_{1/2}$, thrombin inhibitors must be delivered by infusion. Efficacy requires monitoring of Ecarin clotting time (ECT). These agents are not reversed by protamine or platelet factor 4. Clinical experience of using these agents as alternatives to heparin for CPB is relatively limited.

Ancrod

Purified from venom of *Malaysian Pit Viper*, ancrod reduces fibrinogen levels over 24–48 h. Anticoagulation can be reversed by cryoprecipitate and platelet administration. Predicting therapeutic levels and preventing coagulation protein consumption are both problematic.

Danaparoid

This heparinoid, factor Xa inhibitor, is widely used in the management of patients with HITS in the ICU setting. The relatively long elimination $t_{1/2}$, the lack of point-of-care monitor of anti-Xa activity and the absence of an antagonist make the drug less attractive as a heparin substitute in theatre.

Iloprost

Stable analogue of prostacyclin, iloprost is a potent inhibitor of platelet function with thrombolytic properties. Unlike epoprostenol, it is stable at room temperature and resistant to normal light. Short terminal $t_{1/2}$ (15–20 min) combined with potential benefits to RV function, make this the anti-coagulant of choice for cardiac surgery in HITS. The dose required for CPB causes predictable hypotension which responds to vasoconstrictors.

Protamine

Protamine is peptide found in high concentrations in DNA. It carries positive charge due to high content of arginine amino acids. Pharmacological preparations are derived from salmon sperm. Protamine is the routinely used reversal agent for heparin.

Action
- Cationic protamine reverses anionic heparin by a simple acid–base interaction.

Dose
- Standard dose is 3 mg kg^{-1}.
- Vials contain protamine 1%; therefore dose by volume is = 0.3 ml kg^{-1}. The volume of administered protamine (10 mg ml^{-1}) therefore equals the volume of administered heparin (1000 units ml^{-1}).

Problems
- *Common* hypotension if rapidly administered too rapidly, direct myocardial depression or histamine release, normally transient and systemic hypotension – mediated by thromboxane.

- *Rare* IgE-mediated severe anaphylactic reactions:
  – Increased incidence of previous exposure to porcine insulin, fish allergy and vasectomy.
- *Rare* Pulmonary hypertension (PHT), RV failure and systemic hypotension; mediated by thromboxane.

Protamine alternatives

Heparinase and recombinant PF4 are potential alternatives to protamine for reversing systemic heparinization in patients with protamine allergy or PHT.

Heparinase

Heparinase, produced by Gram-negative *Flavobacterium*, metabolizes heparin by cleaving alpha-glycosidic linkages to produce fragments that are unable to activate AT. Full heparin reversal takes 5 min compared to the immediate reversal produced by protamine. Given that heparinase is a foreign protein derived from bacteria, protamine-like anaphylactic reactions are theoretically possible on re-exposure. Phase III studies are in progress.

Platelet factor 4

PF4 is a naturally occurring heparin-neutralizing agent found on platelets, whose major role is to neutralize vascular heparans by ionic binding following endothelial injury. Platelet transfusions contain insufficient PF4 to reverse full heparinization. A recombinant form of PF4, synthesised from *Escherichia coli*, has potential clinical applications.

Antifibrinolytics

The lysine analogues; *trans*-amino-methylcyclohexanoic (tranexamic) acid (TA) and 6-aminohexanoic (epsilon-aminocaproic) acid (EACA) bind to plasminogen and prevent tPA-mediated release of active plasmin. The prevention of plasminogen binding to fibrin via lysine-binding sites results in a fibrin polymer with greater resistance to fibrinolysis. TA is 10 times more potent than EACA. Loading dose should be given at start of surgery, as agents are more effective as prophylactic agents than treatment of fibrinolysis.

TA dosage is 10–15 mg kg^{-1} before and after CPB. TA is cheap and has low risk : benefit ratio. Possible increased risk of deep vein thrombosis (DVT) and pulmonary embolism (PE) postoperatively – patients are frequently given LMWH postoperatively. EACA, ubiquitous in the USA, is not currently licensed in the UK.

Aprotinin

Aprotinin is a polypeptide (58 amino acids, MW ~6.5 kDa) with non-specific, serine protease inhibitory properties and is derived from bovine lung and first investigated in the 1930s as a treatment for acute pancreatitis. Aprotinin has a broad spectrum of activity against serine proteases including: trypsin, plasmin, tPA and both tissue and plasma kallidinogenase (kallikrein). Aprotinin inhibits pro-inflammatory cytokine release and maintains glycoprotein homoeostasis. It reduces platelet glycoprotein (GpIb, GpIIb/IIIa) loss and prevents the expression of proinflammatory adhesive glycoproteins in granulocytes. Commercially available solutions contain 10,000 KIU ml^{-1} (kallikrein inhibitory units), equivalent to aprotinin 1.4 mg ml^{-1} or 215 nmol l^{-1}.

Indications
- Patients at high risk of major blood loss during and following open heart surgery:
  - infective endocarditis,
  - re-operation through a previous median sternotomy,
  - blood dyscrasias and coagulopathy,
  - hyperplasminaemia.
- Blood conservation during open heart surgery:
  - Jehovah's Witnesses,
  - rare blood groups who require open heart surgery.
- Heart–lung transplantation (unlicensed).

Dose
- 'Full-dose' or Munich/Hammersmith regimen for adults:
  - 2 million KIU loading dose,
  - 2 million KIU into CPB pump,
  - 0.5 million KIU per hour by infusion.
- 'Half-dose' and other lower-dose regimens are widely utilized.

Problems
- A shift in haemostatic balance towards a prothrombotic state has lead to concerns about reduced graft patency and increased rates of perioperative MI after CABG surgery.
- Anaphylactoid reactions: incidence without pre-exposure ~1 : 1400. Incidence ~3% per re-exposure, greater if within 6 months of last exposure. Previous exposure to aprotinin-containing fibrin sealants may increase risk. Administration of a test dose (10,000 KIU) is recommended in all cases *before* loading pump.
- Renal dysfunction: over 95% of administered dose stored and metabolised in proximal renal tubules. Transient renal dysfunction follows aprotinin administration. Doubts persist about its safety in aortic surgery and deep hypothermic circulatory arrest (DHCA).
- Cost >£240 per case (compared with ~£5 per case for TA).
- Interference with celite-ACT monitoring.

Desmopressin

Desamino-8-arginine vasopressin (DDAVP) is a longer-acting analogue of vasopressin with no vasoconstrictor effect. Despite increasing von Willebrand's factor (v-WF) and factor VIII levels, studies in cardiac surgery have failed to demonstrate a reduction in blood loss or transfusion requirements. Although DDAVP is rarely given to patients taking aspirin prior to CABG surgery, it may be of use when bleeding is due to confirmed or suspected platelet dysfunction (i.e. uraemia). Suggested dose (unlicensed indication): 0.3 μg kg^{-1} over 20 min.

Key points

- Unfractionated heparin remains the most commonly used anticoagulant for CPB.
- Unfractionated and LMWHs may induce immune thrombocytopenia and thrombosis.
- All heparin substitutes have limitations.
- Although hypotension almost invariably follows protamine administration, life-threatening complications are rare.
- Aprotinin is the most effective agent for reducing blood loss *and* transfusion requirements in cardiac surgery.

Further reading

Pifarré R (Ed.). *New Anticoagulants for the Cardiovascular Patient*. Philadelphia: Hanley & Belfus, Inc., 1997.

M. Prabhu

Terminology

Derivatives of opium have been used by mankind since the 4th century BC, and its analgesic and sedative properties were well known by the 16th century. The perioperative use of opioids has increased significantly since the 1940s, and they remain the mainstay of treatment for moderate to severe pain. The products include:

- *Opioid* Any substance producing morphine-like effects that are blocked by antagonists.
- *Opiate* Morphine-like drugs that bear close structural similarity to morphine.
- *Opium* Extract of the juice of the poppy *Papaver somniferum* containing many morphine-like alkaloids.

Opioids have widespread actions mediated by both opioid and non-opioid (e.g. muscarinic and dopaminergic) receptors. Opioid receptors are distributed in distinct patterns throughout the central and peripheral nervous systems, and have been historically classified into three main types: delta (δ), kappa (κ) and mu (μ). More recently, the International Union of Pharmacology (IUPHAR) has re-classified these as OP_1, OP_2 and OP_3, respectively. The dyphoria and hypertonia associated with opioids were originally thought to be mediated by a fourth receptor namely the sigma (σ) receptor. The σ-receptor system is now recognized as a separate entity with a wide variety of ligands.

Receptor types and their mediated effects:

- *OP_1 or Delta (δ)* Spinal analgesia, μ-receptor modulation.
- *OP_2 or Kappa (κ)* Spinal analgesia, sedation, miosis, diuresis.
- *OP_3 or Mu (μ)* Analgesia (μ_1), respiratory depression, dependence, pruritis, nausea, vomiting (μ_2).

Based on receptor physiology, opioids can be classified as:

- Agonists (e.g. morphine).
- Antagonists (e.g. naloxone).

- Partial agonist–antagonist (e.g. buprenorphine and pentazocine).

Based on structure–function relationships, opioids have been classified as:

- Phenanthrenes (morphine and codeine).
- Benzyisoquinolines (papaverine and noscapine) which incidentally lack opioid activity.
- Semisynthetics (diamorphine) – modification of the morphine molecule.
- Synthetics:
  - Benzomorphinan (methadone and pentazocine).
  - Phenylpiperidines (fentanyl, alfentanil, sufentanil and remifentanil).

Of the opioids currently available, morphine and the phenylpiperidines are the most commonly used in cardiac anaesthesia.

Indications

> **The indications are given as follows:**
>
> Perioperative analgesia
> Premedication
> Conscious sedation
> Attenuate stress response
> Anxiolysis

Routes of administration

> **Commonly utilised routes of administration include:**
>
> Intramuscular (morphine)
> Intrathecal (morphine)
> Epidural (fentanyl)
> Oral (methadone)
> IV (fentanyl and remifentanil)

Pharmacodynamics

Pharmacodynamic properties of commonly used opioids are shown in Table 13.1.

Table 13.1 Pharmacodynamics

Drug	Analgesia	Sedation	Respiratory depression	Tolerance dependence	Physical	Emesis
Morphine	++	++	++	++	++	++
Alfentanil	++	+	+	No data	No data	No data
Fentanyl	++	+	+	No data	No data	+
Sufentanil	+++	No data	++	No data	No data	No data
Remifentanil	+++	++	++	No data	No data	++

Cardiovascular effects

Morphine

In 1969, Lowenstein *et al.* advocated the use of high-dose ($1–3\,\mathrm{mg\,kg^{-1}}$) morphine in patients undergoing valve surgery on the grounds that it had minimal impact on the cardiovascular system. Subsequent use of the technique in patients with ischaemic heart disease however, resulted in unpredictable haemodynamic responses.

Morphine causes a dose-dependent fall in SVR secondary to both histamine release and a direct action on vascular smooth muscle. Although the effect is relatively minor, in comparison with other anaesthetic agents, it is potentiated by nitric oxide (NO) and may be profound in haemodynamically unstable patients. It has no direct effect on coronary blood flow (CBF). Vagal activation and a direct depressant action on the SA node typically induce a bradycardia, although significant myocardial depression is associated with doses far in excess of those used in clinical practice.

Fentanyl

Owing to its superior haemodynamic profile, high-dose ($50–150\,\mathrm{\mu g\,kg^{-1}}$) fentanyl was used as a sole agent for cardiac anaesthesia in the late 1970s. Unfortunately, dose-dependent bradycardia, chest wall rigidity, awareness and the need for prolonged postoperative mechanical ventilation tempered enthusiasm for the technique. To date no drug fulfils the criteria for use as a sole agent in cardiac anaesthesia. For this reason, intermediate-dose ($10–15\,\mathrm{\mu g\,kg^{-1}}$) fentanyl remains the mainstay of balanced cardiac anaesthesia in many centres.

Sufentanil

Sufentanil is more lipophilic, 5–10 times more potent, and has a smaller volume of distribution than fentanyl. High-dose sufentanil ($15\,\mathrm{\mu g\,kg^{-1}}$ and fentanyl ($100\,\mathrm{\mu g\,kg^{-1}}$) anaesthesia are virtually

indistinguishable. This agent is currently not available in the UK.

Alfentanil

The shorter $t_{1/2}$ and smaller volume of distribution (compared to fentanyl) favour the administration of alfentanil as a loading dose ($20–50\,\mathrm{\mu g\,kg^{-1}}$) followed by a continuous infusion ($0.25–2.5\,\mathrm{\mu g\,kg^{-1}min^{-1}}$). Alfentanil is considered to be less cardiovascularly stable, and studies in cardiac surgical patients suggest that it offers no particular advantage over fentanyl.

Remifentanil

This ultra-short-acting agent ($t_{1/2} \sim 3\,\mathrm{min}$) was introduced in 1993. Unlike other opioids it is metabolized by non-specific plasma and tissue esterases. A loading dose of $1.0\,\mathrm{\mu g\,kg^{-1}}$ (administered over 1–2 min) followed by an infusion of $0.05–1.0\,\mathrm{\mu g\,kg^{-1}min^{-1}}$ is recommended. More rapid administration may produce muscle rigidity, and profound bradycardia and hypotension. Although regarded by some as technically more demanding, its proponents state that maintenance with remifentanil is no more demanding than using a vaporizer. Although the side-effect profiles of remifentanil and fentanyl are similar, shivering and hypertension are more common with remifentanil.

Advantages

- Minimal direct effects on contractility, conduction, automaticity.
- Myocardial sensitivity to catecholamines unchanged.
- Attenuation of the stress response.
- Minimal interaction with autonomic or cardiovascular drug actions.
- Preservation of autoregulation.
- Reduces MAC (effect-site concentration) of volatile and IV anaesthetic agents.
- Postoperative analgesia.
- No organ toxicity.

Disadvantages

- Bradycardia and hypotension during induction.
- Muscular rigidity.
- Risk of awareness.
- Prolonged recovery time.
- Respiratory depression.
- Cough suppression.
- Reduced peristalsis, delayed gastric emptying, increased sphincter tone.
- Nausea and vomiting.
- Pruritis.

Cardiopulmonary bypass

CPB significantly alters the pharmacokinetics of many drugs. The effects of haemodilution and sequestration are balanced in part by a reduction in plasma protein binding and a reduction in elimination. The overall effect is a reduction in opioid concentration at the onset of CPB. During prolonged hypothermic CPB, however, the impact of reduced clearance tends to predominate when opioids are administered by infusion. The influence of CPB on the pharmacology of commonly used drugs is discussed in more detail in Chapter 14.

Further reading

Dollery C. Therapeutic drugs, 2nd edition. Edinburgh: Churchill Livingstone, 1999. ISBN 044 305148 8.

International Narcotics Research Conference. http//:www.inrcworld.org.

Lowenstein E, Hallowell P, Levine FH, Daggett WM, Austen WG, Laver MB. Cardiovascular response to large doses of intravenous morphine in man. *N Engl J Med* 1969; 281(25): 1389–1393.

Miller RD. Anesthesia, 5th edition. Philadelphia: Churchill Livingstone, 2000. ISBN 044 307988 9.

Reynolds JF. *Martindale the Extra Pharmacopoeia*, 13th edition. London: The Pharmaceutical Press, 1993.

Appendix

Summary of pharmacokinetic data for opioids commonly used in cardiac anaesthesia					
	Morphine	Alfentanil	Fentanyl	Sufentanil	Remifentanil
pKa	7.93, 9.63	6.5	8.43	8.01	7.07
Solubility : ethanol	1 : 250	1 : 5	1 : 140	–	–
Solubility : water	1 : 5000	1 : 7	1 : 40	–	–
Octanol/H_2O partition coefficient	6.03	145	955	1.75	17.9
Distribution $t_{1/2}$ (min)	–	3.5	5–12	1.4	1
Elimination $t_{1/2}$ (h)	2	1.2	1–4	3.5	0.15
Clearance (ml kg^{-1} min^{-1})	11.5	7.5	12.8	11.3	40–60
V_d (l kg^{-1})	1.5–4	0.28	3–4	2.9	0.1–0.2
V_d, steady state (l kg^{-1})	1–3	0.996	2.2	1.7	0.3
Protein binding (%)	35	89	80	91	70

V_d, volume of distribution.

EFFECTS OF CPB ON DRUG PHARMACOKINETICS

14

B. Murali

Pharmacokinetics of bypass

The pharmacokinetics of many drugs are significantly altered by CPB. The major factors responsible for this are as follows:

- Haemodilution
- Altered plasma protein binding
- Altered regional blood flow
- Hypothermia
- Acid–base balance
- Isolation of lungs from the circulation
- Drug sequestration in the bypass circuit.

Understanding CPB-induced alterations to pharmacokinetics is important for maintaining plasma concentrations and therapeutic effectiveness.

Haemodilution and plasma protein binding

The onset of CPB is associated with a 40–50% increase in circulating blood volume. Acute haemodilution reduces the concentration of circulating proteins, such as albumin and alpha-1 acid glycoprotein, and the total plasma concentration of any circulating drug. The eventual plasma concentration of a drug is dependent upon plasma protein binding, the volume of distribution and plasma concentration before the onset of CPB.

- *Plasma protein binding* Reduced plasma protein concentration increases unbound drug fraction. Particularly important for highly protein-bound drugs.
- *Volume of distribution* (V_d) Drugs with small V_d undergo proportionately greater dilution than drugs with large V_d where plasma concentrations tend to be maintained by transfer of drug from extravascular compartments.

Hydrolysis of triglycerides secondary to heparin-induced lipase release, leads to a rise in the concentration of free fatty acids that compete with drugs for plasma protein-binding sites – an effect reversed by protamine. A rise in the concentration of the inflammatory response protein, alpha-1 acid glycoprotein, following CPB may increase acidic drug binding.

Hypotension and altered regional blood flow

In addition to low pump flow, hypotension during CPB occurs due to reductions in blood viscosity and SVR. Alterations in renal blood flow reduce glomerular filtration rate and renal clearance. Alterations in hepatic blood flow reduce the elimination of drugs with high hepatic extraction ratio.

The circulating concentration of drugs may be reduced further during CPB as pH-sensitive drugs may become 'trapped' in poorly perfused (acidotic) tissues. Following the resumption of normal cardiac output and peripheral perfusion, the trapped proportion is released to the circulation – thus increasing the plasma concentration.

Hypothermia

Hypothermia alters blood flow to and within the kidneys and liver, alters ligand–receptor-binding affinities and reduces the rate of enzymatic reactions. The combination of reduced excretory organ drug delivery, altered enzyme binding and slowed drug metabolism and biotransformation results in reduced elimination and increased plasma drug concentrations.

Acid–base balance

Hypocarbia and alkalosis tend to increase the potency of lipophilic drugs, such as fentanyl, whereas hypercarbia and acidosis tend to increase the potency of hydrophilic drugs, such as morphine.

Lung isolation

The lungs act as reservoir for basic drugs such as local anaesthetics, opioids, catecholamines and induction agents such as propofol and thiopental. During CPB, when the lungs are effectively isolated from the circulation, pulmonary sequestration is reduced so that drugs administered during this time may result in higher plasma concentrations. Re-establishment of pulmonary perfusion tends to liberate sequestered drugs and increase their systemic concentration.

Specific drugs

Propofol

- Decreased total concentration on initiation of CPB.
- Small increase in free fraction (haemodilution and decreased protein binding).
- Decreased plasma clearance due to sequestration in CPB circuit.
- Gradual increase in plasma concentration during CPB (due to reduced metabolism and elimination).
- Heparin-induced increase in free fraction.

Etomidate

- Decreased concentrations on initiation of CPB due to haemodilution.
- Subsequent increased plasma levels due to reduced metabolism.
- Decreased levels on termination of CPB (increased metabolism – increase in hepatic blood flow).

Thiopental

- Abrupt decrease in total plasma concentration ~50% on initiation of CPB.
- Increased free fraction ~50% thereafter.
  - The net effect is maintained or slight increase free fraction.
- The total post-CPB concentration is lower than the pre-CPB concentration due to a fall in protein-bound fraction.
- Redistributes to muscle and fat. Sequestered in CPB circuit.

Ketamine

- Concentrations fall by ~33% immediately after onset of CPB.
- Concentrations return to pre-CPB levels by the end of CPB.

Benzodiazepines

- Decreased total concentration at onset of CPB.
- Elimination $t_{1/2}$ prolonged post-CPB.
- Increased post-CPB total concentrations due to redistribution.

Opioids

- Decreased total concentration (fentanyl ~53%, sufentanil ~34% and alfentanil ~55%) at onset of CPB. Effect limited for drugs with greater V_d. Increased free fraction.

- Extracorporeal and pulmonary sequestration proportional to lipid solubility.
- Infusion during CPB results in cumulation (Decreased hepatic elimination and hypothermia).
- Elimination $t_{1/2}$ prolonged post-CPB.
- Constant remifentanil concentration may be achieved by decreasing infusion rate by 30% for every 5°C decrease in temperature.

Muscle relaxants

- Requirements decreased by hypothermia (increase in muscle sensitivity).
- Decreased concentration at onset of CPB. Increased concentrations when given by infusion due to decrease in clearance.
- Hoffman degradation slowed by hypothermia (atracurium).

Antimicrobials

- Haemodilution may result in subtherapeutic levels.
- Clearance reduced during CPB.

Glyceryl trinitrate

- Increased clearance on CPB – substantial sequestration in circuit.

Lidocaine

- High first-pass metabolism.
- Decreased total concentration at onset of CPB. Free fraction remains therapeutic.
- Decreased free fraction post-CPB due to increase in alpha-1 acid glycoprotein binding.
- Decreased clearance and decreased V_d post-CPB.

Propranolol

- High first-pass metabolism following oral administration.
- Decreased concentration at onset of CPB.
- Decreased metabolism during hypothermia.
- Heparin administration doubles free fraction.
- Decreased free fraction post-CPB due to increase in alpha-1 acid glycoprotein binding.

Phosphodiesterase inhibitors

- Low protein binding and hepatic clearance result in minimal alteration to pharmacokinetic profile.

Calcium antagonists

- Haemodilution may result in subtherapeutic levels.

Digoxin

- Decreased concentration at onset of CPB.
- Levels normalize post-CPB – high V_d and low plasma protein binding.

Volatile agents

The effect of hypothermic CPB on the uptake of volatile anaesthetics administered via the oxygenator is dependent on three factors:

- *Blood–gas solubility* Solubility in blood increases as temperature falls.
- *Tissue–gas solubility* Solubility in tissues increases as temperature falls.
- *Oxygenator uptake* Extracorporeal sequestration.

The MAC of volatile anaesthetic agents during CPB may be lower due to increased distribution to the brain. Hypothermia decreases MAC and volatile anaesthetic requirements. Conversely, rewarming decreases the concentration of volatile anaesthetic agents.

While increasing gas flow to the oxygenator increases the uptake of volatile agents *in vitro*, changes in pump flow rate have no impact on uptake. This is quite different from the non-CPB setting where CO has a major impact on the pulmonary uptake of volatile agents.

The 'wash-in' (uptake) and 'wash-out' (elimination) of volatile anaesthetic agents during CPB is inversely proportional to blood–gas solubility. Therefore relatively insoluble agents (e.g. isoflurane; partition coefficient 1.4 at 37°C) are more rapidly taken up and eliminated than more soluble agents (e.g. enflurane and halothane; partition coefficients 1.4 and ~2.4, respectively, at 37°C).

Key points

- A number of physical and chemical factors account for the alteration of drug pharmacokinetics during CPB.
- Changes in the plasma concentration of drugs, secondary to increased volume of distribution, are often balanced by a reduction in plasma protein binding.
- Hypothermia and altered regional blood flow reduce drug metabolism and elimination.
- Hypothermia simultaneously increases the blood concentration of volatile anaesthetic agents and reduces MAC.

Further reading

Mets B. The pharmacokinetics of anaesthetic drugs and adjuvants during Cardiopulmonary bypass. *Acta Anaesthesiol Scand* 2000; **44(3)**: 261–273.

DIAGNOSIS OF CARDIAC DISEASE

SECTION

3

J.E. Arrowsmith

Despite the widespread availability of investigational tests and imaging techniques for the diagnosis and management of cardiac disease, eliciting a comprehensive history and performing a systematic physical examination remain essential clinical skills.

Symptoms

The presence or absence of specific symptoms should be sought in a systematic fashion. Symptoms should be described in terms of their nature (using the patient's own words), onset, duration and progression, as well any modifying factors or associations:

Nature	Description, anatomic site, radiation
Onset	Acute versus chronic
Progression	Static, rapid versus gradual worsening
Modifying factors	Provoking, Exacerbating, Relieving
Associations	Related symptoms
Duration	Intermittent versus continuous

Overall functional status

Originally published in 1928, the *NYHA Functional Capacity Classification* provides as assessment of the impact of symptoms (dyspnoea, angina, fatigue and palpitation) on physical activity (Table 15.1). An objective assessment of severity of cardiovascular disease, added in 1994, recognizes the fact that severity of symptoms (i.e. functional capacity) may not reflect the severity of underlying cardiovascular disease.

Dyspnoea

The sensation of uncomfortable breathing. It is essential to make the distinction between cardiac and respiratory causes. Mechanisms include: hypoxia, hypercarbia, bronchoconstriction, bronchial mucosal oedema, reduced lung compliance (increased work of breathing), reflex hyperventilation and reduced vital capacity (hydrothorax, ascites and pregnancy).

Cardiac causes include: elevated pulmonary venous pressure, reduced pulmonary blood flow (right to left shunt), and low CO (RV failure). An acute onset may suggest papillary muscle or MV chordal rupture,

Table 15.1 The *NYHA Classification of Functional Capacity* (first published 1928) and American Heart Association (AHA) objective assessment (http://www.americanheart.org)

Functional capacity	Objective assessment
Class I: Patients with cardiac disease but without resulting limitation of physical activity. Ordinary physical activity does not cause undue fatigue, palpitation, dyspnoea or anginal pain.	A: No objective evidence of cardiovascular disease
Class II: Patients with cardiac disease resulting in slight limitation of physical activity. They are comfortable at rest. Ordinary physical activity results in fatigue, palpitation, dyspnoea or anginal pain.	B: Objective evidence of minimal cardiovascular disease
Class III: Patients with cardiac disease resulting in marked limitation of physical activity. They are comfortable at rest. Less than ordinary activity results in fatigue, palpitation, dyspnoea or anginal pain.	C: Objective evidence of moderately severe cardiovascular disease
Class IV: Patients with cardiac disease resulting in inability to carry on any physical activity without discomfort. Symptoms of heart failure or the anginal syndrome may be present even at rest. If physical activity is undertaken, discomfort is increased.	D: Objective evidence of severe cardiovascular disease

Examples: Class I-D, asymptomatic patient with an aortic gradient >100 mmHg; Class IV-A, angina at rest with normal coronary arteries; Class IV-D, cardiogenic shock.

whereas a more insidious onset may suggest gradually worsening ventricular function.

- *Associated symptoms*: especially chest pain, palpitation, diaphoresis and (pre-) syncope.
- *Postural*: supine (orthopnoea and paroxysmal noctural dyspnoea) and other (atrial myxoma).

Haemoptysis

Not uncommon in cardiac disease. Frank haemoptysis may occur in MS (bronchial/pulmonary vein rupture) and pulmonary infarction. In pulmonary oedema, the sputum is frothy and often streaked with blood. Pulmonary causes include: tuberculosis (TB), bronchiectasis and cancer.

Chest pain

The aetiology may be cardiac (ischaemic and non-ischaemic) or non-cardiac. Enquiry should be made about the quality, location, radiation, timing and duration of pain, as well as any provoking, exacerbating or relieving factors and associated symptoms.

Non-ischaemic cardiac causes include: aortic dissection ('tearing' central pain radiating to back), MV prolapse (sharp infra-mammary pain), pericarditis (dull central chest pain worsened on leaning forward) and pulmonary embolus (pleuritic pain worse on inspiration).

Non-cardiac causes include: oesophagitis and oesophageal spasm (relieved by nitrates), biliary and pancreatic disorders, pleural inflammation and musculoskeletal disorders of the chest wall and spine.

Angina pectoris

Typically described as 'choking', 'tightening' or 'heaviness'. Levine's sign (hand clenched against the chest) may be present. Usually diffuse in nature, located to midchest or xisternum with radiation to the left chest and arm, epigastrium, back or jaw. Typically lasting <10 min (duration >20 min may indicate acute coronary syndrome – infarction or unstable angina). Provoked by exertion, cold exposure, eating and emotional stress. May be worsened, or paradoxically relieved, by continuing exertion. Relieved by cessation of activity or nitrates. The CCS Angina Scale is shown in Table 15.2.

Syncope

Transient loss or near loss (pre-syncope) of consciousness secondary to reduced cerebral blood flow – low CO or cerebral perfusion pressure. The patient may describe 'drop attacks', a 'funny turn', dizziness or tinnitus. The presence of associated symptoms, such as a premonitory aura, palpitation or chest pain should be actively sought. The differential diagnosis includes: postural hypotension, neurological disorders and cardiac disease.

Postural hypotension may be drug induced (e.g. β-blockers and vasodilators), vasovagal (e.g. micturitional), orthostatic (>20 mmHg fall in systolic BP on standing) or secondary to aortocaval compression when supine in pregnancy. DM and Parkinson's disease may cause autonomic dysfunction.

A witnessed seizure may indicate epilepsy as the cause, whereas pre-syncope associated with transient dysphasia, blindness (amaurosis fugax) or paresis suggests a thromboembolic or vasculopathic cause.

Stokes–Adams attacks

Stokes–Adams attacks include sinus arrest, heart block and VT.

Exertional syncope

Exertional syncope may suggest AS, coronary artery disease, pulmonary hypertension (PHT) or a congenital

---

Table 15.2 The CCS Angina Scale	
Grade	**Activity**
I	*Ordinary physical activity does not cause angina*: e.g. walking or climbing stairs. Angina occurs with strenuous/rapid/prolonged exertion at work/recreation.
II	*Slight limitation of ordinary activity*: e.g. angina occurs walking/climbing stairs after meals, in cold, in wind, under emotional stress, or only during the few hours after awakening, walking more than two blocks on the level or climbing more than one flight of stairs at a normal pace and in normal conditions.
III	*Marked limitation of ordinary physical activity*: e.g. angina occurs walking one to two blocks on the level and climbing one flight of stairs at a normal pace and in normal conditions.
IV	*Inability to carry on any physical activity without discomfort*: angina syndrome *may* be present at rest.

From Campeau L. *Circulation* 1976; **54**: 522, with permission from Lippincott, Williams & Wilkins.

anomaly of coronary artery anatomy. A family history of syncope may indicate hypertrophic obstructive cardiomyopathy or an inherited cardiac conduction defect (e.g. long QT syndrome or Wolf–Parkinson–White syndrome).

Oedema

'Anasarca', the accumulation of interstitial fluid in dependent areas such as the lower limbs and sacral area. Sodium and water retention may occur in cardiac failure, renal failure and malnutrition. Facial oedema may suggest myxoedema or SVC obstruction.

Palpitations

Awareness of heartbeat. 'Thumping' sensation in chest, neck or back; 'missed', 'jumping' or 'extra' beats or 'racing' of the heart. A common symptom in the absence of cardiac disease. May indicate significant dysrhythmia or abnormal cardiac function. Any relationship to exertion or ingestion of alcohol, caffeine or nicotine should be sought, as should symptoms suggestive of thyrotoxicosis.

Fatigue

A distinction should be made between lethargy or general malaise, and effort tolerance limited by chest pain, dyspnoea, claudication or leg weakness. As static measures of cardiac (ventricular) performance often give no indication of functional reserve, it is essential to obtain a measure of maximal functional capacity and the rapidity of any decline. The Duke Activity Status Index (DASI) is shown in Table 66.2.

Miscellaneous

These include nausea, anorexia, dry mouth (disopyramide), nocturia/polyuria (diuretics), cough (ACE inhibitors), xanthopsia (digoxin toxicity), tinnitus and vertigo (chinchonism), headache (nitrates), photosensitivity (amiodarone), nightmares (propranolol) and abdominal swelling/pain (ascites/hepatomegally).

Physical signs

Physical examination is conducted with the patient supine and reclining at 45°. The patient may be required to turn to the left, sit forward, stand or perform isometric exercise.

Observation (inspection)

General appearance

Conscious level, nutritional status, diaphoresis, xanthelasmata, systolic head nodding (de Musset's sign – AR) and signs of conditions associated with cardiac disease (Marfan's, Cushing's, and Downs syndromes, acromegaly, systemic lupus erythematosus, rheumatoid arthritis, ankylosing spondylitis and muscular dystrophies).

Skin

Cyanosis, orange fingers (tobacco use), anaemia, jaundice (hepatic congestion), malar flush, erythema (pressure sores, cardioversion burns), haemorrhagic palmar/plantar lesions (Janeway's lesions and endocarditis), bruising and phlebitis (venepuncture, IV therapy and drug abuse).

Surgical scars

These include sternotomy (cardiac surgery), thoracotomy (mitral valvotomy, repair of coarctation or patent ductus arteriosus (PDA), subclavian (pacemaker or cardiodefibrillator insertion), cervical (carotid endarterectomy), antecubital (coronary angiography) and abdominal (aortic aneurysm repair).

Nail beds

Clubbing, cyanosis, splinter haemorrhages, arterial pulsation (Quinke's sign – AR) and Osler's nodes (tender fingertip nodules – endocarditis).

Cyanosis

Cyanosis is blue skin discolouration. It may be peripheral (hypovolaemia, low CO) or central (mucous membranes). The latter indicates a deoxygenated Hb concentration $>5\,g\,dl^{-1}$. May not be manifested in severe anaemia.

Respiratory rate

Tachypnoea may indicate anxiety or underlying dyspnoea. Episodic (Cheyne–Stokes) breathing is suggestive of severe cardiac failure.

Neck

Goitre, carotid abrupt carotid distension and collapse (Corrigan's sign – AR), and jugular veins.

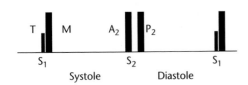

Figure 15.1 Normal heart sounds. *First sound* (S_1) = closure of TV and MV (loudest). Splitting not usually audible. *Second sound* (S_2) = closure of AV followed by PV. Splitting increased on inspiration and with PHT, PS and RBBB as PV closure delayed. ASD causes fixed splitting. Paradoxical splitting (increased on expiration) with AS, LBBB and hypertension secondary to delayed AV closure.

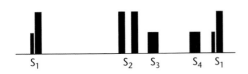

Figure 15.2 *Third sound* (S_3) = rapid early diastolic filling. May be normal in young, otherwise pathological. Present in LV/RV failure, MR, TR, pregnancy and anaemia. Shorter and earlier in diastole in constrictive pericarditis. *Fourth sound* (S_4) = late diastolic filling (atrial systole). Always pathological. Presence of S_4 precludes AF and severe MS.

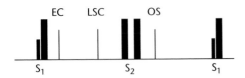

Figure 15.3 *Ejection click* (EC): AS, PS and PHT. *Late systolic click* (LSC): MV prolapse. *Opening snap* (OS): MS. Audible over whole precordium, indicates mobile MV leaflets, louder on expiration. Pneumothorax may produce systolic 'clicking'.

Jugular veins

Pressure level and waveform Level rarely 2 cm above sternal angle when patient reclined at 45° and falls on inspiration. Inspiratory rise suggests pericardial constriction (Kussmaul's sign). Elevated by anxiety, pregnancy, anaemia, exercise, right heart failure and SVC obstruction (non-pulsatile). Giant *a*-wave (TS, PS and RVH), cannon *a*-wave (complete heart block (CHB), VT, junctional rhythm, pacing anomaly), systolic *cv*-wave (TR), slow *y*-descent (TS), sharp/short *y*-descent (pericardial constriction).

Mouth

Foetor oris, mucous membrane dryness, state of dentition, palate and systolic uvular pulsation (Müller's sign – AR).

Fundi

Hypertensive and diabetic changes, and Roth spots (endocarditis).

Palpation

Skin

- Temperature, capillary refill and pitting oedema.

Pulse

- Rate, rhythm, character/volume (bounding, anacrotic, collapsing, thready, irregular), respiratory variation, condition of vessel, radio–femoral delay.
- Pulsus alternans: amplitude varies on alternate beats – indicative of severe LV dysfunction.
- Pulsus bisferiens: combined anacrotic and collapsing pulse. Irregular pulse may indicate AF, sinus dysrhythmia, multiple atrial and ventricular premature (ectopic) beats (APBs/VPBs, respectively) or SVT with variable atrioventricular (AV) block.
- 'Waterhammer' pulse of AR detected by palpating radial artery as arm is elevated – more easily appreciated in calf muscles when elevating leg.
- An arteriovenous fistula (dialysis, severe Paget's bone disease, PDA) may also produce a collapsing pulse.
- Delayed/absent femoral pulses (coarctation, dissection and AAA).
- Tracheal deviation, carotid thrill, radiated cardiac thrill.
- Suprasternal/manubrial pulsation (coarctation).

Precordium

- Apex beat is impulse of ventricular systole normally felt in fifth intercostal space (ICS) in mid-clavicular line. S_4 may be palpable in LVH.
- Thrills in MR, VSD, AS, PS, MS and PDA.
- Left parasternal (RV) heave in PS, PHT, MS.

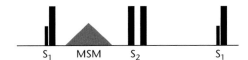

Figure 15.4 Mid (ejection) systolic murmur (MSM). Follows AV/PV opening (crescendo–decrescendo). May be innocent (grade ≤ III) or due to AV sclerosis, increased pulmonary blood flow (ASD, TAPVD), AS (harsh MSM in aortic area, spilt S_2, soft A_2) or PS (soft P_2, opening click, louder on inspiration).

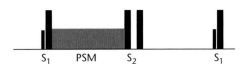

Figure 15.5 Pan (holo) systolic murmur (PSM). High-pitched apical PSM radiating to axilla with soft S_1 and S_3 in MR. Mid or late systolic click suggests MV prolapse. 'Musical' PSM, louder on inspiration, at left lower sternal edge (LLSE) in TR. Harsh PSM at LLSE with thrill suggests VSD.

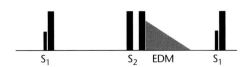

Figure 15.6 Early (immediate) diastolic murmur. *AR* – 'blowing' decrescendo murmur at LLSE ± superimposed S_3. Murmur of functional MS (Austin Flint) may be present. *PR* – decrescendo murmur at left upper sternal edge (LUSE), louder on inspiration. Graham Steell (PR) murmur associated with MS and PHT.

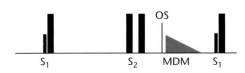

Figure 15.7 Mid diastolic murmur (MDM). *MS* – rumbling apical MDM radiating to axilla, louder on expiration, loud P_2. Duration severity. In severe MS the OS occurs earlier (<70 mS after P_2) and is softer/inaudible. *TR* – louder on inspiration. MDM may be caused by MV/TV thickening in rheumatic endocarditis (Carey Coombs) or by increased bloodflow in VSD, PDA (MV), ASD (TV) and TAPVD (TV).

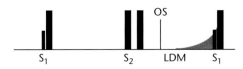

Figure 15.8 Late diastolic murmur (LDM) or (presystolic eccentuation). *MS* – MV flow in late diastole + atrial systole (S_4). OS typically >100 mS after P_2 in mild MS.

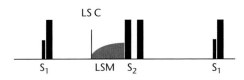

Figure 15.9 Late systolic murmur (LSM). MR/MV prolapse. May only be apparent after exercise.

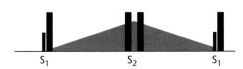

Figure 15.10 Continuous murmur. PDA ('machinery' murmur at LUSE with loud P_2), pulmonary arteriovenous fistula or surgical conduit (e.g. Blalock-Taussig, Waterston, Fontan).

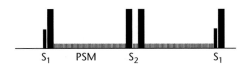

Figure 15.11 Venous hum. Partial obstruction of neck veins (especially in children). Obliterated by digital compression of veins. Important to differentiate from PDA.

Lung fields

- Vocal fremitus.

Abdomen

- Hepatic enlargement/pulsation, splenomegaly (endocarditis), ascites.

Percussion

Precordium

A crude estimate of cardiac size. Area of dullness increased by pericardial effusion and decreased by emphysema.

Lung fields

Pleural effusion, lobar collapse and pneumothorax.

Abdomen

Hepatomegaly and ascites.

Auscultation

Listen all over. Bell best for low frequencies, rigid diaphragm best for high frequencies. Murmurs exaggerated by inspiration (right heart origin), expiration (left heart origin), posture (left lateral, sitting forward), squatting, standing and isometric exercise (MR in mitral valve prolapse). Classical anatomical areas for auscultation of individual valves unreliable.

Peripheral vessels

- *Brachial arteries* BP measurement (by sphygmomanometer), estimation of respiratory paradox.
- *Carotid arteries* Bruit, radiated murmurs.
- *Femoral arteries* Traube's sign (booming systolic and diastolic 'pistol shot' sounds over the artery in AR), Duroziez's sign (diastolic flow murmur heard in AR when artery partially compressed by stethoscope diaphragm).

Lungs

- Vesicular (normal) breath sounds.
- Bronchial breath sounds, crackles (crepitations) and wheeze (rales and rhonchi).

- Whispering pectoriloquy, broncophony and aegeophony.

Heart sounds *(Figs 15.1–3)*

Low-pitched sounds of short duration believed to be created by opening and closure of valve leaflets, and the 'shuddering' of tissues placed under sudden tension. Amplitude reduced by obesity, emphysema, pericardial effusion, AS, PS, low CO and dextrocardia; increased by hyperdynamic circulation and in arterial hypertension/PHT; and varies in AF and CHB.

Cardiac murmurs *(Figs 15.4–11)*

Murmurs are vibrations caused by turbulent blood flow – more likely with high velocity blood flow, low blood viscosity and an abrupt change in vessel/chamber diameter. These are characterized by relationship to cardiac and respiratory cycles, location, radiation, acoustic quality and intensity.

Grading of Cardiac Murmurs	
Grade	**Characteristics**
1/6	Only just audible, even under good auscultatory conditions
2/6	Soft
3/6	Moderately loud
4/6	Loud
5/6	Very loud
6/6	Audible with stethoscope lifted from chest wall

Other sounds

Other sounds include venous hum, friction rub and cardiorespiratory.

Further reading

Burton JL. *Aids to Postgraduate Medicine*, 4th edition. London: Churchill Livingstone, 1983.

Mason S, Swash M. *Hutchinson's Clinical Methods*, 17th edition. London: Baillière Tindall, 1980.

C.P. Searl & R. Coulden

A diagnosis of cardiac disease can often be made from history and physical examination alone. The purpose of further investigation is summarized in Table 16.1.

Electrocardiography

The ECG represents the vector sum of cardiomyocyte depolarization and repolarization. An ECG provides information about the state of the myocardium and its conducting system, as well as the impact of metabolic derangements, drug and extracardiac pathology.

Continuous ambulatory or 'Holter' ECG monitoring for periods up to 24 h allowing transient phenomena (e.g. dysrhythmias and ST segment changes) to be recorded and analysed. Low HR variability, a risk factor for sudden death and ventricular dysrhythmias following MI, can be detected using this method. The condition which produce abnormalities in the ECG are given in Table 16.2. The predicted sites for ischaemia are given in Table 16.3 along with the localization of leads.

Chest radiography

Posteroanterior and lateral CXRs (Figure 16.1) are routinely obtained before cardiac surgery. As well as providing a useful preoperative 'baseline' against which to judge postoperative examinations, the presence of existing abnormalities can be confirmed, and new abnormalities documented. The assessment of the preoperative CXR in cardiac surgical patients is given in Table 16.4.

Echocardiography

Echocardiography provides qualitative and quantitative assessment of cardiac structure and function, with both the transthoracic and transoesophageal approaches having a place in preoperative diagnosis. Transthoracic echocardiography (TTE) is truly non-invasive and can be performed in the clinic setting. It is particularly useful for imaging anterior cardiac structures (e.g. LV apex) but the ribs, obesity and

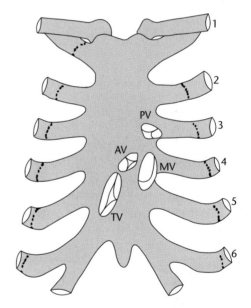

Figure 16.1 Orientation of heart valves in relation to skeletal structures visible on a plain posteroanterior CXR.

Table 16.1 The rationale for non-invasive investigations in cardiac surgical patients and methods commonly used

Rationale	Methods
Define the precise nature and extent of disease	ECG, CXR, Echocardiography
Determine the prognostic significance of disease	Physical and pharmacological stress testing
Formulate and guide treatment plans	Myocardial perfusion imaging
Guide further non-invasive and invasive investigations	Radionucleotide ventriculography

Table 16.2 Conditions that produce abnormalities in the ECG

General		Rate, rhythm, axis
AV conduction	1°HB	PR > 200 ms
	2°HB	Mobitz I: PR interval gradually increases (Wenkebach)
		Mobitz II: PR interval fixed
	3°HB	Complete AV dissociation
Intraventricular conduction	LBBB	QRS >120 ms, delayed LV activation produces late R-waves in I, AVL and V5–V6, loss of q-wave in V3–V6, deep S_{V1}, tall R_{V6}
	LAHB	QRS ~100 ms, left-axis deviation, rS complexes in II, III, aVF; small q in I and/or aVL.
	LPHB	QRS ~100 ms, right-axis deviation
	RBBB	QRS > 120 ms, delayed RV activation produces late R (rSR) waves in V1–V2, q-wave preserved in V3–V6, deep broad S_{V6}; if left/right-axis deviation also present = bifascicular block
Ischaemia/infarction		Q-waves (>3 mm, >30 ms), loss of R-wave progression, ST elevation/depression, T-wave inversion
Chamber hypertrophy/ enlargement	LVH	$R_{V5} + S_{V1} > 35$ mm
	RVH	Dominant R_{V1} (>5 mm)
Electrolyte disturbances	↑ K+	T-wave peaking, QRS widening
	↓ K+	T-wave flattening, ST depression, U-wave
	↑ Ca2+	↓ QT and ST intervals
	↓ Ca2+	↑ QT interval
	↑ Mg2+	↑ PR interval, QRS widening, ↓ QT interval

Table 16.3 ECG localization of ischaemia

Predicted site of ischaemia	ECG leads
Inferior	II, III, aVF
Inferolateral	II, III, aVF, V5, V6
Inferoseptal	II, III, aVF, V1–V3
Anterior	V1–V4 ± V5
Anterolateral	I, aVL, V5, V6
Lateral	aVL, V5, V6
Posterior	Reciprocal changes in V1–V2

Table 16.4 Assessment of the preoperative CXR in cardiac surgical patients

Cardiac silhouette
- Cardiothoracic ratio ('normal' ≤50%)
- LA enlargement
- Calcification – LV wall, valvular, pericardial
- Prostheses/pacing wires

Mediastinal silhouette
- Calcification – aortic arch
- Mediastinal widening
- Tracheal deviation

Hila
- Pulmonary arteries and veins
- Lympadenopathy and other masses

Lung fields
- Upper lobe blood diversion
- Interlobular septal (Kerley B) lines
- Perihilar ('bats wing') consolidation

Diaphragm
- Pleural effusion

Skeleton
- Sternal wires – previous surgery
- Rib notching
- Retrosternal space – in redo-surgery

pulmonary emphysema, may degrade image quality. On the other hand, TOE is semi-invasive, usually requires patient sedation and yields superior images of posterior structures (e.g. left atrium (LA), LA appendage and MV). It should be borne in mind that echocardiography is, to some extent, operator dependent. TOE is discussed in more detail in Chapters 24 and 25.

Tissue doppler

Tissue Doppler imaging uses the same principles as colour flow Doppler mapping. As cardiac structures move around 10 times slower than blood cells and have greater (+40 dB) reflectivity, it is possible to obtain high-resolution tissue Doppler images free of significant artefact originating from the blood pool.

Myocardial tissue Doppler imaging uses standard colour coding to depict both speed and direction of movement, allowing semi-quantitative assessment of myocardial motion during both systole and diastole. The enhancement in temporal resolution obtained with M-mode tissue Doppler (in comparison to a two-dimensional (2D) representation) allows differences in endocardial and epicardial velocity to be mapped.

Myocardial contrast echo

Echocardiography is particularly suited to the evaluation of myocardial perfusion as it has very good spatial resolution (superior to single positron emission computed tomography (SPECT) and positron emission tomography (PET) but not as good as MRI) and extremely good temporal resolution (30–200 Hz), which exceeds that of other imaging technologies. It is also relatively inexpensive. Myocardial contrast echocardiography (MCE) has evolved from the use of agitated saline solutions, through first generation of contrast agents containing air, to newer contrast agents containing higher-molecular-weight gases, such as perfluoropropane, which improve microbubble persistence. These newer agents are capable of transpulmonary passage and opacification of the left heart chambers and myocardial microcirculation after IV administration. MCE can provide information about the integrity and functional status of the myocardial microvasculature as the microbubbles remain in the microcirculation (unlike the contrast agents used for SPECT, PET and MRI which rely on myocyte uptake).

Exercise stress testing

As the term implies, physical or exercise stress testing consists of cardiovascular monitoring while the patient exercises on a static cycle or treadmill. Typically ECG and intermittent BP measurement are used, although TTE may also be used. Exercise testing can be safely performed in the outpatient setting by trained personnel and is relatively inexpensive (Table 16.5).

Treadmill testing using the Bruce protocol, or one of its many modifications, is the most commonly used form exercise testing. This protocol has been the most extensively validated and specifies how the intensity of exercise progresses during the test (Table 16.6).

The development of ECG changes, dysrhythmias or a blunted BP response is suggestive of myocardial ischaemia. Testing is halted at this point and the test reported as positive (Figure 16.2). Testing has relatively low specificity and sensitivity (60–70%).

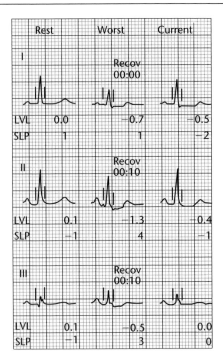

Figure 16.2 Sample exercise ECG showing leads I, II and III at rest before the test, a peak exercise and during recovery. During exercise 1.3-mm ST segment depression is seen in lead II.

Table 16.5 Contraindications to exercise stress testing

Disabilities preventing exercise
- Neurological and musculoskeletal disease
- Peripheral vascular disease
- Pulmonary disease

Conditions precluding attainment of adequate target HR
- β-blockers
- Atrio-ventricular conduction abnormalities

Medical conditions conferring significant risk
- Aortic stenosis
- Unstable coronary syndromes

Pharmacological stress testing

As an alternative to exercise, temporary pacing or drugs such as dobutamine can be used to 'stress' the cardiovascular system. In this situation, when patient's movement is minimal, TTE monitoring is more practical. Echocardiographic evidence of a regional wall motion abnormality (RWMA) that is not present at rest is highly suggestive of myocardial ischaemia. Stress echocardiography can also be used to determine the severity of LVOT obstruction in hypertropic obstructive cardiomyopathy (HOCM). Stress echocardiography has high specificity, avoids the use of ionizing radiation and provides additional information about cardiac structure and function.

Nuclear Cardiology

Nuclear cardiology non-invasive techniques allow assessment of coronary blood flow, myocardial metabolism and ventricular function. Gamma-emitting radioisotopes are used as 'tracers' and images are

---

Table 16.6 The Bruce treadmill protocol and an example of one of the many modifications described

Stage	Bruce protocol		Modified protocol		Duration (min)
	Speed (mph)	Grade (%)	Speed (mph)	Grade (%)	
1	1.7	10	1.7	0	3
2	2.5	12	1.7	5	3
3	3.4	14	1.7	10	3
4	4.2	16	2.5	12	3
5	5.0	18	3.4	14	3
6	5.5	20	4.2	16	3
7	6.0	22	5.0	18	3
8			5.5	20	3
9			6.0	22	3
10			6.5	24	3

The target HR for the test is 220 minus age in years. For example, the test would be halted (regardless of ECG changes) for a patient aged 50 when a HR of 170 had been achieved.

acquired with a gamma camera using simple (planar) scintigraphy, PET or SPECT. The most frequently used tracers are thallium (^{201}Tl) and technetium (^{99m}Tc).

The characteristics of ^{99m}Tc allow for repeated examinations on consecutive days with superior image quality for a lower overall radiation dose (Table 16.7).

Table 16.7 The properties of ^{201}Tl and ^{99m}Tc

	^{201}Tl	^{99m}Tc
	K$^+$ analogue	–
Half-life (h)	72	6
Gamma emission energy (keV)	68–80	140
Myocardial uptake (%)	~4	<1.5
Redistribution	Significant	None

Ventriculography

A small quantity of blood is removed and mixed with a gamma-emitting radioisotope that binds to erythrocytes (e.g. sodium pertechnetate; Na^{99m}TcO$_4$) and re-injected into the patient. A tin compound (e.g. stannous chloride) is used to improve erythrocyte adhesion. A gamma camera is then placed over the precordium and continuous ECG monitoring used to time the acquisition of images over several hundred cardiac cycles. As each cardiac cycle is divided into 8–16 epochs or 'gates', the procedure is often referred to as a gated blood pool or multi-gated acquisition

(MUGA) imaging (Figure 16.3). The rate of gamma emission is proportional to the volume of blood within the ventricles. Although an absolute measure of end-diastolic volume (EDV) and SV cannot be made, ventricular *ejection fraction* (EF) can be accurately measured for both ventricles using the formula:

$$EF = (EDV - ESV)/EDV$$

where ESV = end-systolic volume.

The absolute margin of error is in the order of 5% – this means that the technique is less able to detect changes in left ventricular ejection fraction (LVEF) in patients with poor LV function. The technique cannot be used in pregnant or breast-feeding women, and dysrhythmias, such as AF, interfere with image acquisition.

Perfusion imaging

Perfusion imaging is based on the principle that the distribution of radiolabelled tracers within myocardium is directly proportional to coronary blood flow. Tracer uptake is impaired or absent in areas of myocardial ischaemia. By comparing tracer distribution at rest and under conditions of 'stress', coronary flow reserve and myocardial viability can be assessed (Figure 16.4).

Although myocardial stress can be induced by exercise, it is more usual to use a coronary vasodilator (e.g. adenosine or dipyrimadole) or an inotrope (e.g. dobutamine), which divert blood from areas fed by stenosed arteries to other regions (see Figure 7.4). The tracer agent is injected at peak stress and myocardial imaging performed. As ^{201}Tl does not bind to cardiomyocytes, immediate or 'first-pass' imaging must be

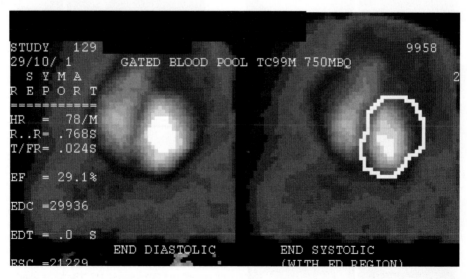

Figure 16.3 Multi-gated angiographic ventriculography. In the example shown, the outline of the LV end-diastolic image (left) is superimposed on the LV end-systolic image (right). The LVEF is 29%.

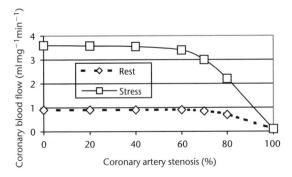

Figure 16.4 The effect of coronary artery stenosis on coronary blood flow at rest and during stress. Redrawn from Gould and Lipscomb. *Am J Cardiol* 1974; 34: 48–55, with permission from Elsevier.

Table 16.8 Testing for presence of viable myocardium, particularly important in patients with LV dysfunction

Perfusion defect	Significance
Fixed	Defect on stress and rest study Fixed RWMA Indicates myocardial infarction
Reversible	Defect on stress study only Reversible RWMA Indicates reversible ischaemia/viable myocardium

If viable myocardium is present patients may gain functional and prognostic benefit from revascularization.

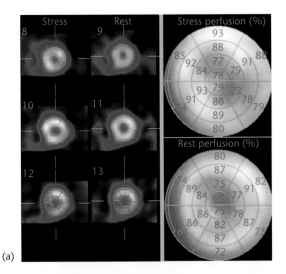

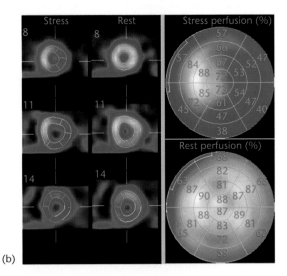

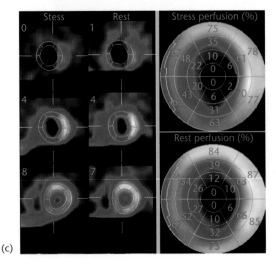

Figure 16.5 Short-axis ^{99m}Tc-MIBI images through the LV following stress and at rest in a normal heart (a) in extensive lateral and inferior wall reversible ischaemia (b) and MI (c). Normal LV uptake on SPECT appears as a yellow 'donut', with ischaemia producing a defect, which may reverse at rest or be fixed indicating infarction. Images on the right of each figure (so-called 'bulls-eye' plots) show nested short-axis 'donuts' for the whole LV (apex at the centre and base at the periphery). This allows easy comparison of the entire LV at rest and following stress. The large fixed black hole on the bulls-eye plots (c) indicates an extensive apical infarct that also involves the distal anterior and inferior walls.

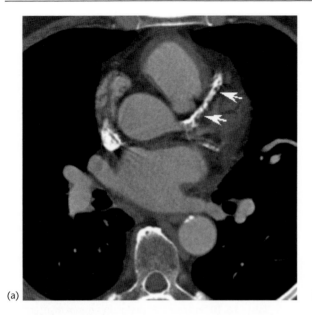
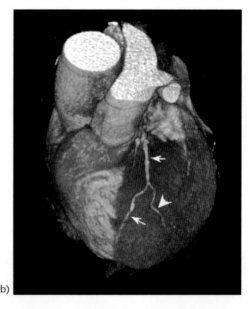

Figure 16.6 (a) ECG triggered transaxial CT slice through the proximal coronary arteries without IV contrast. Dense calcification in the LAD (white arrows) indicates atheroma. The extent and severity of calcification correlates with the extent of atheroma and hence risk of a cardiac event but it does not correlate with the severity of the underlying stenosis. (b) Three-dimensional (3D) reconstruction of proximal LAD (white arrows) and a large diagonal (arrowhead) from an ECG triggered CT volume data set acquired following IV contrast injection with a 16-slice CT scanner. The LAD shows diffuse irregularity but no significant stenosis.

undertaken before 'wash-out' takes place. In contrast, ^{99m}Tc chelated with methoxyisobutyl isonitrile (^{99m}Tc-MIBI), irreversibly binds to cardiomyocytes. As ^{99m}Tc-MIBI is concentrated in the liver and excreted in the bile, imaging is undertaken after the tracer has cleared the liver ~1 h after injection. Images are acquired with a stationary camera (i.e. planar) or using SPECT, where the camera moves around the patient in a 180° arc.

In stable angina, myocardial perfusion imaging is superior to stress ECG testing for detecting flow-limiting coronary stenoses. A negative perfusion study in a patient with chest pain confers <1% risk of cardiac death or MI. Cardiac risk associated with a positive perfusion study is a function of the number and size of defects. Left main stem disease is more often associated with multiple, rather than single large defects. High lung uptake, a marker of severe disease, indicates a poor prognosis (Figure 16.5).

Conventional ^{201}Tl imaging is a more sensitive indicator of hibernating myocardium. Late redistribution (~4 h) may reveal areas of myocardial perfusion that were not immediately obvious (i.e. considered fixed) 1–2 h after injection.

Metabolism imaging

Using PET it is possible to measure myocardial uptake of radiolabelled substrate (e.g. ^{18}fluorodeoxyglucose,

^{18}FDG) – an accurate indicator of metabolically active and thus viable myocardium. PET imaging is expensive but produces images with high spatial resolution. More recently, ^{18}FDG–SPECT and 15-(p-^{123}iodophenyl)-3-(R,S)-methylpentadecanoic acid (BMIPP)–SPECT have been used to demonstrate the presence of viable myocardium.

Computed tomography

Easy access to the patient, the ability to perform a rapid examination and good spatial resolution make CT the imaging technique of choice for patients with acute aortic or pulmonary vascular disease.

Contrast-enhanced gated CT coronary angiography using either electron-beam CT (EB-CT) or multi-slice CT (MS-CT) can image the major branches of the coronary tree and any luminal narrowings (Table 16.9). Although CT coronary angiography has been shown in experienced centres to have a good sensitivity, specificity and negative predictive value in the assessment of coronary artery disease, it remains experimental in this application (Figure 16.6).

Magnetic resonance imaging

MRI does not involve the use of ionizing radiation. A powerful magnetic field is used to line up the protons

Table 16.9 Characteristics of electron beam-CT and multi-slice-CT

EB-CT

- High temporal resolution
- Used to quantify coronary calcium/plaque load
- No contrast media required
- Cannot identify/localize coronary arteries

MS-CT

- The newer technique of MS (helical) CT can provide images of the beating heart in diagnostic quality. This may facilitate the broader application of cardiac and coronary CT. At present there is much more experience in imaging the heart with EB-CT than with MS-CT.

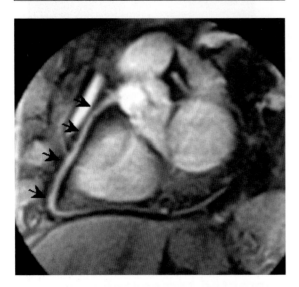

Figure 16.7 MR angiogram of the right coronary artery (RCA) from origin to crux as it runs in the atrioventricular groove. Cardiac and respiratory motion was eliminated using ECG triggering and breath holding, but intravascular contrast was provided by flow. No IV contrast enhancement was necessary.

in the hydrogen atoms in the body. A radio-frequency emission distorts this line-up and as the atoms return to their previous position they give off energy that is then detected and reconstituted to form an image (Figure 16.7).

In contrast to CT, an MRI examination may last 60 min. Patient access is limited, specialized anaesthetic and monitoring equipment is required, and the technique cannot be used for obese patients (>130 kg) and those with severe claustrophobia (~5%). Although spatial resolution is inferior to that obtained with CT, contrast resolution is superior. MRI is currently used in the diagnosis of pericardial and aortic disease, cardiac masses, congenital heart disease and RV dysplasia. It can be used to measure LV size and mass, and to

assess global and regional function. Valvular function can also be interrogated.

A number of techniques have been developed to overcome substantial difficulties in imaging coronary arteries. Diastolic gating with ultra-fast sequences reduces cardiac motion. Breath-holding techniques or respiratory gating can overcome movement artefact due to respiration. The signal-to-noise ratio can be increased by the use of contrast agents (e.g. gadolinium-DPTA, Gd-DPTA).

Perfusion imaging

Cardiac MRI offers potential advantages over radioisotope techniques as it provides superior spatial resolution and does not require ionizing radiation. MRI provides a variety of methods of obtaining information on residual viability after MI (Table 16.10).

Table 16.10 Indirect MRI perfusion signs of myocardial viability

- Absence of increased signal intensity on spin echo images
- Absence of late Gd-DPTA enhancement in a myocardial region involved in a recent infarct
- Any sign of wall thickening at rest
- Wall thickening after stimulation by low dose dobutamine
- Preserved wall thickness.

Key points

- The ECG gives a snapshot of the electrical activity of the heart, giving information about the state of the myocardium and its conducting system.
- Myocardial perfusion imaging may identify ischaemic myocardium that would benefit from revascularization.
- [201]Tl is a potassium analogue with a long half-life that does not bind to cardiomyocytes and is rapidly washed out of the myocardium.
- ^{99m}Tc-MIBI has a short half-life and binds irreversibly to cardiomyocytes providing a 'snapshot' of myocardial perfusion that can be imaged later.

Further reading

http://www.cardiolite.com

Kaul S. Myocardial contrast echocardiography: basic principles. *Prog Cardiovasc Dis* 2001; **44(1)**: 1–11.

Kramer CM. Current and future applications of cardiovascular magnetic resonance imaging. *Cardiol Rev* 2000; **8(4)**: 216–222.

C.P. Searl

Cardiac catheterization

Cardiac catheterization was originally developed as a means to measure pressures within the heart chambers and great vessels. The introduction of radio-opaque contrast media lead to the development of ventriculography and coronary angiography. These invasive procedures involve exposure to contrast media and ionizing radiation, and may be accompanied by both minor and life-threatening complications. Despite the development of new, non-invasive techniques (e.g. radionucleotide perfusion imaging and MRI), cardiac catheterization remains the most widely used method for assessing the severity and distribution of coronary artery disease.

Left heart

Thin radio-opaque catheters (Figure 17.1), introduced via the femoral, brachial or radial artery, are used to instrument the heart via the aorta. The choice of access site is both patient and operator dependent.

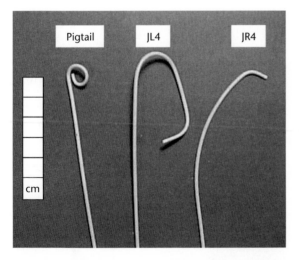

Figure 17.1 Commonly used adult (6F) cardiac catheters. Pigtail: for ventriculography. Judkins 'left' (JL4): left coronary artery (LCA). Judkins 'right' (JR4): right coronary artery (RCA).

Typical LV and aortic pressure traces obtained during Left heart catheterization (LHC) and the LHC procedures are given in Figure 17.2 and Table 17.1, respectively.

Coronary angiography will demonstrate whether the coronary circulation is right or left dominant (i.e. the origin of the posterior descending artery is from the right or left system). It will also define the location and extent of intraluminal filling defects or occlusions, which normally indicate the presence of coronary artery disease. Multiple views are obtained to create a 'map' of the coronary vessels and to characterize lesions in terms of their morphology. A reduction in luminal diameter > 75% (>50% in the left main stem) is considered to be significant (Figures 17.3–17.6).

Local vascular complications, angina and dysrhythmias are common. Life-threatening complications are more common in patients with left main stem disease, AS and peripheral vascular disease (Table 17.2).

Right heart

Thin radio–opaque catheters, introduced via the femoral, internal jugular or median basilic vein, are used to instrument the heart via the cavae. The choice of access site is both patient and operator dependent. Right heart catheterization (RHC) is combined with LHC in approximately 10% patients – arguably too

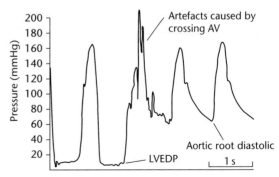

Figure 17.2 Typical LV and aortic root pressure traces obtained during left heart catheterization.

Table 17.1 Left heart catheterization procedures

Technique	Procedure	Information obtained
Manometry	Pressure measurements are made with the catheter in aortic root and LV cavity	Aortic valve gradient, LVEDP
Angiography	The ostia or the coronary arteries, vein grafts or internal mammary artery are selectively cannulated and contrast injected	Coronary anatomy, left or right dominance, location and severity of stenotic lesions, presence of collateral circulation, patency of bypass grafts
Ventriculogram	A pigtail catheter is advanced across AV into LV; 40–60 ml contrast is rapidly injected	Ventricular size and function; LV ejection fraction; LV aneurysm; severity of mitral regurgitation
Aortogram	A catheter is placed in the aortic root; contrast is injected manually	Severity of aortic regurgitation

In the past, real-time images were recorded onto cine film. Digital media such as CD-ROM have superseded this method of data storage.

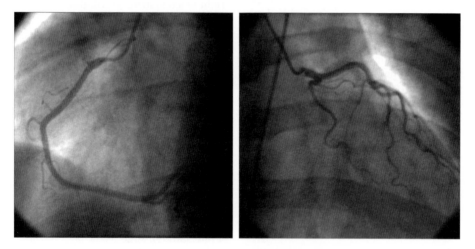

Figure 17.3 Normal right and left coronary angiograms (right anterior oblique views).

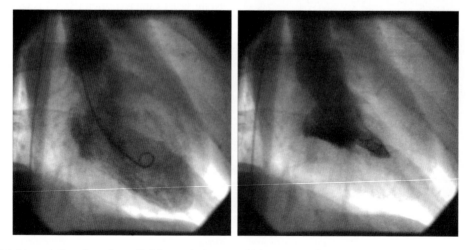

Figure 17.4 Normal diastolic and systolic left ventriculograms (right anterior oblique views).

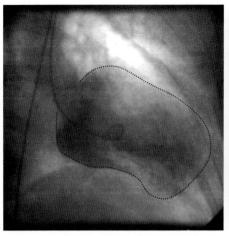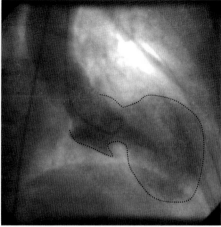

Figure 17.5 Diastolic and systolic left ventriculograms (right anterior oblique views) demonstrating LV cavity enlargement and a large apical aneurysm.

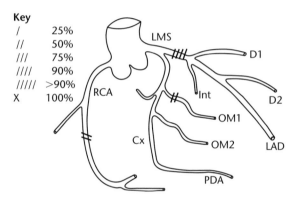

Key

/	25%
//	50%
///	75%
////	90%
/////	>90%
X	100%

Figure 17.6 An example of a coronary angiogram report showing left dominance, severe proximal LAD disease and mild disease in the mid-RCA and the first obtuse marginal branch (OM1) of the circumflex artery (Cx). PDA, Posterior descending artery; Int., intermediate.

Table 17.2 Complications of left heart catheterization

Site	Examples
Access site	Bleeding, haematoma, infection pseudo-aneurysm vascular injury – distal limb ischaemia;
Vascular	Aortic dissection; renal, mesenteric, cerebral embolization
Cardiac	Coronary dissection/occlusion; MI; dysrhythmia – including VF
General	Vasovagal syncope contrast-induced nephrotoxicity allergic reactions to contrast

infrequent given the relatively high incidence of pulmonary hypertension in cardiac disease.

The most common indication for RHC is breathlessness of unknown origin. It forms an essential part of the diagnostic 'work-up' of patients with congenital heart disease, MV disease, restrictive cardiomyopathy and constrictive pericarditis. In the setting of cardiac transplantation, RHC is performed preoperatively, to measure pulmonary vascular resistance and transpulmonary gradient, and postoperatively, to assess graft function and obtain endomyocardial biopsies. Conventional pulmonary angiography requires the placement of a catheter in the right heart.

The complications of RHC are the same as those for central venous cannulation and PA catheter insertion. Additionally, haemodynamic instability, allergic reactions and nephrotoxicity may occur when contrast media are used.

Table 17.3 shows the measurements obtained during LHC and RHC.

Intravascular ultrasound

An ultrasound transducer mounted at the tip of a coronary catheter can now be used to allow three-dimensional (3D) visualization of coronary plaques from within the artery and provides information about plaque composition and structure that cannot be obtained from routine angiography (Figure 17.7).

Table 17.3 Measurements obtained during LHC and RHC, and normal values

	Parameter	Measurement	Normal values
Left	Systemic arterial/aortic pressure	S/D (M)	<140/90 (105) mmHg
	LV pressure	S/D$_E$	<140/12 mmHg
Right	RA pressure	(M)	(<6) mmHg
	RV pressure	S/D$_E$	<25/5 mmHg
	PA pressure	S/D (M)	25/12 (22) mmHg
	PAWP	(M)	12 mmHg
	Cardiac index		2.5–4.2 l min^{-1} m^{-2}
	End-diastolic volume index		<100 ml m^{-2}
	DaVO$_2$		<5.0 ml dl^{-1}
	PVR		~100 dyne s cm^{-5}
	SVR		800–1200 dyne s cm^{-5}

S/D (M), systolic/diastolic (mean); D$_E$; end-diastolic.

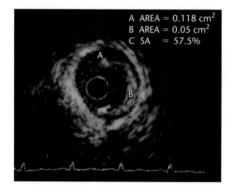
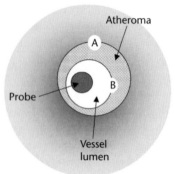

Figure 17.7 Intravascular ultrasound. In the example shown, the vessel area (A) is 0.118 cm^2 and the luminal area (B) is 0.05 cm^2.

Intravascular ultrasound studies may demonstrate extensive disease that has not been demonstrated on conventional angiography and so may assist in the investigation of patients with symptoms and signs highly suggestive of coronary artery disease but 'normal' coronary angiograms. Intravascular ultrasound can also be used to demonstrate vessel patency following coronary angioplasty and stenting.

Doppler

Intracoronary Doppler wires have been developed that have a small piezoelectric cell mounted at the tip to allow assessment of coronary flow velocity. The Doppler wire is positioned distal to the diseased segment and a baseline recording is made of the peak blood flow velocity. Hyperaemia is then induced using intracoronary adenosine to maximize blood flow and the ratio of basal to maximal blood flow is determined – the coronary flow reserve. A ratio of <2 indicates a haemodynamically significant stenosis.

Key points

- Cardiac catheterization remains the gold standard for imaging the coronary arteries.
- Serious cardiovascular complications are rare but may be life threatening.

Further reading

Bashore TM, Bates ER, Berger PB, Clark DA, Cusma JT, Dehmer GJ *et al.* American College of Cardiology/Society for Cardiac Angiography and Interventions Clinical Expert Consensus Document on cardiac catheterization laboratory standards. A report of the American College of Cardiology Task Force on Clinical Expert Consensus Documents. *J Am Coll Cardiol* 2001; **37(8)**: 2170–2214.

Gerber TC, Kuzo RS, Karstaedt N, Lane GE, Morin RL, Sheedy PF 2nd, *et al.* Current results and new developments of coronary angiography with use of contrast-enhanced computed tomography of the heart. *Mayo Clin Proc* 2002; **77(1)**: 55–71.

CARDIAC SURGERY FOR ANAESTHETISTS

S.A.M. Nashef

It is questionable (and politically incorrect) whether doctors should 'select' patients for procedures. What actually happens is that doctors decide if they are prepared to offer a procedure to a patient who then decides whether or not to go ahead. Both of these steps involve a similar thought process, the basis for which is outlined in this chapter.

For any medical treatment to be of use, it should either improve symptoms or improve prognosis. This applies to all medical intervention, from the prescription of a paracetamol tablet to open heart surgery. A treatment that improves neither symptoms nor prognosis is as useful as an ashtray on a motorbike. The decision to proceed with a cardiac operation is therefore based on weighing the advantages (symptomatic and/or prognostic) against the main disadvantage – the risks of death and complications. If the doctor believes it is worthwhile on this basis, the operation is offered. If the patient thinks it worthwhile, the operation is accepted. Both need information to make a decision.

Symptomatic indications

Symptomatic indications are easy. As most patients prefer to take a tablet rather than have a surgeon to cut them with a knife; the symptomatic indication is always the same whatever the surgery: *failure of medical treatment* adequately to control symptoms.

Prognostic indications

Prognostic indications are little more complicated and differ between the various cardiac conditions. Some lesions have such an obvious impact on prognosis that the surgical option is virtually mandatory unless the risk is truly prohibitive. An example would be acute aortic dissection involving the ascending aorta. This carries a cumulative mortality of 1% for every hour of conservative treatment, so that by 2 days nearly half the patients would have expired. Most decisions, however, are not as clear-cut, and the

risks of conservative management need to be assessed carefully and weighed against the risks of surgery. In some areas there are clear guidelines based on quite good evidence, whereas in others, the indications are still poorly defined.

Ischaemic heart disease

The evidence for ischaemic heart disease (IHD) comes from two aging but still valid studies carried out in North America and Europe. The American Coronary Artery Surgery Study (CASS) and a similar European study randomized patients with angina to continuing medical treatment or CABG surgery. Follow-up included patients who refused randomization. With passing time, those treated surgically began to show a survival advantage. This was particularly marked in these groups, listed in descending order of prognostic importance.

Survival benefit	Indication
+++	Left main stem coronary artery stenosis (>50%)
++	Proximal stenosis (>50%) of the three major coronary arteries ('Triple vessel disease')
+	Stenosis (>50%) of two major coronary arteries *including* a high-grade stenosis of the proximal LAD

The presence of LV dysfunction increased the prognostic advantage of surgery over medical treatment in all categories.

Coronary angiography is essential to the assessment of the prognostic implications of IHD, and makes decision-making relatively straightforward. On prognostic grounds alone, a young otherwise fit patient with a 90% left main stenosis should be offered surgery, whereas an old, unfit diabetic arthropath with single vessel disease affecting only a branch of the circumflex coronary artery should not.

Aortic valve disease

The symptomatic indication is failure of medical treatment to control symptoms. The prognostic indication depends on the lesion.

Stenosis

Strangely enough, prognosis here is directly related to symptoms! Patients are usually deemed to have significant AS when the gradient across the valve exceeds 40 mmHg. Most of these patients, however, will continue to be asymptomatic for years. Sudden death or decompensation in asymptomatic patients with AS is as rare as hens' teeth. Indeed, it has been stated that the commonest cause of death in asymptomatic AS is valve replacement! When symptoms begin, however, the picture changes quite dramatically, with death or decompensation becoming a distinct possibility within a matter of months from the onset of symptoms (angina, dyspnoea or exertional syncope). The best time to operate is the day before symptoms appear! The obvious impossibility of such a practice means that most surgeons will treat the onset of symptoms as an indication for relatively urgent surgery.

Regurgitation

Here too, many patients are asymptomatic. The trouble with AR is that it can be difficult to predict the likelihood of future decompensation. Some hearts tolerate substantial amount of regurgitation for life, whereas others dilate and fail. Most clinicians use a combination of three factors to determine the prognostic indication:

- severity of regurgitation,
- echocardiographic evidence of LV dilatation,
- LV strain pattern on ECG.

Mitral valve disease

The symptomatic indication is failure of medical treatment to control symptoms. The prognostic indication depends on the lesion.

The traditional teaching about MV disease is that it becomes haemodynamically important when symptoms worsen, so that there is rarely an indication to offer mitral surgery to the asymptomatic patient. The improved results obtained with MV repair in particular and with mitral surgery in general have led many surgeons to challenge this accepted wisdom. The prognostic sequelae of untreated MS and MR are different: MS causes pulmonary hypertension

(PHT) and MR results in LV dilatation and dysfunction. In both cases, delaying surgery until these complications have become established reduces long-term prognosis. Current thinking is that mitral lesions should be treated on prognostic grounds if there is evidence of early development of PHT or early LV dysfunction (as shown by dilatation on echocardiography) even if symptoms are well controlled on medical treatment. Fortunately, in most patients, these developments tend to go in tandem with symptomatic deterioration, thus making decisions relatively easy.

Risk assessment

Having defined the symptomatic and prognostic indications for surgery, a method of quantifying operative risk is required. Fortunately – thanks to statistics, registers and the work of many individuals – the calculation of risk in cardiac surgery has moved from guesswork to an almost exact science. Michael

Table 18.1 The Parsonnet (1989) additive risk stratification model

Factor	Points
Age	
70–74	7
74–79	12
≥80	20
Diabetes	3
Hypertension	3
Morbid obesity	3
Female	1
LV function (LVEF %)	
Good (≥50)	0
Moderate (30–49)	2
Poor (<30)	4
LV aneurysm	5
Redo procedure	
First	5
Second	10
Preoperative intra-aortic balloon	2
Catheter laboratory complication	10
On dialysis	10
'Catastrophic state'	10–50
'Rare conditions'	2–10
Valve surgery	
Mitral	5
PA pressure ≥ 60 mmHg	3
Aortic	5
AV gradient > 120 mmHg	2
With CABG	2

LVEF, left ventricular ejection fraction.

Crichton, began his 1969 novel *A Case of Need* with the immortal words 'all heart surgeons are bastards' and went on to describe the surgeon in the novel as an 'eight-percenter', meaning his operative mortality was 8% (good for 1969). The message is that for over 30 years cardiac surgical mortality has been measured and incorporated into decisions about clinical care. Crude mortality, however, is not enough and even journalists understand that the risk profile of the patient has as much to do with outcome as the quality of surgical care.

In the late 1980s, Victor Parsonnet, a New Jersey surgeon, published a landmark paper on a method of assessing risk of death in adult cardiac surgery. Using uni- and multivariate logistic regression analysis he identified 14 independent risk factors and assigned them points or 'weights' (Table 18.1). Addition of these weights yielded a number, which was equivalent to the percentage chance of death. The so-called Parsonnet Score was adopted by many centres throughout the world and is still in use today. Most units and surgeons, however, will 'outperform' Parsonnet predictions. In British cardiac surgery, for example, mortality today is about half that predicted by the Parsonnet score.

Although Parsonnet has been refined, updated versions have been neither widely validated nor widely used. Nowadays, a reasonable prediction of risk can be obtained by dividing the Parsonnet score by two.

Many other models of measuring risk in adult cardiac surgery have been developed, but the author is particularly (and understandably) biased towards the European System for Cardiac Operative Risk Evaluation (EuroSCORE). Apart from the appealing acronym, the system is more accurate and up-to-date than Parsonnet and has been fully validated in both Europe and America. It too is an additive system (add up the points to get the percent predicted mortality) but is much less subjective and much more powerfully discriminatory than Parsonnet (Table 18.2). Additive systems tend to 'underscore' very high-risk patients who are better served by using the full logistic equation – a complex calculation which cannot be done at the bedside on the back of an envelope. The EuroSCORE project group offer both additive and logistic risk calculators (online and downloadable at www.euroscore.org) to those with an obsessional commitment to accurate risk prediction.

Table 18.2 The EuroSCORE (1999)

	Comments	Points
General factors		
Age	Per 5 years or part thereof over 60	1
Sex	Female	1
Chronic pulmonary disease	Long-term use of bronchodilators or steroids for lung disease	1
Extracardiac arteriopathy	*Any one or more of the following*: claudication, carotid occlusion or >50% stenosis, previous or planned intervention on the abdominal aorta, limb arteries or carotids	2
Neurological dysfunction	Severely affecting ambulation or day-to-day functioning	2
Previous cardiac surgery	Requiring opening of the pericardium	3
Serum creatinine	>200 µmol l^{-1} preoperatively	2
Active endocarditis	Patient still under antibiotic treatment for endocarditis at the time of surgery	3
Critical preoperative state	*Any one or more of the following*: VT or VF or aborted sudden death, preoperative cardiac massage, preoperative ventilation before arrival in the anaesthetic room, preoperative inotropic support, IABP or preoperative ARF (anuria or oliguria <10 ml h^{-1})	3
Cardiac factors		
Unstable angina	Rest angina requiring IV nitrates until arrival in the anaesthetic room	2
LV dysfunction	Moderate (LVEF 30–50%)	1
	Poor (LVEF <30%)	3
Recent myocardial infarct	Within 90 days	2
Pulmonary hypertension	Systolic PA pressure >60 mmHg	2
Operative factors		
Emergency	Carried out on referral before the beginning of the next working day	2
Other than isolated CABG	Major cardiac procedure other than or in addition to CABG	2
Surgery on thoracic aorta	For disorder of ascending arch or descending aorta	3
Postinfarct septal rupture		4

Conclusion

Determining the indications for and risks of surgery are now a piece of cake. It's so simple, even a cardiac surgeon can do it.

Step	Process
1	Work out the likely benefit (symptomatic and prognostic)
2	Work out the likely risk (Parsonnet or preferably EuroSCORE)
3	Weigh the risk against the benefit
4	Make a decision

Key points

- Surgery is indicated on symptomatic grounds when symptoms are not adequately controlled by maximal medical therapy.

- Surgery is indicated on prognostic grounds in situations, such as severe MR and left main stem coronary disease, regardless of the severity of symptoms.
- The use of validated risk models, such as EuroSCORE, allows rapid risk assessment at the point of care.

Further reading

CASS Principal investigators and their associates. Myocardial infarction and mortality in the coronary artery surgery study (CASS) randomized trial. *N Engl J Med* 1984; **310(12)**: 750–758.

Parsonnet V, Dean D, Bernstein AD. A method of uniform stratification of risk for evaluating the results of surgery in acquired adult heart disease. *Circulation* 1989; **79(6 Pt 2)**: I3–I12.

Nashef SA, Roques F, Michel P, Gauducheau E, Lemeshow S, Salamon R. European system for cardiac operative risk evaluation (EuroSCORE). *Eur J Cardiothorac Surg* 1999; **16(1)**: 9–13.

Roques F, Michel P, Goldstone AR, Nashef SA. The logistic EuroSCORE. *Eur Heart J* 2003; **24(9)**: 881–882.

S.A.M. Nashef

Despite the romantic notions attached to it, the heart is a muscular pump. When it 'goes wrong', the cause is usually a faulty valve or a blocked pipe. Although it seems obvious that the management of plumbing or mechanical faults should be surgical, patients with these problems remained almost exclusively under the care of physicians during the first half of the 20th century.

Early obstacles

Knowledge of the obstacles that delayed the development of heart surgery is useful. Firstly, surgeons took some time to appreciate that lungs cannot breathe by themselves without an intact chest. Early attempts at thoracic surgery on spontaneously breathing patients anaesthetized with chloroform and ether were doomed to failure.

The development of endotracheal intubation (1910s), muscle relaxants and positive pressure ventilation (1940s) allowed some operations to be undertaken on the beating heart. Closed mitral valvotomy, was carried out 'blind', by inserting a finger or an instrument into the LA or LV to stretch, cut or tear open the fused rheumatic, stenotic valve. Closure of ASDs was undertaken by clamping the venae cavae (inflow occlusion), which rendered the heart bloodless and motionless for a short period of time. The RA was then quickly opened, the lesion repaired with indecent haste and the atrium closed with obscene rapidity. Prayers were then said for the heart to resume beating and for the brain to be intact. This approach resulted in some interesting complications, such as unintentional closure of the IVC orifice, the coronary sinus or worse: the tricuspid valve. It also explains why the first generation of cardiac surgeons became legends of surgical bravado. The reputation still lingers, but in fact the specialty and its practitioners are now as worthy (and as dull) as accountants.

Breakthroughs

In the 1950s, two important developments took place. The first was the realization of the concept of an artificial heart (and lungs) to support the patient while the heart was being operated. The second was the exploration of systemic cooling to allow longer periods of cardiac standstill. Both had the same aim, that is to prolong the time available to fix a heart problem, and both had limited success. Cooling gave the surgeon some time to manoeuvre but was tedious and messy – the patient being lowered into an ice bath or sprinkled with ice–cold water. The early heart–lung machine was complicated,

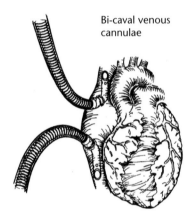

Bi-caval venous cannulae

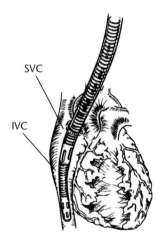

SVC

IVC

Figure 19.1 Techniques of venous cannulation. Bicaval (top) using simple armoured cannulae and unicaval (bottom) using an armoured two-stage cannula. Courtesy of Medtronic Ltd. and reproduced with permission.

unreliable and needed some 20 units of blood to prime it, and although effective as an oxygenator, produced considerable aeroembolism and defibrination. As neither on its own was particularly user-friendly or safe, early cardiac surgery employed both techniques, with topical cooling providing a margin of safety in the likely event of pump failure. Nowadays, heart–lung machines are so reliable and perfusionists so obsessional that pump malfunction is extremely rare. Surgeons who still use active systemic cooling in *routine* cardiac surgery do so out of nostalgia and force of habit.

Cardiopulmonary bypass

Myocardial protection

Most cardiac operations rely on the heart–lung machine which protects *the patient*, while the heart is being operated (see Chapter 45). During CPB, the heart beats empty, but the coronary arteries are still perfused from the aorta, which itself is perfused by the heart–lung machine. Opening the coronary arteries or the aorta results in a gush of blood, making surgery impossible. Clamping the aorta between the site of insertion of the aortic cannula and the origin of the coronary arteries produces a bloodless field, and makes intricate surgery possible. Clamping the aorta would cause the heart to become globally ischaemic unless steps are taken to protect *the heart itself* (see Chapter 20).

Setting up

Most operations proceed along a pre-ordained path, so that cardiac surgery, if performed well, should be as predictable and boring as possible. After induction of anaesthesia, skin preparation and draping, a median sternotomy is performed. Traditionally, the anaesthetist deflates the lungs before the sternal saw divides the sternum, to reduce the risk of opening the pleura (if it is opened, it is not a big deal). Where needed, conduits for coronary bypass are harvested from the leg, arm or chest. The patient is then fully heparinized and the ACT used to confirm the adequacy of anticoagulation. Most cardiac units have rigid protocols for administering heparin. Purse-string sutures are inserted into the aorta to secure the cannula, which will deliver oxygenated blood from the heart–lung machine (the wise anaesthetist stands well back during aortic cannulation and decannulation). Further purse-string sutures are inserted into the RA to secure the cannula or cannulae, which drain venous blood into the heart–lung machine. There may be one atriocaval cannula or two separate caval cannulae (Figure 19.1).

Once everybody is happy with the ACT and the conduits are ready, the patient is 'put on bypass'. This is done by unclamping the 'venous' or RA cannula and allowing it to drain RA blood into the oxygenator by simple gravity or siphonage. Oxygenated blood is then pumped into the aorta and the ventilator is switched off. During the first few minutes of the bypass time, the surgeon may make preparations for the operation, such as inspecting and preparing the coronary graft targets, inserting vents into the LV, LA, PA or aorta (to drain any residual intracardiac blood), or carrying out preliminary dissection and mobilization to achieve better exposure.

The juicy bits

The surgeon begins the central component of the operation by cross-clamping the aorta. This marks the beginning of the 'cross-clamp' time. The heart is now ischaemic and there should be little time wasted in subsequent manoeuvres. There is usually an increase in efficiency and a decrease in idle chatter at this point. Appropriate myocardial protection (Chapter 20) is achieved, usually by cardioplegia administration via the aortic root (this segment of aorta is now blocked by the clamp distally and the AV proximally so the solution can only flow down the coronaries). The heart stops and the 'cardiac' part of the operation begins.

Coronary surgery

In a coronary operation, the target coronary artery is opened longitudinally with a sharp fine blade, distal to any stenosis. The arteriotomy is extended with fine scissors, and the distal coronary anastomosis or 'bottom end' is constructed with fine continuous sutures joining the end of the conduit (saphenous vein, radial artery or mammary artery) to the coronary arteriotomy. This is an 'end-to-side' anastomosis. If the same conduit is then used to graft another vessel, a sequential 'side-to-side' anastomosis is performed. Additional cardioplegia may be given down the aortic root or the grafts or both as the case proceeds. The left internal mammary anastomosis, usually to the LAD, is constructed last.

Aortic valve surgery

In AV surgery, the aorta is opened above the sinuses of Valsalva. If the patient has AR, antegrade cardioplegia must be administered directly into the coronary ostia, which are visible through the open aortotomy. Direct administration via the aortic root would simply distend the LV. AVR is carried out by removing the diseased valve, inserting interrupted sutures first into the annulus then into the sewing ring of the prosthesis, sliding the prosthesis on the sutures down into the annulus and tying the sutures. The aorta is then closed with a continuous suture.

Mitral valve surgery

MV surgery needs an incision in the LA, just medial to the right-sided pulmonary veins, and involves quite a bit of retraction of the atrium to gain access. This tends to deform the overlying RA, and is the main reason for using two caval cannulae rather than one atrial cannula for the bypass circuit. Mitral repair involves a number of different manoeuvres, such as leaflet resection, annular plication or annuloplasty. Most units carrying out mitral repair rely heavily on TOE to analyse the nature of the mitral lesion and to confirm the success of the repair. MVR follows the same pattern as AVR. Once the mitral repair or replacement is completed, the left atriotomy is closed with a continuous suture.

De-airing

If a main heart chamber (atrium, aorta, PA or ventricle) has been opened as part of the procedure, it is important to evacuate air from the heart, especially the left side, before the heart is put back into the circulation and the air escapes to the brain. The many deairing methods essentially rely on washing the air out with blood and saline. This may involve a fair amount of vigorous physical activity by the surgeon while the heart and sometimes the entire patient are shaken, stirred and repositioned to optimize the process. This, together with a request for restarting ventilation briefly to expel air from the pulmonary veins, is usually sufficient to rouse the sleepiest anaesthetist from deepest torpor. It is also a reliable signal that the end, though not quite close enough, is now at least in sight.

Clamp-off

The aortic cross-clamp is then removed, allowing perfusion of the coronary arteries and the heart then begins to come to life. If myocardial protection has been optimal, the heart reverts to a normal sinus rhythm. If not, VF is the commonest dysrhythmia seen and internal cardioversion is carried out. Any proximal anastomoses (top ends) of coronary grafts are then carried using a partially occluding or 'side-biting' aortic clamp. The patient is then prepared for 'coming off bypass'. The lungs are ventilated and the perfusionist gradually occludes the RA cannula, thus allowing more blood to return to the heart and be pumped. The arterial pressure line begins to show pulsation as the heart gradually takes over the circulation. The heart–lung machine is then stopped and the atrial or caval cannulae removed.

… and finally

Heparin is reversed using its antidote, protamine, which often produces hypotension. This can be treated by transfusing blood from the pump into the patient via the aortic cannula. Haemostasis is secured (what a long and tedious process these three simple words describe!) and the chest is closed over the appropriate number of drains and epicardial pacing wires. The patient is then transferred to a critical care area for postoperative monitoring.

Off-pump surgery

In an effort to avoid the potential adverse effects of the heart–lung machine, many surgeons now perform coronary surgery without it, using clever contraptions to steady the bit of heart they are working on. Early reports suggest that it is feasible in some, if not most coronary patients, and may reduce complications in high-risk patients. There is no cannulation, extracorporeal circulation or cross-clamping of the aorta. The absence of CPB means that these operations are more demanding of the anaesthetist, who will need to work constantly on optimizing haemodynamics as the heart is mobilized, retracted and stabilized while continuing to support the circulation (see Chapter 30).

Developments

Efforts to reduce the invasiveness of cardiac surgery continue apace. Minimally invasive coronary surgery can allow the left internal mammary artery to be grafted to the LAD through a small anterior thoracotomy without bypass. Percutaneous CPB with endoscopic surgery allows some operations to be carried out without dividing the sternum. Equipment has been developed which replaces the surgeon's hands within the chest with small, robotic 'hands' controlled by the surgeon from outside, another room or even another continent! The reader may wish to speculate on the motivation for all these developments at a time when cardiac surgery is phenomenally successful and has an enviable safety record. Are we motivated by a true desire to help the patients by reducing the invasiveness of our procedure, a desperate attempt to claw back from the cardiologists the large number of patients now treated by percutaneous intervention or do surgeons, like little boys, get bored with their predictable old 'toys' and want new ones?

Key points

- Most routine cardiac surgical procedures follow a predictable and well-defined path.
- The principle aims of the surgeon are to complete the surgical procedure in the shortest ischaemic time possible and secure haemostasis following CPB.
- Time invested in thorough de-airing and coronary reperfusion is generally rewarded with interest.

MYOCARDIAL PROTECTION

20

D.P. Jenkins

The majority of cardiac surgical procedures depend on the intentional interruption of coronary artery blood flow by cross clamping the aorta. This greatly facilitates surgery by producing a bloodless field, a flaccid heart and by reducing the risk of air embolism. Myocardial ischaemia – the obvious disadvantage – can be limited by using protective techniques.

Historical perspective

Developments in the management of the myocardium during cardiac surgery have probably had more impact on perioperative mortality and morbidity than any other innovation. The term 'myocardial management' is a better term than 'myocardial protection' as it encompasses the whole strategy employed.

In the early days of cardiac surgery it was not appreciated that the heart could suffer ischaemic injury as a direct result of the operative procedure. In the 1960s, myocardial necrosis was considered neither a complication of heart surgery nor a cause of postoperative shock. The advent of coronary artery bypass surgery a decade later focused the minds of surgeons on intraoperative myocardial ischaemia. Complete prevention of ischaemia/reperfusion injury is impossible; if the ischaemic time is long enough all myocytes will die (transmural infarction). Effective myocardial management provides a sufficiently long period in which to perform the procedure by using techniques to delay the onset of myocardial injury.

Despite the introduction and widespread use of a number of protective techniques (Figure 20.1), morbidity and mortality were relatively high compared with today's standards. It soon became obvious that there was a temporal limit to unmodified ischaemic arrest. Techniques that did not interrupt coronary blood flow were only safe if coronary perfusion was maintained at near physiological levels in a beating heart. The principle of hypothermia (reduced metabolic rate/tissue oxygen demand) has nevertheless persisted and moderate whole body hypothermia and varying degrees of topical hypothermia are still used in the majority of centres.

Specific myocardial protection using cardioplegic solutions to create elective cardiac arrest was first investigated in the 1950s, but did not become widely accepted until the constituents of the solutions were modified and systematically tested in the laboratory. More recent developments have focused on modification of reperfusion to reduce injury (Buckberg), and the type and route of administration of cardioplegia.

Contemporary practice

Although the majority of cardiac surgeons use some form of cardioplegia for myocardial protection, there are almost as many variations as practising surgeons. The main reason is that no single method of myocardial management has been proven to be superior under all conditions. The literature contains many trials comparing different methods of myocardial management

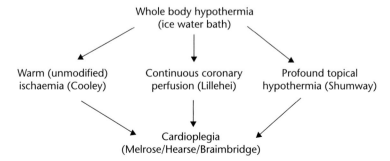

Figure 20.1 The evolution of myocardial management techniques. Whole body hypothermia was used to induce circulatory arrest (rather than protect the myocardium) before the advent of CPB systems. Variability in the degree of cooling and rewarming limited the efficacy of topical hypothermia.

during heart surgery, but in most cases there is very little clinically relevant difference between the strategies. This may, in part, be explained by the deliberate recruitment of low-risk patients and inadequate statistical power.

Essential to all methods of myocardial management is attention to detail and careful observation of the heart throughout surgery. It is important to realize that the ability of one surgeon to obtain good results with a particular myocardial management technique does not necessarily mean that another surgeon or institution can achieve similar results.

Cardioplegic arrest

Rationale

Cardioplegia induces rapid cessation of electromechanical activity (diastolic arrest) in the ischaemic heart, preventing wasteful energy consumption and reducing metabolite accumulation. It provides a predictable and 'safe' period of cardiac flaccidity and a bloodless field. It is frequently used during coronary revascularization and remains the preferred protection method for longer intra-cardiac procedures.

The constituents of modern cardioplegia solutions vary, (Table 20.1) although most use K^+ as the arresting agent with varying concentrations of Ca^{2+}, glucose, buffers and Mg^{2+}. Many additives have been tried to increase the protection afforded including, insulin, amino acids (glutamate and aspartate), adenosine analogues and K^+-channel opening drugs. Cardioplegia has been proven in many experimental preparations and in clinical studies to give good myocardial protection. As the myocardium continues to receive a limited amount of non-coronary (bronchial and pericardial) collateral blood flow, cardioplegic solution is gradually washed out over 20–30 min after which further cardioplegia is required.

Cold versus warm

Following the institution of CPB, cardioplegia is usually administered through the coronary arteries (i.e. antegrade) via an aortic root cannula following application of the aortic cross-clamp (AXC), directly into the coronary ostia or via a partially fashioned bypass graft (Figures 20.2 and 20.3). Typically 1000 ml are given over 3 min at a pressure of 70–80 mmHg. The risk of LV distension contraindicates cardioplegia administration via a root cannula in aortic regurgitation. Cold (4–10 °C) cardioplegia is frequently supplemented by direct cardiac cooling with ice slush, cold saline or a cold jacket.

The observation that hyperkalaemic arrest alone is responsible for most of the reduction in myocyte metabolic demand achieved by cardioplegia has raised doubts about the need for cardiac cooling. Warm blood cardioplegia solutions provide excellent protection and appear to restore energy stores more quickly than cold solutions. Warm blood cardioplegia induction or a terminal infusion of warm blood before AXC release (a 'hot shot') is advocated by some surgeons. Some groups have extended this evidence by using warm blood cardioplegia throughout, although at 37 °C almost continuous infusion is necessary to sustain arrest. Others have tried to combine the benefits of all temperatures and there is a growing literature on the benefit of 'tepid' (29 °C) cardioplegia. Here the differences in overall technique become important; when warmer solutions are used, the cardioplegia is repeated relatively often whereas those surgeons who give a single dose of cardioplegia use more profound topical cooling.

Blood versus crystalloid

Over the last decade, blood cardioplegia has gradually replaced crystalloid solutions in most centres. There

Table 20.1 Composition of commonly used cardioplegic solutions with concentrations in mmol l^{-1}

	St Thomas' 2 (STS2)	Plegivex® (STS1)	Ringer's	Birmingham
Na^+	110	147	147	
K^+	16	20	4	80
Ca^{2+}	1.2	2	2.25	
Mg^{2+}	16	16		20
Cl^-	160	204	155.5	
$NaHCO_3$	10			
Procaine HCl		1		

Recipes for blood cardioplegia include: 4 parts blood to 1 part crystalloid (Ringer's 500 ml + STS2 25–50 ml); blood 500 ml + STS2 10 ml and blood 250 ml + Birmingham 50 ml.

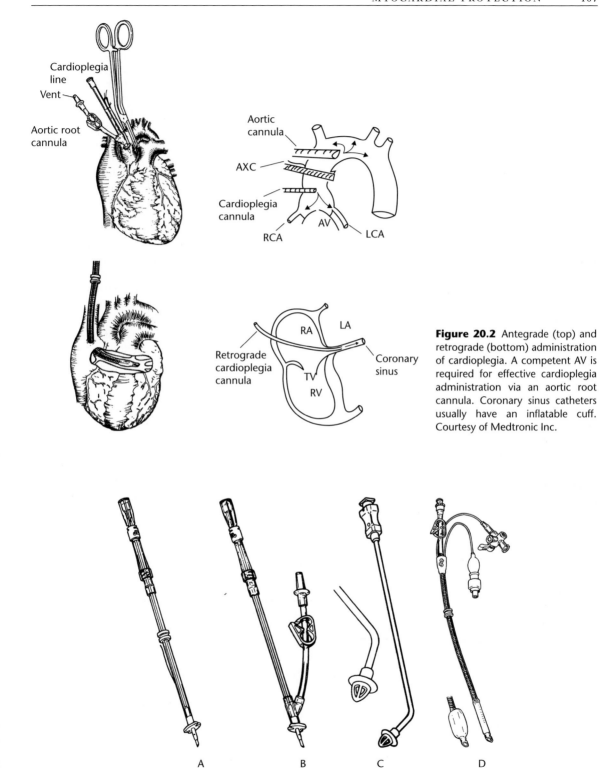

Figure 20.2 Antegrade (top) and retrograde (bottom) administration of cardioplegia. A competent AV is required for effective cardioplegia administration via an aortic root cannula. Coronary sinus catheters usually have an inflatable cuff. Courtesy of Medtronic Inc.

Figure 20.3 Examples of cardioplegia administration cannulae. A: Aortic root cannula. B: Combined aortic root cannula and vent. C: Ostial cannula for direct coronary administration (with close-up of tip). D: Elongated balloon-tipped retrograde cardioplegia cannula (with balloon deflated and inflated). Courtesy of Medtronic Inc.

are some theoretical reasons for this change including, improved buffering capacity, free radical scavenging by erythrocytes and oxygen carriage. There is also some evidence of superior myocardial preservation with blood compared with crystalloid cardioplegia, especially in patients with impaired ventricular function and those undergoing longer ischaemic times.

Antegrade versus retrograde

One of the disadvantages of cardioplegia is the potential failure of adequate distribution to the whole myocardium. This hazard is particularly relevant to patients undergoing redo–revascularization with atheromatous vein grafts and extensive native coronary disease. This problem can be partly overcome by delivering the cardioplegia by another route. The coronary sinus can be cannulated relatively easily with a specifically designed cannula, allowing cardioplegia to be administered via the coronary sinus in a retrograde manner to perfuse the myocardial capillaries (Figure 20.2). This has the advantage of perfusing areas of myocardium not reached by the antegrade coronary route and also flushing out any embolic matter from diseased vein grafts. It also means that cardioplegia can be repeated regularly during complex aortic and mitral valve procedures without interrupting the flow of surgery. During retrograde perfusion the aortic root must be vented to prevent distension and care should be taken to avoid damage to the coronary sinus. There is some evidence that the right ventricle is not perfused adequately by retrograde infusion alone and in practice some surgeons now use a combination of both antegrade and retrograde cardioplegia to maximize the benefits of both routes.

Reperfusion

The reperfusion phase following ischaemia is crucial to recovery. As stated above, the term ischaemia / reperfusion injury is the most accurate description because capillary endothelial and myocyte damage occur on reperfusion. It is, therefore, logical that modification of the reperfusion phase may influence myocardial recovery. The infusion of warm blood cardioplegia prior to AXC release and the avoidance of excessive coronary perfusion pressure during the first few minutes of reperfusion may reduce endothelial injury.

Intermittent ischaemia and reperfusion

Rationale

This technique relies on the fact that the heart is able to tolerate brief periods of ischaemia (up to 15 min)

without appreciable deleterious effects and that repeated episodes of ischaemia are also tolerated as long as there is a brief period of reperfusion in between. This method of 'myocardial management', in which no myocardial 'protective' agents are used, is particularly suited to CABG surgery where distal and proximal anastomoses can be alternated. The technique has been in use clinically since the 1970s and is still the preferred method for CABG surgery in a minority of centres today. It is probable that the more recent understanding of endogenous myocardial protection and ischaemic preconditioning is the reason the method is successful. Published series of patients operated on in these centres have revealed outcomes at least as good as those obtained by cardioplegia. Trials comparing intermittent ischaemia with cardioplegia have revealed little difference in outcome. Compared with the cardioplegic techniques, intermittent ischaemia and reperfusion is simpler and allows sequential revascularization of each coronary artery as the operation progresses. However, repeated clamping and declamping the aorta increases the risk of embolization and stroke in patients with atheromatous disease.

Technique

The aorta is cross-clamped and the heart is electrically fibrillated to render it quiescent and allow easier operating conditions. A distal coronary artery anastomosis is then constructed, taking around 10 min under normal circumstances. The AXC is then removed and the heart defibrillated to allow reperfusion of the beating heart for at least 5 min while the proximal aortic anastomosis is constructed. A brief exposure to low voltage alternating current is used to induce VF that serves to reduce motion. The energy consumption of fibrillating myocardium has been shown to be greater than normally beating myocardium in laboratory canine experiments. Moderate systemic hypothermia is often used to sustain fibrillation. It is essential that good venous drainage is obtained to prevent ventricular distension and some surgeons continue to decompress the heart with an LV apical or pulmonary venous vent.

Off-pump revascularization

The same principles apply to 'off pump' revascularization when CABG is performed on the beating heart without CPB. Here the ischaemic insult affects only one region of the heart at a time as an individual coronary artery is snared and temporarily occluded for the construction of the distal anastomosis. In this method the local area being operated on is stabilized with a mechanical device but the remainder of the heart is beating to sustain the circulation.

Inadequate protection

Measurement of the success of myocardial management strategies in clinical practice is an inexact science. In some patients it may be obvious post-operatively that something has gone wrong; difficulty weaning from CPB, the need for intra-aortic balloon pump or inotropic support, ECG changes and elevation of cardiac-specific enzymes and proteins. In others the signs are subtler; dysrhythmia, low–cardiac output due to stunned myocardium, delayed myocardial fibrosis leading to lower ejection fraction. However, it can be difficult to separate the influence of pre-morbid state, the technical result of the surgical repair and the myocardial management on the eventual outcome. In the future it is likely that older and sicker patients will require technically more difficult and extensive cardiac surgery and therefore myocardial management will continue to have a very important influence on outcome.

Key points

- No single method of myocardial management has been shown to be superior under all conditions.
- The active arresting ingredient of most cardioplegia solutions in potassium.

- Ventricular distension should be avoided at all costs.
- Retrograde cardioplegia infusion may incompletely protect the right ventricle.
- Inadequate myocardial protection may have life-threatening consequences in both the immediate and long term.

Further reading

Vinten-Johansen J, Thourani VH. Myocardial protection: an overview. *J Extra Corpor Technol* 2000; **32(1)**: 38–48.

Amrani M, Yacoub MH, Royston D. Myocardial protection for cardiac surgery: classical views and new trends. *Int Anesthesiol Clin* 1999; **37(2)**: 39–53.

Schlensak C, Doenst T, Beyersdorf F. Clinical experience with blood cardioplegia. *Thorac Cardiovasc Surg* 1998; **46(Suppl 2)**: 282–285.

Harlan BJ, Starr A, Harwin FM. *Manual of Cardiac Surgery*. Berlin: Springer-Verlag, 1994. ISBN 3540942203.

STUNNING, HIBERNATION AND PRECONDITIONING

21

W.E. Johnston

Myocardial ischaemia

Without reperfusion, acute coronary occlusion causes necrosis, the extent of which is determined by the size of the area at risk, collateral perfusion, regional metabolic oxygen demands at the onset of ischaemia and duration of ischaemia. With timely reperfusion, however, the myocardium may survive but can display contractile dysfunction (e.g. stunning and hibernation) or preconditioning.

Stunning
- Transient systolic and diastolic dysfunction persisting after reperfusion.
- Duration of stunning $\gg$ duration of ischaemia.
- Ameliorated by pretreatment and reversed by inotropes.

Hibernation
- Regional wall motion abnormalities caused by chronic hypoperfusion.
- Cardiomyocyte dedifferentiation and interstitial fibrosis.
- Mechanism: adaptive versus apoptotic?
- Recovery rate/extent a severity of cardiomyocyte alteration and fibrosis.

Preconditioning
- Exposure to a brief stimulus reduces subsequent injury from a sustained period of lethal ischaemia.
- Characterized by early and delayed windows of protection.
- May be triggered by physical and pharmacological factors.

Myocardial stunning

Myocardial stunning is transient contractile dysfunction that persists after reperfusion despite the absence of irreversible damage. The duration of stunning greatly exceeds the period of antecedent ischaemia; temporary occlusion for 15 min can cause contraction abnormalities for up to 24 h. Stunning can cause both systolic and diastolic dysfunction and is diagnosed by a persistent contractile abnormality that gradually reverses over time with normal coronary perfusion. The mechanisms of myocardial stunning are attributed to oxygen free radical (OFR) damage, altered intracellular calcium (Ca_i^{2+}) homoeostasis or both. With reperfusion, OFRs are produced, causing sarcolemmal damage and a greater influx of Ca^{2+}. Ca_i^{2+} activates endogenous proteases (e.g. calpains) that decrease myofibrillar Ca^{2+} responsiveness. If the burst of Ca_i^{2+} during early reperfusion is prevented, stunning does not occur. Diastolic dysfunction may be secondary to Ca_i^{2+}-induced relaxation impairment. In experimental animals, stunning can be minimized by pretreatment with antioxidants, OFR scavengers and Ca^{2+} antagonists. The contractile dysfunction from myocardial stunning can, however, be reversed with inotropes without potentiating further myocyte damage, which makes pretreatment unnecessary.

Myocardial hibernation

Myocardial hibernation is a term first used to describe chronic wall motion abnormalities in patients with ischaemic heart disease (IHD) without infarction.

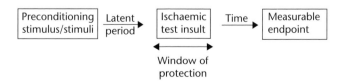

Figure 21.1 Experimental scheme for inducing a preconditioning response. Following the preconditioning stimulus, a time window of protection exists during which the amount of tissue injury from an otherwise lethal ischaemic insult is attenuated.

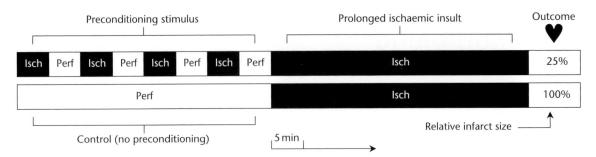

Figure 21.2 Canine model of myocardial preconditioning described by Murry *et al.* Four, 5 min periods of circumflex artery occlusion, each separated by 5-min reperfusion, reduced infarct area by 75% following a subsequent 40-min occlusion. Despite 50% more ischaemia, infarct size was significantly reduced in preconditioned animals. Preconditioning could not attenuate damage after 180 min of ischaemia, indicating that the time course of myocyte death could be delayed but not prevented. Isch, ischaemia; Perf, perfusion.

This entity represents a new equilibrium of the heart in response to chronic hypoperfusion with reduced contractility and regional oxygen consumption so that myocytes remain viable (i.e. a 'smart heart'). Consequently, despite a persistent reduction in perfusion, a new energy balance is achieved whereby myocardial lactate extraction and intracellular high-energy phosphate concentrations normalize. Chronic hibernation may not be an adaptive process but simply a result of repeated ischaemic episodes that cause repetitive myocardial stunning and eventually cell death.

Hibernating myocardium undergoes morphologic changes with loss of sarcomeres and reduced mitochondrium and sarcoplasmic reticulum size. Remaining sarcomeres have greater glucose uptake, causing glycogen deposition within the myocardium. This pattern of dedifferentiation does not appear to be as stable as originally thought and may represent apoptotic death. With restoration of coronary perfusion, the rate of functional and morphologic recovery is linked to the severity of cardiomyocyte alteration and interstitial fibrosis. Dobutamine echocardiography can be used to assess the reversibility of contractile dysfunction in patients scheduled for myocardial revascularization. Improvement in contractility is inversely proportional to the degree of myocardial fibrosis.

The diagnosis of hibernating myocardium requires:

- reduced coronary perfusion,
- regional contractile dysfunction,
- viable myocardium with intact cell membranes or ongoing metabolism.

Similar to stunning, hibernating myocardium has inotrope-recruitable reserves but, unlike stunning, any improvement in contractility may occur at the expense of greater lactate production and myocyte necrosis. Hibernation can be temporized with afterload reduction, but the definitive treatment remains revascularization.

Myocardial preconditioning

Myocardial preconditioning describes the phenomenon whereby exposure to a brief stimulus can reduce the subsequent injury from a sustained period of lethal ischaemia. The experimental model for inducing myocardial preconditioning consists of a preconditioning stimulus (i.e. repetitive episodes of brief ischaemia) followed by reperfusion (Figure 21.1).

During the ensuing finite window of cardioprotection, the injury from a lethal test ischaemic insult can be attenuated. Sufficient time for reperfusion after the test ischaemia is necessary to permit accurate functional or histologic assessment of the injury. Each component of this scheme can impact the amount of protection, and marked species variability exists. Myocardial ischaemic preconditioning has been found in immature animals although the intensity of the preconditioning response diminishes with the animal's age. Tolerance to preconditioning can occur after multiple repetitive ischaemic stimuli. The traditional model of myocardial preconditioning by repetitive episodes of sublethal ischaemia, as described by Murry and colleagues in 1986, is shown in Figure 21.2.

The benefits of ischaemic preconditioning – reduction in infarct size, contractile dysfunction, dysrhythmias, loss of coronary vasodilator reserve and leucocyte adhesion – have been described in rats, rabbits, pigs, dogs and sheep. In humans, early myocardial preconditioning has been demonstrated using different indices, such as cardiac event rate after pre-infarction angina, severity of chest pain and ECG changes during coronary

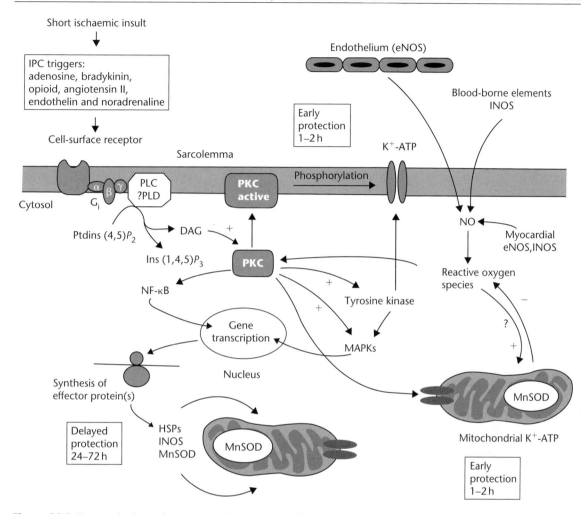

Figure 21.3 Proposed scheme for early and delayed preconditioning in the cardiomyocyte (Rubino, 2000).

angioplasty, and myocardial ATP and troponin-T levels during cardiac surgery. For preconditioning with angioplasty, at least two episodes of coronary occlusion, each lasting 120 s, are necessary.

Ischaemic preconditioning

Early preconditioning occurs 5–15 min after the stimulus and lasts for 1–2 h; a delayed or second window of myocardial preconditioning occurs 24 h after the stimulus and lasts up to 72 h. Each pathway has a different mechanism.

Early preconditioning

As seen in Figure 21.3, in the early, or classical, pathway of preconditioning, adenosine formed by ATP dephosphorylation with ischaemia activates phospholipase C (or D) via a G-protein-coupled membrane-bound A_1-receptor. Phospholipase C then cleaves a membrane phospholipid to diacylglycerol, which acts as a second messenger to upregulate cytosolic protein kinase C (PKC) with translocation to the cell membrane and mitochondria. The latent period after the preconditioning stimulus (Figure 21.1) relates to the time required for PKC translocation; the time during which PKC is translocated accounts for the time window or duration of protection. Ischaemia–reperfusion preconditioning causes the release of multiple mediators in addition to adenosine that can activate the membrane G-protein; these endogenous mediators include norepinephrine, bradykinin, endothelin, endogenous opioids and reactive oxygen species. Each receptor may produce a suboptimal signal, but signals from multiple receptors summate to attain the necessary threshold for PKC translocation. During the subsequent test insult, adenosine released by ischaemia activates translocated PKC, causing phosphorylation of potassium (K^+-ATP) channels on the sarcolemma.

As a result, the cell membrane hyperpolarizes, which shortens phase II of the action potential and reduces Ca^{2+} influx, thereby providing cardioprotection. Another pathway is phosphorylation of the K^+-ATP channel on the mitochondria causing electron transfer uncoupling with reduced Ca^{2+} overload and improved water transport. This scheme may be rather simplistic, as multiple interactive mechanisms probably co-exist.

Delayed preconditioning

A delayed or second window of preconditioning results approximately 24 h later with gene transcription, translation and synthesis of endogenous proteins, such as heat shock proteins, proto-oncogenes and antioxidants. PKC activation plays a pivotal role in the development of delayed preconditioning by translocating to the perinuclear region to induce gene expression or by activating mitogen-activated protein kinase (MAPK). Heat shock proteins (HSPs), in particular, act as molecular chaperones by promoting new protein synthesis while at the same time assisting in the degradation of ischaemia-injured proteins. Another important mechanism is intrinsic nitric oxide (NO) synthase with involvement of the K^+-ATP channel. Although not conclusively demonstrated in humans, there is supporting evidence that delayed preconditioning occurs in patients where recent pre-infarction angina improves morbidity after subsequent MI.

Preconditioning triggers

Various physiological and pharmacological triggers can elicit early preconditioning. Physiological triggers vary widely and do not require either myocardial ischaemia within the area at risk or myocardial ischaemia *per se*. For example, occlusion of the circumflex artery can precondition myocytes in the LAD distribution. Myocardial preconditioning can also result from renal, mesenteric and lower limb ischaemia in experimental animals. Early preconditioning can occur via myocardial stretch receptors, as well as by the stress response to tachycardia, haemorrhage and CPB.

Pharmacological preconditioning differs from ischaemic preconditioning, the latter being associated with a cascade of released mediators, which may amplify the preconditioning, signal intensity and cause greater PKC activation. A sufficiently intense preconditioning response may be difficult to achieve pharmacologically with a single drug. For example, a greater degree of myocardial protection results from ischaemic preconditioning than with pharmacological preconditioning using only adenosine. However, adenosine combined with suboptimal ischaemic preconditioning can produce greater myocardial

protection than either stimulus by itself. Pretreatment with dipyridamole or acadesine, both of which increase interstitial adenosine concentration, does not attenuate infarct size by itself, but can substantially potentiate an otherwise suboptimal ischaemic preconditioning stimulus. This finding may account for the lack of efficacy seen with acadesine alone in several studies. Different pharmacological stimuli administered together, such as adenosine and a K^+-ATP channel opener, produces even greater benefit. Unfortunately, many direct PKC activators that are effective experimentally produce toxic side effects in patients.

Administering β-adrenergic agonists or exogenous $CaCl_2$ can induce preconditioning by direct PKC activation. Inhalational anaesthetics, including isoflurane, desflurane and sevoflurane, activate the K^+-ATP channel and offer preconditioning benefit. In dogs, one MAC of isoflurane produces the same preconditioning benefits as four, 5-min coronary occlusions. Opioid (δ_2) activation by morphine produces significant myocardial preconditioning that can be blocked by naloxone pretreatment. K^+-ATP channel openers, such as bimakalim, lower the threshold for PKC activation so that a suboptimal ischaemic or adenosine preconditioning stimulus becomes effective in addition to lengthening the time window of protection. Nicorandil, which combines nitrate therapy with a K^+-ATP channel opener, is effective.

Many preconditioning agents produce undesirable side effects when administered systemically. Adenosine and bradykinin produce bradycardia and hypotension, while norepinephrine, angiotensin and endothelin produce hypertension. Combining preconditioning triggers (e.g. norepinephrine + adenosine) allows lower individual drug doses and attenuates undesirable haemodynamic side effects while providing significant cardioprotection. The most feasible approach for clinical myocardial preconditioning is likely to be a combination of several agents. Another delivery method that avoids some of the systemic side effects is intracoronary injection, but this technique requires direct coronary cannulation.

Combining triggers for early myocardial preconditioning with hypothermia (10°C) or cold cardioplegia does not further enhance cardiomyocyte preservation. However, when uniform cardioplegic delivery is impaired by severe coronary disease or with myocardial hypertrophy, the combination of ischaemic preconditioning and cardioplegia can provide superior protection. For off-pump coronary revascularization, an anaesthetic technique based on experimental studies can be designed to optimally precondition the myocardium prior to coronary occlusion. Such an anaesthetic technique would include the following: preoperative ACE inhibition preoperative ACE inhibition (increase bradykinin), volatile anaesthetic agent (0.5–1.0% isoflurane), morphine sulphate ($0.25–0.5\,\mathrm{mg\,kg^{-1}}$). Coupled with transient (2 min) coronary occlusions prior to revascularization, this approach could provide multi-mediated PKC translocation and preconditioning. Preconditioning is antagonized by hypothermia (increased preconditioning threshold), hyperglycaemia (glucose $> 16\,\mathrm{mmol\,l^{-1}}$), sulphonylureas ($\mathrm{K^+}$-ATP blockers), methylxanthines (A_1 antagonists) and possibly $\mathrm{Ca^{2+}}$ antagonists.

Clinically, the longer window of protection produced by delayed preconditioning is particularly attractive as the preconditioning stimuli can be delivered several days prior to surgery. Delayed myocardial preconditioning can be induced by δ_2-opioids, endotoxin derivatives and NO donors, such as GTN. Chronic alcohol ingestion produces dose-dependent myocardial preconditioning that involves $\mathrm{K^+}$-ATP channel activation and does not show tolerance with prolonged exposure. Lastly, due to different intracellular mechanisms, early and delayed preconditioning agents can be combined for additive benefits – a 2-min infusion of adenosine or phenylephrine provides greater myocardial protection in animals pretreated with endotoxin.

Conclusions

Myocardial ischaemia may progress to infarction, but not all ischaemic episodes are detrimental in terms of myocardial salvage. Recent advances in our understanding of organ preconditioning have potential relevance for the patient undergoing planned or anticipated ischaemic intervals in the operating room. For the heart, both early and delayed preconditioning responses can be elicited to provide significant cardiomyocyte protection. Potential combinations of early with delayed preconditioning responses, physiological with pharmacological stimuli and various drugs combinations, represent appealing approaches to improve myocardial salvage after ischaemia.

Key points

- The use of inotropes to improve the performance of stunned myocardium does not induce cardiomyocyte damage.
- Identification of hibernating myocardium is the key to achieving functional improvement with myocardial revascularization.
- Ischaemic preconditioning has been demonstrated in many species and many organs.
- Pre-infarction angina may result in a smaller infarct as a result of ischaemic preconditioning.
- Preconditioning can be induced with isoflurane and morphine and antagonized by hyperglycaemia and sulphonylureas (e.g. glibenclamide).

Further reading

Heusch G, Schulz R. The biology of myocardial hibernation. *Trends Cardiovasc Med 2000*; **10(3)**: 108–114.

Kloner RA, Jennings RB. Consequences of brief ischemia: stunning, preconditioning, and their clinical implications: part 1. *Circulation* 2001; **104(24)**: 2981–2989.

Kloner RA, Jennings RB. Consequences of brief ischemia: stunning, preconditioning, and their clinical implications: part 2. *Circulation* 2001; **104(25)**: 3158–3167.

Murry CE, Jennings RB, Reimer KA. Preconditioning with ischemia: a delay of lethal cell injury in ischemic myocardium. *Circulation* 1986; **74(5)**: 1124–1136.

Rubino A, Yellon DM. Ischaemic preconditioning of the vasculature: an overlooked phenomenon for protecting the heart? *Trends Pharmacol Sci* 2000; **21(6)**: 225–230.

Yellon DM, Baxter GF. Protecting the ischaemic and reperfused myocardium in acute myocardial infarction: distant dream or near reality? *Heart* 2000; **83(4)**: 381–387.

PROSTHETIC HEART VALVES 22

K. Grixti

Since the first prosthetic heart valve was implanted in 1952 more than 100 different designs have been introduced. Each device has unique characteristics in terms of durability, thrombogenicity, transvalvular gradient and propensity to cause haemolysis.

Table 22.1 Classification of implantable heart valves	
Mechanical	Caged ball
	Caged disc
	Single leaflet tilting disc
	Twin leaflet
Bioprosthetic*	Porcine heterograft (xenograft)
	Bovine pericardial
Homograft (HG)	Human HG (allograft)
	Pulmonary autograft

* Bioprosthetic valves incorporate both biological and synthetic materials.

Mechanical valves

The first valves were of the *caged-ball* type (Figure 22.1) and were adapted from valves used in industry. They consisted of a small ball held in place by a closed or semi-closed metal cage. The characteristic feature of these valves was non-central flow, with blood flow having to change direction as it flows around

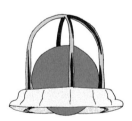

Figure 22.1 Ball in cage valves. **Starr-Edwards** (shown): Still available and occasionally used. Smallest orifice for given annulus size. Cage fractures cause ball embolism and fulminant regurgitation. **Smeloff-Cutter**: Smaller ball than Starr-Edwards valve. Device has both distal and proximal semi-closed cages. Lipid accumulation caused swelling of the ball. Withdrawn from market.

the ball. This causes a loss of momentum with the heart having to work harder for a given output. The complex flow pattern led to haemolysis and increased thrombogenicity.

The next progression was the *caged disc* valve (e.g. Beall, Cross-Jones and Kay-Shiley), which substituted a flat disc for the ball used in previous designs. All designs have been discontinued and withdrawn from use.

The mid-1960s saw the development of *tilting disc* valves, consisting of a polymer disc held in place by struts which enabled them to 'flip' open during forward flow (Figure 22.2). The larger effective orifice area, for a given valve size, significantly improved flow and reduced haemolysis and thrombosis. Early designs were reliable and very durable. Attempts to increase the opening angle in some models led to an increase in strut fracture rate.

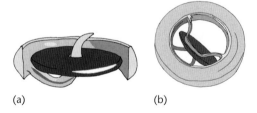

(a)   (b)

Figure 22.2 Single leaflet and single disc valves. (a) **Medtronic-Hall**: Most commonly used valve of this type today. Extremely durable. Very low failure rate. Central hole in disc through which passes gooseneck-shaped central strut. (b) **Bjork-Shiley**: Early models reliable and extensively used. Design *improvement* enabling disc to open at 70° caused increased strut failure rate in larger sizes. All models withdrawn from US market.

In 1979 the *bileaflet* valve (Figure 22.3), consisting of two semi-lunar leaflets designed to open nearly parallel (80–85°) to blood flow, was introduced. The flow characteristics of these durable valves were superior to previous designs. Despite having regurgitant 'washing-jets', which reduce stasis and thrombosis, anticoagulation is still required. The bileaflet mechanical valve is considered by many to be the gold standard and is the most commonly implanted mechanical valve.

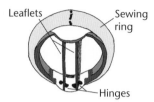

Figure 22.3 Bileaflet valves. **St Jude Medical** (shown): Low profile. Various models available. Most commonly used bileaflet valve. One central and two peripheral washing-jets. **ATS**: Quieter valve sounds. Can be rotated within sewing ring. Less thrombogenic than St Jude. **On X**: Supra-annular implantation site. Elongated flared entry channel to reduce entry turbulence.

Bioprosthetic valves

Bioprosthetic (xenograft) valves are derived from porcine valves or bovine pericardium harvested during commercial meat processing and treated with glutaraldehyde. Mimicking native valve design with biocompatible materials allows central blood flow,

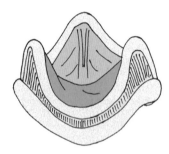

Figure 22.4 Stented bioprosthetic valves. **Hancock**: Porcine valve with plastic stent and planar sewing ring. Bovine pericardial model withdrawn. **Carpentier-Edwards** (shown): Porcine and bovine pericardial types available. Saddle-shaped sewing ring. **Ionescu-Shiley**: Bovine pericardial. Excellent haemodynamics but inferior durability. Withdrawn from market.

negligible red cell trauma and obviates the need for long-term anticoagulation. Disadvantages include a tendency to calcification and degeneration, particularly in younger patients. Most xenografts are mounted on supporting, U-shaped stents which reduces the effective orifice area for a given valve size (Figure 22.4).

In order to overcome this problem, *stentless* AVs have been produced in which the valve leaflets are left attached to the aorta (Figure 22.5). Stentless valves have a significantly increased effective orifice area and offer excellent haemodynamic characteristics – important when replacing a small valve. The valve is usually trimmed for sub-coronary implantation but can be used as a valved root replacement with coronary reimplantation. As stentless valves are deformable, sizing may be difficult and implantation requires considerable surgical skill. Claims that the use of stentless valves reduces operative mortality and improves long-term survival are currently being evaluated in prospective randomized studies.

Homograft valves

Homografts (HGs) are obtained from two sources: cadavers and tissue explanted during transplantation surgery. They are cryopreserved in liquid nitrogen and must be thawed before use. Rigorous virological donor screening is undertaken to reduce the risk of cross infection. The aortic valve and root is the most commonly used HG, although both pulmonary and mitral HGs are available. The principle indications for aortic HG use are: the young patient (particularly females of childbearing age) and surgery for endocarditis.

The Ross procedure, described in 1967, involves using the patient's own PV (an autograft) to replace a diseased AV (Figure 22.6). The PV is then replaced by a pulmonary HG. The technique obviates the need for long-term anticoagulation and, in theory, reduces the risk of valvular calcification. The procedure does,

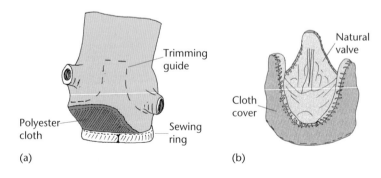

(a)   (b)

Figure 22.5 Stentless bioprosthetic valves. (a) **Edwards Prima Plus** (left): Porcine. Removal of phospholipids reduces post-implantation Ca^{2+} uptake. **Toronto SPV®** (right): Porcine. Polyester cloth separates valve from native aortic wall.

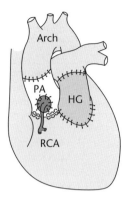

Figure 22.6 The Ross procedure. The patient's pulmonary trunk is excised and used to replace the AV and aortic root. A pulmonary HG is then used to replace the pulmonary trunk. The coronary arteries are then reimplanted into the autograft. RCA, right coronary artery.

however, require considerable surgical skill and entails lengthy CPB and ischaemic times.

Anticoagulation and antimicrobial prophylaxis

All patients with mechanical prosthetic valves should receive life-long anticoagulation. In contrast to the US guidelines (Table 22.2), the combination of aspirin and warfarin in UK practice is unusual. In addition, warfarin is not routinely used after bioprosthetic valve implantation.

Current guidelines for antimicrobial prophylaxis are discussed in Chapter 64.

Complications of valve replacement

The majority of problems associated with prosthetic heart valves are mechanical. Infection and anticoagulation-related complications account for the remainder (Table 22.3):

- Mechanical
  - Thrombosis
  - Thromboembolism
  - Haemolysis
  - Paravalvular leak
  - Persistent valve gradient
  - Device failure
- Infective
  - Endocarditis
- Other
  - Complications of anticoagulation
  - Noise

Thrombosis

Prosthetic valve thrombosis has an incidence of one case every 15–100 patient years and is invariably due to inadequate anticoagulation. Mechanical valves are prone to thrombosis, although the caged-ball and tilting disc valves are more vulnerable than bileaflet types. Bioprosthetic valve thrombosis is rare.

Table 22.2 Antithrombotic therapy for prosthetic heart valves

Valve type	Clinical setting	Warfarin		Aspirin
		INR 2–3	INR 2.5–3.5	(80–100 mg)
Mechanical	First 3 months after replacement		✓	✓
	After first 3 months			
	AVR	✓		✓
	AVR + additional factor(s)		✓	✓
	MVR		✓	✓
	MVR + additional factor(s)		✓	✓
Bioprosthetic	First 3 months after replacement		✓	✓
	After first 3 months			
	AVR			✓
	AVR + additional factor(s)	✓		✓
	MVR			✓
	MVR + additional factor(s)		✓	✓

American College of Cardiology/American Heart Association Task Force on Practice Guidelines (1998). Additional risk factors include: AF, LV dysfunction, hypercoagulable states and a history of thromboembolism.

Table 22.3 The Veterans Affairs Cooperative Study. Probability of death due to any cause, any valve-related complication and individual valve-related complications 11 years after randomization, according to type and location of replacement valve historical data on valve outcomes. Hammermeister *et al*, 1993.

	AV		MV	
	Mechanical	Bioprosthesis	Mechanical	Bioprosthesis
Death (any cause)	0.53	0.59	0.64	0.67
Valve complications	0.62	0.64	0.71	0.79
Systemic embolism	0.16	0.15	0.18	0.15
Haemorrhage	0.43	0.24*	0.41	0.28*
Endocarditis	0.07	0.08	0.11	0.17
Valve thrombosis	0.02	0.01	0.01	0.01
Perivalvular leak	0.04	0.02	0.17	0.09
Repeat surgery	0.07	0.16	0.21	0.47
Structural valve failure	0.00	0.15†	0.00	0.36†

*Risk of bleeding significantly higher with mechanical valve ($P < 0.02$).
†Risk of structural failure significantly higher with bioprosthetic valve ($P < 0.001$).

Valve thrombosis may result in functional stenosis, regurgitation or both. Auscultation may reveal decreased prosthetic heart sounds and a new murmur. Echocardiography is used to confirm the diagnosis, determine the extent of thrombosis, assess valve motion and quantify the haemodynamic impact.

Management varies from centre to centre. In general, the stable patient with minimal (<5 mm thick) thrombus is treated with either IV heparin or a thrombolytic. This strategy is more successful in patients with a bileaflet valve in the aortic position with symptoms of <2 weeks duration. Unstable patients and those with extensive thrombosis require more aggressive treatment. Thrombolytics, which carry a significant risk ($\approx$20%) of thrombo-embolism, may be the only option in the moribund patient. Surgical thrombectomy is associated with a high rate of recurrent thrombosis and valve replacement carries significant mortality.

Embolism

The incidence of systemic embolization in anticoagulated patients with mechanical valves is $\approx$1% per year. The most common clinical manifestation is neurological with the clinical spectrum ranging from TIA to fatal stroke. Transcranial Doppler (TCD) studies suggest that a significant number of patients have frequent asymptomatic cerebral microemboli.

In addition to thrombolytic therapy, the risk factors for embolism are the same as those for valve thrombosis– MV or multiple valve prostheses, caged-ball valves, AF, patient age >70 years and severe LV dysfunction.

Table 22.4 Causative organisms implicated in infective endocarditis following valve surgery

Early (<60 days)
Staphylococcus epidermidis and *aureus*
Gram-negative organisms, Diphtheroids
Fungi, Mycobacteria, Legionella

Late (>60 days)
Streptococci
Staphylococcus epidermidis

Haemorrhage

The risks associated with long-term anticoagulation should not be underestimated. The risk of life-threatening intracranial and GI bleeding increases exponentially with age.

Endocarditis

Infective endocarditis is a multi-organ disease. There tends to be a relationship between the time since surgery and the causative organism (Table 22.4). Early infections are due to intraoperative contamination and skin flora (i.e. direct) whereas later infections are commonly due to bacteraemia from dental infections and non-cardiac operative sites (indirect).

It may be difficult to make the diagnosis of endocarditis, and a high index of suspicion is required. Both pathological and clinical criteria are used. Pathological criteria include culture of microorganisms from an intracardiac abscess or an embolized vegetation. A histological diagnosis may be made from a vegetation or

Table 22.5 The Duke clinical criteria for diagnosis of infective endocarditis includes two major criteria; one major plus three minor criteria or five minor criteria. Durack, 1994.

Major criteria

1. Positive blood cultures for infective endocarditis by:
   (a) Typical micro-organisms consistent with infective endocarditis or
   (b) Persistently positive blood cultures
2. Evidence of endocardial involvement
   (a) Positive echocardiogram for endocarditis:
      – Oscillating intracardiac mass – on valve or supporting structures, in path of regurgitant jet, or on implanted material
      – Abscess
      – New partial dehiscence of prosthetic valve
   (b) New valvular regurgitation (worsening or change of a pre-existing murmur is not sufficient for diagnosis)

Minor criteria

1. Predisposing heart condition or IV drug abuse
2. Fever $\geqslant 38°C$
3. Vascular phenomenon:
   (a) Major arterial emboli, septic pulmonary infarcts, mycotic aneurysm, intracranial haemorrhage, conjunctival haemorrhages and Janeway's lesions
4. Immunologic phenomena:
   (a) Glomerulonephritis, Osler's nodes, Roth's spots and positive rheumatoid factor
5. Microbiological evidence:
   (a) Positive blood culture but not meeting major criteria or
   (b) Serologic evidence of active infection with organism consistent with infective endocarditis
6. Echocardiographic findings consistent with infective endocarditis but not sufficient to meet major criteria

intracardiac abscess. The presence of major and minor clinical criteria permits a clinical diagnosis of definite endocarditis to be made (Table 22.5).

The principle indications for surgery are: valve dysfunction, conduction abnormalities, abscess or fistula formation and embolic phenomena. Whenever possible surgery is deferred until after several weeks of antimicrobial therapy. This facilitates surgery and reduces the likelihood of reinfection and multi-organ failure.

Haemolysis

This is a rare complication, usually associated with caged-ball prostheses or a small paravalvular leak. It can be sub-clinical or manifest as anaemia and mild jaundice. The increase in blood flow velocity, associated with decreased blood viscosity, accelerates the rate of haemolysis. Markers of haemolysis include: anaemia, haptoglobinaemia, a reticulocytosis and an elevated serum lactate dehydrogenase. Management is guided by both the rate of haemolysis and the magnitude of any haemodynamic disturbance.

Paravalvular leak

This uncommon complication may result from endocarditis, poor valve design or primary implantation failure. The diagnosis is confirmed by the finding of a regurgitant jet that lies *outside* the valve sewing ring on angiography or echocardiography. It is important to exclude endocarditis. The timing of surgical correction is guided by both the rate of haemolysis and the magnitude of any haemodynamic disturbance.

Valve degeneration

Primary mechanical valve failure – even after 15–20 years – is extremely rare. In contrast, some bioprosthetic AVs may begin to degenerate as early as 8 years after implantation, and after 15 years more than 20% will have failed. Mitral bioprostheses fare even worse; with degeneration evident as early as 6 years and a >40% failure rate at 15 years.

Key points

- Bileaflet mechanical valves are commonly used for AV replacement in young patients because device durability outweighs the risks associated with anticoagulation.
- Whenever possible, mechanical valves should be avoided in women of child bearing age.
- Bioprosthetic valves are indicated in elderly patients where the risks of anticoagulation are more important than device durability.

- Stentless valves offer the greatest effective orifice area and the least transvalvular gradient for a given annulus size – particularly useful in patients with a small annulus.

Further reading

ACC/AHA guidelines for the management of patients with valvular heart disease. A report of the American College of Cardiology/American Heart Association. Task Force on Practice Guidelines (Committee on Management of Patients with Valvular Heart Disease). *J Am Coll Cardiol* 1998; **32(5)**: 1486–1588.

DeWall RA, Qasim N, Carr L. Evolution of mechanical heart valves. *Ann Thorac Surg* 2000; **69(5)**: 1612–1621.

Durack DT, Lukes AS, Bright DK. New criteria for diagnosis of infective endocarditis: utilization of specific echocardiographic findings. Duke Endocarditis Service. *Am J Med* 1994; **96(3)**: 200–209.

Hammermeister KE, Sethi GK, Henderson WG, Oprian C, Kim T, Rahimtoola S. A comparison of outcomes in men 11 years after heart-valve replacement with a mechanical valve or bioprosthesis. Veterans Affairs Cooperative Study on Valvular Heart Disease. *N Engl J Med* 1993; **328(18)**: 1289–1296.

MONITORING

M.J.T. Lanzinger & J.B. Mark

The PA catheter (PAC) (Figure 23.1) was introduced into clinical practice in 1970 by Swan and Ganz. PAC monitoring is considered to be helpful in the management of haemodynamically unstable patients, where right heart pressures cannot be assumed to predict left heart pressures, or when empirical treatment is unsuccessful and additional haemodynamic data are needed.

The features of a standard adult PAC include:

- *Proximal lumen* Opening 30 cm from the catheter tip for CVP measurement/fluid administration.
- *Distal lumen* Opening at the catheter tip for PAP monitoring.
- *Balloon lumen* For inflation/deflation of a 1.5-ml balloon at the catheter tip used to facilitate catheter placement.
- *Thermistor* Temperature-dependent resistor embedded near the tip for blood temperature measurement.

Placement

Normal waveforms that should be encountered during positioning of the PAC are displayed in Figure 23.2. Negotiation of the TV and PV during placement may

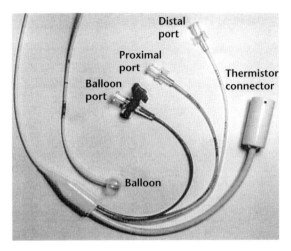

Figure 23.1 Features of a standard adult PAC.

be aided by the use of head-down and right lateral postures, respectively.

Complications

In addition to the recognized complications of central venous cannulation, the incidence of minor

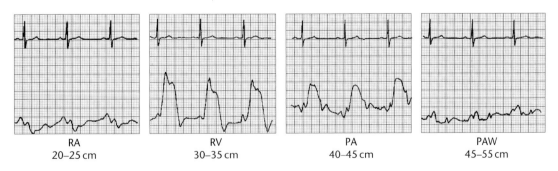

RA	RV	PA	PAW
20–25 cm	30–35 cm	40–45 cm	45–55 cm

Figure 23.2 *Waveforms during PAC insertion and distance from skin insertion.* In the SVC and RA, a CVP waveform is recorded. After crossing the TV, an RV pressure tracing is recognized by the sudden increase in systolic pressure, the wide pulse pressure and the low diastolic pressure that approximates CVP. With passage through the RVOT (often accompanied by ventricular dysrhythmias) and across the PV, the catheter records PAP characterized by the sudden step-up in the diastolic pressure. The diastolic pressure of PA exceeds that of RV, but the pressure values may not be easily distinguishable. The waveforms, however, are characteristic for each; diastolic filling of the RV produces a steady increase in diastolic pressure. In contrast, a steady decrease in diastolic pressure is seen in the PA, as blood flows towards the LA. When the catheter reaches the wedge position, the waveform resembles a CVP trace. The PAWP is a delayed representation of LA pressure dampened by the interposed pulmonary vascular bed. Mean PAWP is *always* lower than mean PAP.

complications associated with PAC insertion and use is as high as 50%, though major morbidity is uncommon (Table 23.1). PA rupture, heralded by haemoptysis, is the most serious complication, often resulting in fatal exsanguination or hypoxaemia. As medical management carries the risk of PA pseudo-aneurysm formation and secondary hemorrhage, definitive surgical treatment (i.e. lung resection) is required.

Monitoring artefacts

The most common pressure measurement artefact is a sharp pressure spike recorded immediately following the ECG R-wave and caused by the multidimensional motion of PAC within the heart during early systole. A second common measurement artefact, 'over-wedging', appears as a continually rising pressure devoid of pulsatile detail. It occurs when the catheter tip is located in an inappropriately small distal vessel and occluded by the vessel wall or the prolapsed balloon during wedging.

If the catheter tip is positioned in lung zones where alveolar pressure exceeds PAP (West zone I) or pulmonary venous pressure (West zone II), the PAC will measure alveolar pressure rather than intravascular pressure. These conditions should be suspected when the pressure trace varies markedly with respiration, and PAWP appears to be greater than PA diastolic pressure (PADP). These observations suggest that the PAC is malpositioned and that the PAWP is artefactually elevated.

Interpretation of pressure recordings

The PAWP waveform is morphologically similar to the CVP trace. Due to the transmission delay from the LA to the wedged PAC, the pressure waves appear delayed in relation to the ECG (Figure 23.2). In general, CVP

waveform components (Table 23.2) reflect right heart events, and PAWP waveforms reflect analogous left heart pathophysiology.

Estimation of left ventricular preload

PAWP is used to estimate LV preload, but absolute values alone may be misleading. The adequacy of ventricular preload is better estimated by measuring the response to a rapid fluid challenge (250–500 ml), since this also provides physiological information about the ventricular pressure–volume relationship. As an alternative to PAWP, both CVP and PADP may be used to estimate cardiac filling. Figure 23.3 displays the confounding physiological factors involved when using these surrogates for ventricular preload.

Waveform abnormalities and pathophysiology

Retrograde systolic filling of the LA through an incompetent MV results in tall *cv*-waves in the PAWP

Table 23.2 CVP waveform components

Component	Cardiac phase	Mechanical event
a-wave	End diastole	RA contraction
c-wave	Early systole	Isovolumic ventricular contraction; TV moving towards the RA
x-descent	Early/mid-systole	RA relaxation; RV ejection
v-wave	Late systole	RA filling
y-descent	Early diastole	Outflow from RA to RV

Table 23.1 Complications of pulmonary artery catheter monitoring

Arrhythmias	Transient: 50%. Sustained: 3%
Transient RBBB	Incidence: 5%
Complete heart block	Rare – pre-existing LBBB increases risk
Thrombus formation	Platelet aggregation begins within hours
Infection	Increased incidence after 3 days
Pulmonary infarction	Prolonged wedging of balloon or catheter tip
PA rupture	Incidence: 0.02–0.2%. Mortality: 50%
Other: myocardial perforation; air embolism; catheter coiling or knotting; balloon rupture/embolism; misinterpretation of data	

trace (Figure 23.4). Impeded LV filling in MS results in an elevated mean PAWP, a tall end–diastolic *a*-wave, and a slurred or absent early diastolic y-descent. In restrictive LV diastolic dysfunction, the PAWP y-descent will be steep and of short duration, due to rapid early filling that abruptly ceases (see Figure 39.4). The *a*-wave is absent in the presence of AF.

LV ischaemia causes impaired diastolic relaxation of the ventricle, increasing LVEDP and thereby raising LA pressure (LAP) and PAWP. In the setting of systemic arterial hypotension, this increase in PAWP suggests severe systolic dysfunction. Myocardial ischaemia may also cause 'functional' MR with cv-waves in the PAWP trace. When myocardial ischaemia predominantly affects RV, rather than LV function, CVP may be greater than PAWP.

Canon a waves are seen in both the CVP and PAWP traces in the presence of AV dysynchrony during ventricular pacing, junctional rhythm or complete heart block (CHB).

Cardiac output monitoring

The thermodilution technique of CO measurement has become the *de facto* clinical standard. The method measures RV blood flow and assumes that this equals LV output. The method assumes that there is no loss of thermal energy between injection and detection sites, complete mixing of the thermal indicator with blood, accurate discrimination of temperature change from baseline, and constant flow during the dilution curve. Large left-to-right or right-to-left shunts lead to an overestimation or underestimation of systemic CO, respectively. In the presence of severe TR, CO is usually underestimated due to recirculation of the thermal signal, but it may be overestimated, depending on the severity of valvular regurgitation and the magnitude of the CO.

Although the Stewart–Hamilton equation appears complex, CO can be more simply considered to be the quotient of *thermal input energy* and the *area under the PA temperature curve*:

$$Q = \frac{V_i(T_b - T_i)}{\int_0^\infty \Delta T_b \,(t)\,dt} \times \frac{S_i \cdot C_i}{S_b \cdot C_b} \times k$$

The Stewart–Hamilton Equation

where Q is the CO; V_i, injectate volume (ml); T_b, blood temperature; T_i, injectate temperature; S_i, injectate specific gravity (kg^{-1}); S_b, blood specific gravity; C_i, injectate specific heat capacity (J kg^{-1} °C^{-1}) C_b, blood

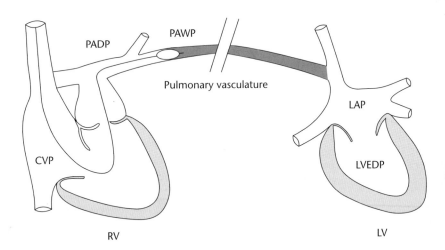

Figure 23.3 *Estimating cardiac filling with the PAC.* The schematic shows the PAC wedging in a proximal PA to measure indirectly downstreaming left heart filling pressures. The PADP provides an estimate of LA pressure and LV filling pressure (LVEDP), as pressure in the PA at the end of diastole usually equilibrates with downstream pressure in the LA. In critically ill patients, when the RV and LV may have different diastolic pressure–volume curves, the PADP offers a more accurate estimate of LV preload than the CVP. PAWP is measured closest to the LA, and therefore is subject to the least interference and error. Whenever 'upstream' pressures are used to estimate the LV filling, confounding factors may invalidate the estimate. Although LV compliance, HR, MV disease, PVR and alveolar pressure are key factors, RV compliance and TV and PV disease may also play a role. PAWP overestimates LVEDP when alveolar pressure exceeds intravascular pressure, in MS, in pulmonary hypertension and in the presence of tachycardia. In AR, LV filling is underestimated, because all PAC measurements are isolated from the continued retrograde inflow into the LV following MV closure.

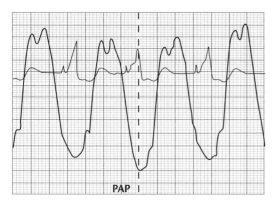 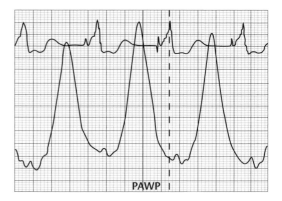

Figure 23.4 MR is associated with tall v-waves in the PAWP trace, which begin in early systole and are more properly termed regurgitant *CV*-waves. This abnormal wave is generated during ventricular systole and obliterates the systolic x-descent in the PAWP waveform. The height of the regurgitant wave is influenced by the severity of MR as well as LA volume and compliance. Tall PAWP v-waves may also be seen in patients with hypervolaemia, congestive heart failure and VSD. In these cases, the v-wave is caused by increased LA volume or exaggerated antegrade filling of the LA.

specific heat capacity and the integral function that of blood temperature versus time (°C, min).

For intermittent bolus determination of CO, a 10 ml bolus of (room temperature or iced) fluid is injected into the RA and the subsequent blood temperature measured by the thermistor at the tip of the PAC.

Continuous CO (CCO) monitoring involves the release of small quantities of heat from a 10-cm thermal filament incorporated into the RV portion of the PAC. The temperature changes induced are one order of magnitude lower than those achieved with intermittent administration of a bolus of cold fluid causing a reduction in signal-to-noise ratio. One solution to this problem is to turn the input power on and off in a pseudo-random sequence. Resulting temperature fluctuations are recorded and a computer cross correlates input power with detected temperature to produce a computed wash-out curve. Typically, the displayed value for CO is updated every 30 s and represents the average CO over the previous 3–6 min.

Mixed venous oximetry

Continuous measurement of SvO_2 can provide a real-time indication of changes in the circulation. Changes in SvO_2 are directly proportional to changes in CO when arterial oxygen saturation, oxygen consumption and Hb concentration remain stable. Furthermore, SvO_2 provides a global indication of the balance of oxygen delivery and consumption.

Key points

- The pressure waveforms and ECG should be continuously displayed to validate absolute values and examine the timing of cardiac events.
- During diastole; RV pressure increases and PA pressure decreases.
- If used during cardiac surgery, the PAC should be withdrawn 5–10 cm prior to the onset of CPB to reduce the risk of catheter migration, pulmonary infarction and pulmonary artery rupture.

Further reading

Mark JB. *Atlas of Cardiovascular Monitoring*. New York: Churchill Livingstone, 1998.

Mark JB. Cardiovascular monitoring. In: Miller RD (Ed.), *Anesthesia*. Philadelphia: Churchill Livingstone, 2000; pp. 1117–1206.

Sandham JD, Hull RD, Brant RF, Knox L, Pineo GF, Doig CJ *et al*. A randomized,controlled trial of the use of pulmonary-artery catheters in high-risk surgical patients. *N Engl J Med* 2003; **348(1)**: 5–14.

TRANSOESOPHAGEAL ECHOCARDIOGRAPHY 24

R.M.O. Hall

The growth in use of perioperative TOE over the last decade has been such that TOE is now considered to be a core component of modern cardiac anaesthesia and intensive care. Its value as a monitor is complementary to traditional invasive pressure measurements and in some aspects is superior to them. This chapter will cover the physics of ultrasound, the principles of Doppler ultrasound, imaging modes, the format of a basic TOE examination and indications for TOE. The perioperative assessment of cardiac function using TOE is discussed in the next chapter.

Ultrasound physics

Ultrasound is sound whose frequency is above the audible range. Humans can hear sound with a frequency that is between 20 and 20,000 Hz, hence ultrasound is any sound with a frequency greater than 20 kHz. Medically useful ultrasound however is usually in the range of 1–10 MHz.

The 'wave-like' properties of ultrasound can be described in terms of frequency, wavelength, velocity and amplitude (Table 24.1). Ultrasound causes alternating rarification and compression of tissues that are propagated through the tissue at the speed of sound.

The ultrasound wavelength in blood is 0.3 mm for a 5-MHz probe and 0.6 mm for a 2.5-MHz probe. The two-point discrimination (spacial resolution) of ultrasound is dependent upon wavelength as the minimum distance that can be resolved between two objects is one wavelength (Figure 24.1).

A 1-MHz probe will be unable to distinguish between two structures less than 1.5 mm apart, whereas a 5-MHz probe can resolve structures 0.3 mm apart. Thus, as ultrasound wavelength shortens, image detail (resolution) increases.

As with radio waves, where short wave (very high frequency (VHF)) broadcasts have a smaller range than long wave, ultrasound tissue penetration decreases as frequency increases. In clinical practice, the maximum

Table 24.1 Sound velocity in lung, blood and bone

Tissue	Sound velocity (m s^{-1})
Lung (air)	300
Blood	1540
Bone	4000

Velocity = Frequency × wavelength ($C = f\lambda$).

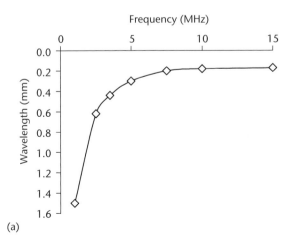

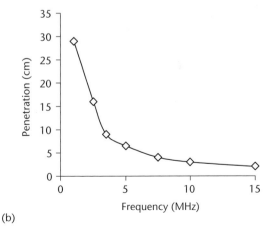

Figure 24.1 The inverse relationship between (a) frequency and wavelength (spacial resolution) and (b) frequency and tissue penetration.

tissue penetration (attenuation) depth is equivalent to 200 wavelengths. The practical implication is that TOE is better at imaging structures that are closely related to the oesophagus such as the LA and MV. Although anterior structures, such as the LV apex, are poorly imaged from the oesophagus, they are accessible with TTE.

Modern medical ultrasound equipment employs a series of piezo-electric crystals to alternately emit and receive ultrasound waves. A small number ($\sim$1%) of emitted waves are reflected back at interfaces between tissues of varying acoustic density. Given that ultrasound travels 1cm in 13 µs, knowledge of the time interval between emission and reception allows the distance to the reflective interface to be calculated. Ultrasound waves reflected from interfaces at varying depths will be received at different times, which can be displayed as points a line. The strength (amplitude) of the reflected wave is represented by the size of the point. This is the basis of B-mode echo.

Current imaging techniques are based on B-mode imaging. In M-mode, a single B-mode 'line' is sampled at a VHF ($1000\,\mathrm{s}^{-1}$) and the information is then displayed with depth information on the y-axis and time on the x-axis. While this still looks only at one discrete anatomical line, motion of the region examined can be seen.

The classic echo display is two-dimensional (2D) where anatomical information is displayed in near real time. This sector scan is actually made up of multiple B-mode lines. As the equipment is bound to the speed of sound, the speed at which the image can be updated (the frame rate) is inversely proportional to the scan depth and angle.

Factors increasing the strength of returning signal are greater transmitted amplitude and an angle of incidence close to 90°.

Modern TOE probes resemble a flexible gastroscope and contain arrays of piezo-electric that can emit ultrasound at varying frequencies.

Doppler ultrasound

When sound waves are reflected from a moving target the wavelength of the reflected sound is altered in proportion to the velocity of the target. The resulting change in frequency, first described by Doppler and known as the *Doppler shift*, forms the basis of the vehicle 'speed traps'. The same principle can be employed by using ultrasound to measure the velocity of blood within the heart.

When the direction of blood flow is not parallel to the ultrasound beam, the velocity will be underestimated by a factor equal to the cosine of the incident angle (Figure 24.2). In clinical practice an angle <20° (where the cosine = 0.94) produces acceptably accurate measurements.

Information about blood flow velocity obtained using Doppler ultrasound can be displayed in a number of ways. In PWD, the velocity of blood flow is measured at a precise distance from the ultrasound probe. In CWD, the velocities of blood flow are measured at all points along the ultrasound beam without localization. In *colour flow Doppler*, PWD is used to construct a map of blood flow velocities that is superimposed on the corresponding 2D image.

Once velocity is known it is then possible to estimate pressure gradients using a simplified form of the Bernoulli equation, which describes the relationship

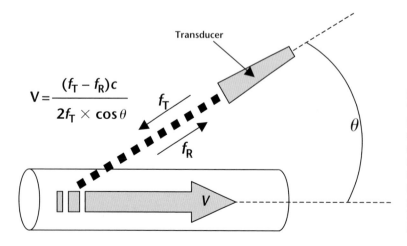

$$V = \frac{(f_T - f_R)c}{2f_T \times \cos\theta}$$

Figure 24.2 The Doppler principle. The mathematical relationship between blood flow velocity, change in frequency of reflected ultrasound, and angle between blood flow and ultrasound vectors. V is the blood flow velocity; f_T, the frequency of transmitted ultrasound; f_R, the frequency of reflected ultrasound and θ, the angle between blood flow and ultrasound beam.

between instantaneous pressure gradient and velocity:

$$\textbf{Pressure gradient} \approx \textbf{4} \times \textbf{Velocity}^2$$

A pressure gradient can be estimated in any part of the heart where a velocity can be measured. For example; if peak flow velocity (using CWD) is $5\,\mathrm{m\,s^{-1}}$ (Figure 24.3), then the estimated peak instantaneous pressure gradient is $100\,\mathrm{mmHg}$ (i.e. 4×5^2). This information can be combined with a direct pressure measurement to estimate the pressure in a second site. RV systolic pressure can be estimated from peak TV regurgitant velocity and RA pressure:

$$\textbf{Peak RV systolic pressure} = \textbf{4} \times (V_{TR})^2 + \textbf{RAP}$$

where V_{TR} is the peak tricuspid regurgitant velocity and RAP is the RA pressure.

Flow can be measured in the great vessels to estimate cardiac output or across a regurgitant valve to assess the severity of the valve pathology. SV can be estimated by multiplying the distance blood travels in a cardiac cycle (*stroke distance*) by the cross-sectional area of the vessel at the *same* point.

As distance is the integral of velocity, the stroke distance can be obtained by integrating the velocity profile with respect to time. The result is known as the *velocity time integral* (VTI) (Figure 24.4).

Basic examination

A complete TOE examination requires some 20 views and includes the heart, the great vessels, and the descending aorta. In practice, however, a satisfactory examination of the heart can be achieved rapidly using only 12 views – four each at the mid-oesophageal (ME) AV level (Figure 24.5), ME MV level (Figure 24.6) and transgastric (TG) level (Figure 24.7).

For teaching purposes at Papworth, we have found that trainees grasp the principles of TOE more quickly

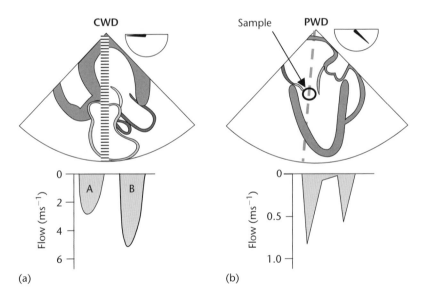

Figure 24.3 Measurement of blood flow velocity.
(a) CWD is used to measure high-velocity flow across the AV in AS. A is mild (peak gradient; 36 mmHg). B is severe (peak gradient; 100 mmHg).
(b) PWD is used to measure diastolic trans-mitral blood flow velocity at the MV leaflet coaptation point. Note that PWD measures much lower velocities than the CWD.

$$\textbf{Stroke volume (ml\,cm}^3\textbf{)} = \textbf{Area}_{\textbf{LVOT}}\,(\textbf{cm}^2) \times \textbf{VTI}_{\textbf{LVOT}}\,(\textbf{cm})$$

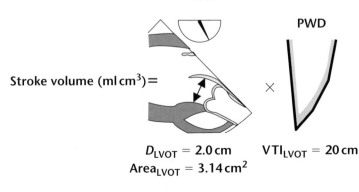

Figure 24.4 Calculation of stroke volume and CO using the VTI. The clear centre of the PWD pattern indicates LVOT flow. If HR is 80 bpm, then cardiac output = 80 × stroke volume (3.14 × 20) ≈ 5000 ml min^{-1}.

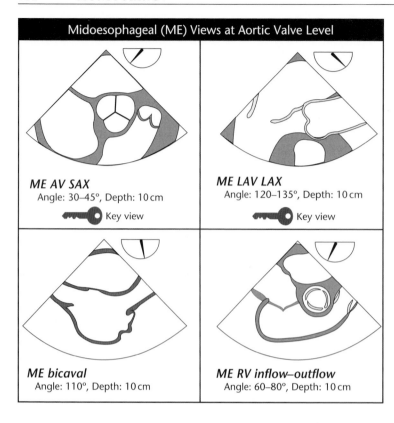

Figure 24.5 ME views at AV level. (a) SAX: angle 30–45° and depth 10 cm. (b) LAX: angle 120–135° and depth 10 cm. (c) Bicaval: angle 110° and depth 10 cm. (d) RV inflow–outflow: angle 60–80° and depth 12 cm.

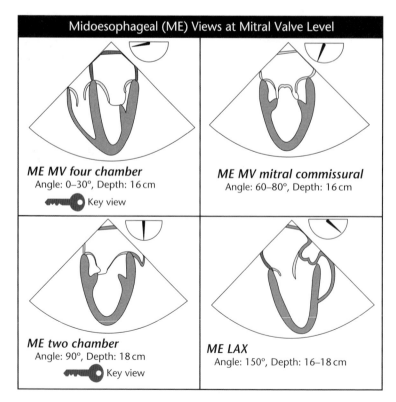

Figure 24.6 ME views at MV level. (a) Four chamber: angle 0–30° and depth 16 cm. (b) Mitral commissural: angle 60–80° and depth 16 cm. (c) Two chamber: angle 90° and depth 18 cm. (d) LAX: angle 150° and depth 16–18 cm.

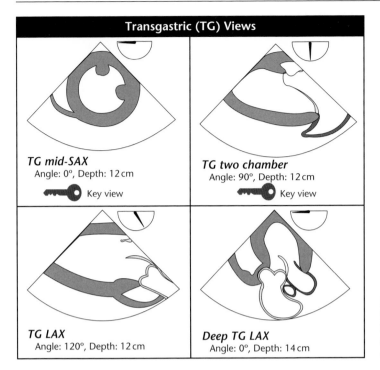

Figure 24.7 TG views. (a) Mid-SAX: angle 0° and depth 12 cm. (b) Two chamber: angle 90° and depth 12 cm. (c) LAX: angle 120° and depth 12 cm. (d) Deep TG LAX: angle 0° and depth 14 cm.

if the examination is initially limited to just six 'key' views using the ME SAX (30°) view of the AV, the so-called '*Mercedes Benz*' view, as a starting point. Once this very basic approach has been mastered, the examination is quickly expanded to 12 views. Only when the trainee has demonstrated competence at this level is the examination expanded to all 20 views. It is essential that the TOE examination be performed in a systematic manner; regardless of the order in which the standard views are obtained.

Although a complete TOE examination should include the confirmation and quantification of known pathological conditions, it is important not to miss undiagnosed lesions. Furthermore, the physiological impact of general anaesthesia should be taken into account when estimating the severity of valvular lesions. Unexpected findings must be reported to the surgical team as they may significantly influence the conduct of the operation.

Indications

The putative benefits of perioperative TOE are largely based on consensus or 'expert' opinion, rather than prospective, randomized controlled trials. Although the evidence that TOE improves outcome is weak, there is accumulating evidence that TOE alters cardiac surgical management (Table 24.2 and 24.3).

Practice standards

The use of TOE is not without risk and may be contraindicated in the presence of oesophageal pathology. As the inexperienced echocardiographer may inappropriately interpolate suboptimal or missing information, the most common complication is misdiagnosis. Frequent sources of error include artefacts (e.g. side lobe and reverberation) that mimic intracardiac structures.

Table 24.2 The impact of perioperative TOE on clinical decision-making

- Undiagnosed ASD/patent foramen ovale
- Undiagnosed valvular pathology in coronary patients
- Undiagnosed 'second-valve' pathology in valve patients
- New regional wall motion abnormalities following revascularization
- Assessment of adequacy of reparative surgical procedures
- Congenital cardiac disease

Table 24.3 American Society of Echocardiography/Society of Cardiovascular Anesthesiologists (ASE/SCA) classification of indications for the use of perioperative TOE

Category	Evidence	Examples
I	Supported by the strongest evidence or expert opinion TOE is frequently useful in improving clinical outcomes	Evaluation of life-threatening instability in theatre or the ICU that is not resolved using standard therapies Valve repair surgery Repair of congenital cardiac lesions Assessment of unstable aortic dissection or aortic aneurysms Surgery for hypertrophic obstructive cardio-myopathy (HOCM) Surgery for endocarditis
II	Supported by weaker evidence or opinion, may be useful clinically	Assessment of prosthetic valve replacement Checking adequacy of de-airing Perioperative use for patients at increased risk of myocardial ischaemia or haemodynamic instability
III	Little current scientific or expert support, infrequently useful	Intraoperative monitoring for emboli during orthopaedic surgery Monitoring for placement of PAFC catheters, balloon pumps or defibrillators

Key points

- Knowledge of the basic physical principles under-lying medical ultrasound is essential for the effective use of perioperative TOE.
- Every TOE examination should be comprehensive, recorded for later inspection and formally inter-preted in a report.
- Considerable time is required to develop com-petency in perioperative TOE.
- There are few contraindication to the use of TOE.
- Physical complications are rare but may be lethal.

Further reading

Practice guidelines for perioperative transesophageal echocardiography. A report by the American Society of Anesthesiologists and the Society of Cardiovascular Anesthesiologists Task Force on Transesophageal Echo-cardiography. *Anesthesiology* 1996; **84(4)**: 986–1006.

Shanewise JS, Cheung AT, Aronson S, Stewart WJ, Weiss RL, Mark JB *et al.* ASE/SCA guidelines for performing a comprehensive intraoperative multiplane transesophageal echocardiography examination: recommendations of the American Society of Echocardiography Council for Intraoperative Echocardiography and the Society of Cardiovascular Anesthesiologists Task Force for Certifica-tion in Perioperative Transesophageal Echocardiography. *Anesth Analg* 1999; **89(4)**: 870–884.

INTRAOPERATIVE ASSESSMENT OF LEFT VENTRICULAR FUNCTION

25

J. Graham & J.H. Mackay

This chapter will discuss the intraoperative assessment of systolic and diastolic myocardial function.

Global systolic function

Preload

Direct inspection and CVP measurement provide useful information about RV filling, while traditionally intraoperative assessment of LV filling has relied on PAWP or direct LA pressure (LAP) measurement. Assumptions made when using PAWP to assess LV filling are summarized in Chapter 23 (see Figure 23.3). The reduction in ventricular compliance (the slope of the LV end-diastolic pressure–volume relationship (EDPVR); see Chapter 4, Figure 4.9), commonly seen in cardiac surgical patients, can have a major impact on PAWP interpretation (Figure 25.1). In the setting of altered LV compliance, TOE allows better assessment of preload.

The standard view most commonly used to assess preload is the transgastric mid–papillary short axis (TG mid-SAX) view (Figure 25.2d).

Apical views underestimate true LV filling and may lead to inappropriate fluid administration. In practice, the assessment of LV filling is often qualitative (by 'eyeballing') using a fixed depth of field (e.g. 12 cm) throughout the study period. More quantitative measures include measurement of LV end-diastolic diameter (LVEDD) using M-mode and LV end-diastolic area (LVEDA) using the two-dimensional (2D) image (Figure 25.3).

Long axis (LAX) views are less useful in the assessment of LV filling for two reasons:

1 Difficulty in visualizing the LV apex.
2 As 90% of normal LV ejection can be ascribed to short axis (SAX) contraction, changes in LV end diastolic volume (LVEDV) produce minimal changes

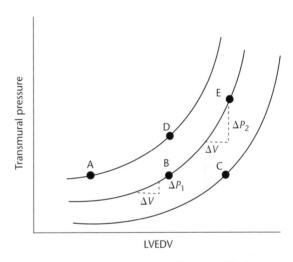

Figure 25.1 LV compliance curves for three differing ventricles. Reduced compliance shifts the curve upwards and to the left. Points A, B and C represent the wide differences in LV filling (LVEDV) that may occur despite identical transmural pressure (PAWP). Hypovolaemia could be missed in the patient with the least compliant ventricle (line AD), if PAWP is the only method used to assess LV filling (from Tuman KJ,1989).

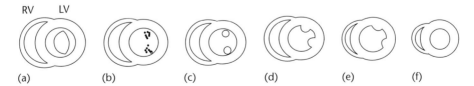

Figure 25.2 Images obtained from SAX views at basal (a and b), mid (c and d) and apical (e and f) levels. If MV or chordae tendinae are seen, the image is too basal (a and b). The probe needs to be advanced and/or anteflexion reduced. If no papillary muscle or valvular apparatus is seen, the image is too apical (f). The probe needs to be withdrawn and/or anteflexion increased. (a) MV level, (b) CT level, (c) high-PM level, (d) mid-PM level, (e) low-PM level and (f) apex level.

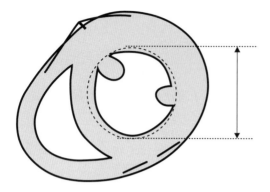

Figure 25.3 Estimation of LVEDA. The papillary muscles are included in the LV cavity outline. End diastole is taken as the peak of the R-wave. Normal (adult) LVEDA is 14–24 cm^2 and normal LVEDD is 3.5–5.5 cm.

in LAX dimensions. SAX views are more sensitive at detecting alterations in end-diastolic volume.

LV filling should be measured at the end of diastole. However, LV end-systolic cavity obliteration, when papillary muscles touch or 'kiss' at the end of systole in the TG mid-SAX view, is a sensitive marker of reduced preload.

Ejection fraction

The 2D echocardiography measurement of LV fractional area change (FAC) is often used as a surrogate measure of ejection fraction. Both LVEDA and the LV end-systolic area (LVESA) are measured from the TG mid-SAX view and FAC calculated using the formula:

$$FAC = \frac{LVEDA - LVESA}{LVEDA}$$

As both CO and LV ejection fraction (LVEF) are load dependent, they do not provide an accurate assessment of contractility.

Cardiac output

SV can be calculated using Doppler ultrasound, by measuring the area under the velocity–time curve (velocity time integral (VTI)) at a point of known diameter where blood flow is largely non-turbulent. Suitable sites include the LVOT and the main PA.

$$SV = VTI \times \pi \times (diameter/2)^2$$
$$CO = HR \times SV$$

The technique is limited by two potential sources of error:

1 A 10% error in measurement of the diameter of LVOT or PA results in a 21% error in SV.
2 If the angle of insonation is >20° to the direction of blood flow, the VTI will be significantly underestimated.

Regional systolic function

Within a few seconds of the onset of severe myocardial ischaemia or total coronary artery occlusion, systolic wall thickening and inward wall (endocardial) motion are reduced in the territory supplied by the coronary artery. As this so-called regional (or segmental) wall motion abnormality (RWMA) precedes ECG changes, TOE is a more sensitive monitor of myocardial ischaemia. Reduced systolic thickening is more important than reduced endocardial motion. The description of regional wall motion is shown in Table 25.1.

Table 25.1 Description of segmental (regional) ventricular wall motion

Class of motion	Wall thickening	Change in radius
1 Normal	Marked	$\downarrow\downarrow\downarrow$ >30%
2 Mild hypokinesis	Moderate	$\downarrow\downarrow$ 10–30%
3 Severe hypokinesis	Minimal	$\downarrow$ <10%
4 Akinesis	None	0%
5 Dyskinesis	Thinning	$\uparrow$

The TG mid-SAX view is particularly useful for detecting RWMA as myocardium supplied by all three major coronary arteries can be visualized (Figure 25.4). The use of additional views improves the likelihood of detecting a RWMA.

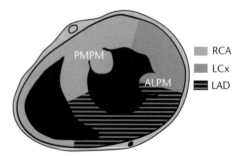

Figure 25.4 Mid-papillary, SAX view of the ventricles illustrating the distribution of coronary artery blood flow. LAD, left anterior descending artery; LCx, left circumflex artery; RCA, right coronary artery;. ALPM, anterolateral papillary muscle; PMPM, posteromedial papillary muscle.

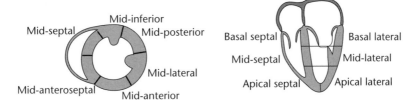

Figure 25.5 The 16-segment LV model. On the left is the TG mid-SAX view with the prefix mid for each of the six segments. On the right is the ME four-chamber view with the lateral and septal walls separated into basal, mid and apical segments.

Mid-oesophageal view	Angle	LV walls imaged	
		Left	**Right**
Four chamber	30°	Septal	Lateral
Two chamber	90°	Inferior	Anterior
Long axis	150°	Posterior	Anteroseptal

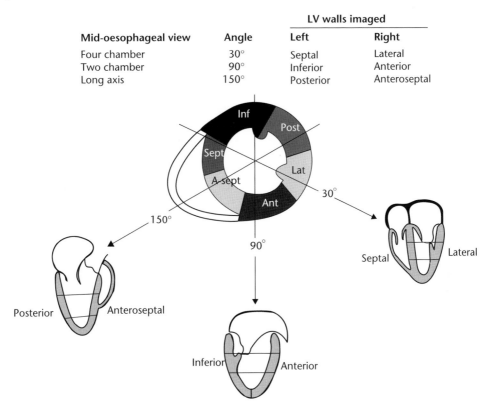

Figure 25.6 Imaging the 16-LV segments from the mid-oesophagus. The lines at 30°, 90° and 150° represent the orientation of the ultrasound imaging plane to SAX view.

For the purposes of assessment, a 16-segment model of the LV is advocated. The model divides the LV into three levels from base to apex. The basal and mid-levels are both circumferentially divided into six segments, while the apical level is divided into four segments (Figure 25.5). The four apical segments are anterior, septal, inferior and lateral.

In theory all of the 16 segments can be visualized from the mid-oesophagus (ME) in the LAX using the 30° (four chamber), 90° (two chamber) and 150° (LAX) views (Figure 25.6). However, in practice, foreshortening (when the imaging plane passes through the middle part of the anterior wall rather than the true apex) makes it difficult to visualize the apical segments.

The hypotensive patient

TOE is very useful in the differential diagnosis of three common causes of acute hypotension in theatre and ICU.

Common causes	LVEDA	LVEF
Hypovolaemia	↓	↑
Low SVR*	Normal	↑
Pump failure	↑	↓

*Severe MR, AR or VSD may mimic a decrease in SVR and should be excluded.

Pump failure is the easiest to diagnose due to increased LVEDA and decreased LVEF. Both hypovolaemia and vasodilatation increase LVEF and may induce LV end systolic cavity obliteration. LVEDA is decreased by hypovolaemia but is usually normal in patients with reduced SVR.

Diastolic function

Normal LV diastolic function allows adequate LV filling with low LVEDP and consists of four phases (see Chapter 4):

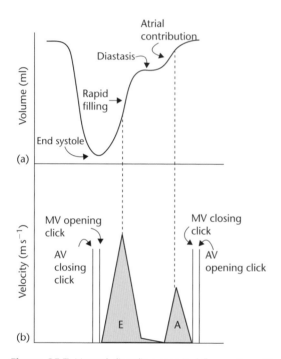

(a)

(b)

Figure 25.7 Normal diastolic transmitral flow pattern. The deceleration time is time between peak E-wave velocity and the point it would pass through if it were to continue to baseline. The E : A ratio is the ratio of peak E-wave to peak A-wave velocity. (a) LV volume (b) LV inflow. (Reprinted with permission from Otto CM, 2000.)

- *Isovolumic relaxation* Between aortic valve closure and MV opening.
- *Early diastolic filling* E-wave (80% LV filling). Initial relaxation is an active process that causes rapid decrease in LV pressure. When LA pressure exceeds LV pressure, MV opening occurs and rapid early diastolic filling commences. The speed of

filling is determined by the rate of myocardial relaxation and LV elastic recoil.
- *Diastasis* LV pressure is equal to LA pressure. Transmitral blood flow ceases.
- *Late diastolic filling* A-wave (20% LV filling). Atrial systole.

The LV with diastolic dysfunction requires a compensatory increase in LA pressure to maintain an adequate CO. Assessment of LV diastolic function by TOE requires examination of both mitral inflow and pulmonary vein blood flow using PWD.

Placing the PWD sampling volume between the tips of the MV leaflets allows the pattern of transmitral blood flow to be examined. The E-wave represents the rapid filling of early diastole. The A-wave represents blood flow during atrial contraction (Figure 25.7).

Withdrawing the probe slightly from the ME AV SAX view, and turning to the left allows the left superior pulmonary vein (LSPV) to be visualized. The so-called 'coumadin ridge', which separates the LSPV from the LA appendage, is a useful landmark. Correct identification of the LSPV can be confirmed by using colour flow Doppler. The PWD sampling volume is then placed in the LSPV as far from the LA as possible. A normal pulmonary venous inflow pattern is shown in Figure 25.8.

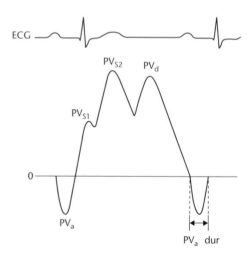

Figure 25.8 Normal pulmonary venous blood flow. During atrial systole, pulmonary venous blood flow (PV_a) transiently reverses. The PV_{S1} peak is caused by atrial relaxation. The PV_{S2} peak is caused by increased pulmonary venous pressure after RV systole. The PV_d peak is produced by rapid early diastolic ventricular filling. (Reprinted with permission from Oh JK, 1997.)

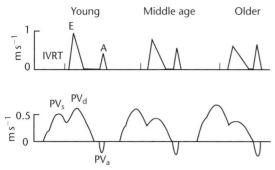

Figure 25.9 Impact of age on mitral inflow and pulmonary flow patterns. (from Oh JK, 1999; with permission.)

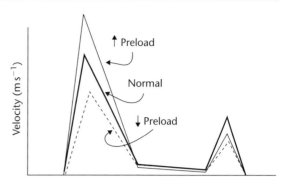

Figure 25.10 Impact of preload on mitral inflow pattern. (from Otto CM, 2000; with permission.)

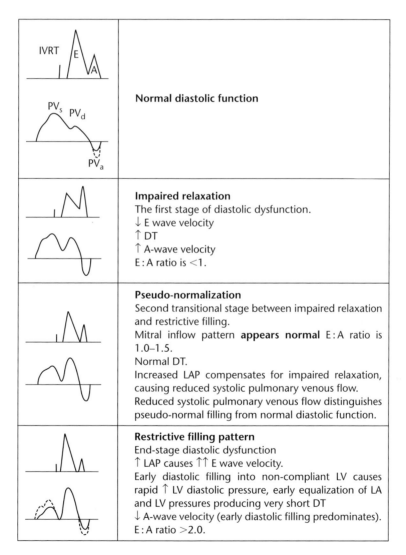

IVRT, E, A, PV$_s$, PV$_d$, PV$_a$ waveform	**Normal diastolic function**
waveform	**Impaired relaxation** The first stage of diastolic dysfunction. ↓ E wave velocity ↑ DT ↑ A-wave velocity E : A ratio is <1.
waveform	**Pseudo-normalization** Second transitional stage between impaired relaxation and restrictive filling. Mitral inflow pattern **appears normal** E : A ratio is 1.0–1.5. Normal DT. Increased LAP compensates for impaired relaxation, causing reduced systolic pulmonary venous flow. Reduced systolic pulmonary venous flow distinguishes pseudo-normal filling from normal diastolic function.
waveform	**Restrictive filling pattern** End-stage diastolic dysfunction ↑ LAP causes ↑↑ E wave velocity. Early diastolic filling into non-compliant LV causes rapid ↑ LV diastolic pressure, early equalization of LA and LV pressures producing very short DT ↓ A-wave velocity (early diastolic filling predominates). E : A ratio >2.0.

Figure 25.11 Typical transmitral flow (top) and pulmonary venous flow (bottom) patterns in normal and abnormal diastolic function.

Factors affecting transmitral and pulmonary venous inflow

1 *HR*   Tachycardia shortens diastole, causing loss of diastasis and fusion of E- and A-waves.

2 *Age*   E : A ratio decreases with age due to progressive reduction in elastic recoil and myocardial relaxation (Figure 25.9). Normal E : A ratio is 1 at age 65, and <1 when age >70. Decreased early diastolic filling with increased age is accompanied by decreased diastolic pulmonary venous flow.

3 *Preload*   Increased LA pressure causes increased E : A ratio and decreased systolic pulmonary flow (Figure 25.10).

Abnormal diastolic function

Elevated LVEDP is the hallmark of diastolic dysfunction. Left ventricles in patients with aortic stenosis and arterial hypertension are examples of primary diastolic dysfunction. Extrinsic compression by tamponade and long-standing systolic dysfunction causes secondary diastolic dysfunction. The importance of diastolic dysfunction after myocardial ischaemia or infarction is frequently underestimated. (Figure 25.11)

Key points

- TOE provides a better estimate of preload than the PAFC in conditions when LV compliance is reduced.

- Although CO can be measured echocardiographically, the PAFC is, in practice, easier to use.
- TOE permits assessment of both global and regional ventricular systolic function.
- Examination of the patterns of pulmonary venous and transmitral blood flow is required to assess LV diastolic function.

Further reading

Oh JK, Appleton CP, Hatle LK, Nishimura RA, Seward JB, Tajik AJ. The noninvasive assessment of left ventricular diastolic function with two-dimensional and Doppler echocardiography. *J Am Soc Echocardiogr* 1997; **10(3)**: 246–270.

Poortmans G, Schupfer G, Roosens C, Poelaert J. Transesophageal echocardiographic evaluation of left ventricular function. *J Cardiothorac Vasc Anesth* 2000; **14(5)**: 588–598.

Shanewise JS, Cheung AT, Aronson S, Stewart WJ, Weiss RL, Mark JB *et al.* ASE/SCA guidelines for performing a comprehensive intraoperative multiplane transesophageal echocardiography examination: recommendations of the American Society of Echocardiography Council for Intraoperative Echocardiography and the Society of Cardiovascular Anesthesiologists Task Force for Certification in Perioperative Transesophageal Echocardiography. *Anesth Analg* 1999; **89(4)**: 870–884.

Tuman TK, Carroll GC, Ivankovich AD. Pitfalls in interpretation of PA catheter data. *J Cardiothorac Anesth* 1989; **3(5)**: 625–641.

NEUROLOGICAL MONITORING 26

J.E. Arrowsmith

Injury to the brain, spinal cord and peripheral nerves represents a significant cause of morbidity and disability after cardiac surgery. Although monitors of neurological function have been available since the 1950s, their use remains uncommon. The reasons are undoubtedly the perception that neuromonitors are large, complex and costly devices that produce spurious results, and merely document neurological injury, rather than allow prevention. Emerging evidence, however, suggests that modern neuromonitoring technologies, particularly when used together, can be used both to predict and to modify clinical outcome.

Neuromonitoring devices can be divided into two broad categories: invasive and non-invasive (Table 26.1).

Clinical monitoring

The risk of neurological injury is reduced by early detection of aortic cannula displacement and venous air entrainment, as well as the avoidance of hypoxia, hypoglycaemia, acidosis, gross anaemia, prolonged cerebral hypoperfusion and cerebral hyperthermia (Figure 26.1).

$$CPP = MAP - (ICP + CVP)$$

It should be borne in mind that cerebral perfusion pressure (CPP) is dependent upon MAP, intracranial pressure (ICP) and CVP. A marked elevation in CVP, even in the presence of a seemingly adequate MAP, may result in significant cerebral hypoperfusion. As continuous invasive haemodynamic monitoring is a key component of cardiac anaesthesia, the accuracy of

Table 26.1 Types of currently available neuromonitors for use in cardiac surgery

Non-invasive
Electroencephalography
Near infrared spectroscopy (NIRS)
Transcranial Doppler (TCD) sonography
Evoked potentials (EPs)

Invasive
Jugular venous oxygen saturation ($S_{JV}O_2$)

the equipment used should be critically assessed at regular intervals.

At temperatures $>30°C$ cerebral autoregulation (flow–metabolism coupling) is essentially preserved so that cerebral blood flow (CBF) across a wide range of MAP is governed by $PaCO_2$. At $PaCO_2$ $<3.0\,kPa$ CBF may be reduced by more than half leading to cerebral ischaemia. At $PaCO_2$ $>9\,kPa$ CBF may be more than doubled, resulting in the delivery of greater numbers of microemboli to the cerebral circulation. At lower temperatures, autoregulation is gradually lost and progressive cerebral 'vasoparesis' renders CBF pressure passive.

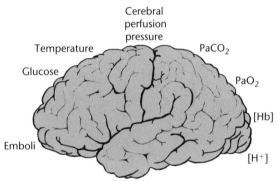

Figure 26.1 Factors affecting cerebral function during cardiac surgery: [Hb]; Hb concentration; [H$^+$]; hydrogen ion concentration.

Electroencephalography

The EEG is a representation of the spontaneous electrical activity of the cerebral cortex recorded through a series of scalp electrodes (Figure 26.2).

The potential differences (typically $20–200\,\mu V$) between pairs of electrodes or between each electrode and a common reference point are displayed continuously on up to 16 channels. The resulting output is usually described in terms of location, amplitude and frequency. EEG frequency is conventionally grouped into one of four bands: δ, θ, α and β (Figure 26.2). A normal awake adult has a posteriorly located, symmetrical EEG frequency of around $9\,Hz$ (i.e. α rhythm).

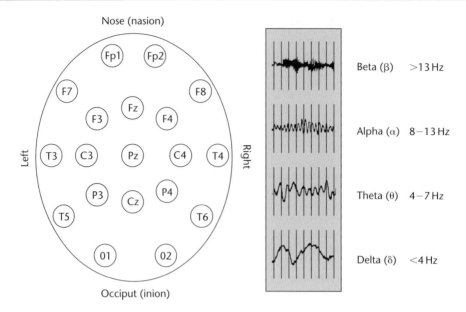

Figure 26.2 The international 10–20 system of EEG electrode placement. F, frontal; C, central; P, parietal; T, temporal; O, occipital. Right-sided placements are indicated by even numbers, left-sided placements by odd numbers and midline placements by Z.

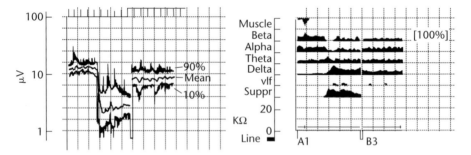

Figure 26.3 Typical CFAM tracing. The left trace displays the log-weighted-mean raw EEG amplitude distribution in μV, 10th and 90th centiles, and maximum and minimum amplitudes. The right trace displays electromyography (muscle), percentage α, β, θ, δ and very low frequency (vlf < 1 Hz) activity, percentage of suppression (Suppr < 1 μV peak to peak) and electrode impedance in kΩ.

Opioids and most anaesthetic agents produce dose-dependent EEG slowing (decreased α and increased δ and θ) culminating in periods of very low EEG amplitude – burst suppression. Nitrous oxide induces high-frequency frontal activity and decreased amplitude. Ketamine increases EEG amplitude at low doses, and slows the EEG at higher doses.

Cerebral hypoxia induces an acute increase in EEG amplitude followed by a reduction in both amplitude and frequency. Persistent EEG abnormalities may be predictive of adverse neurological outcome.

As the interpretation of continuous intraoperative multi-channel EEG monitoring is time consuming, a number of automated processed EEG systems

have been developed. In the cerebral function monitor (CFM), the EEG signal is filtered to remove low-frequency activity and rectified to produce a single trace representing EEG power varying with both amplitude and frequency. The cerebral function analysing monitor (CFAM) overcomes many of the shortcomings of CFM by displaying the signal amplitude and frequency separately (Figure 26.3). A further method of EEG processing is power spectrum analysis.

Evoked potentials

Sensory evoked potentials (SEPs) are the electrical responses of the CNS to peripheral stimulation.

Typically a stimulus is delivered at regular intervals and an averaged evoked response is extracted from background electrical activity. In clinical practice, the stimulus may be visual (VEP), auditory (AEP; Figure 26.4) or somatosensory (SSEP). In contrast, motor-evoked potential (MEP) monitoring employs transcutaneous, transcranial electrical stimulation of the motor cortex and measurement of the evoked electromyography. Use of the MEP technique is precluded by complete neuromuscular blockade.

Lower limb SSEPs, and more recently, MEPs have been used in spinal and major vascular surgery to monitor spinal cord function and prevent postoperative paraplegia.

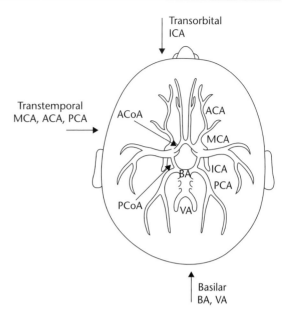

Figure 26.5 TCD ultrasound windows for examination of the basal cerebral arteries (the circle of Willis) – submandibular approach not shown. ACA, anterior cerebral artery; ACoA, anterior communicating artery; MCA, middle cerebral artery; ICA, internal carotid artery; PCoA, posterior communicating artery; BA, basilar artery; PCA, posterior cerebral artery and VA, vertebral arteries.

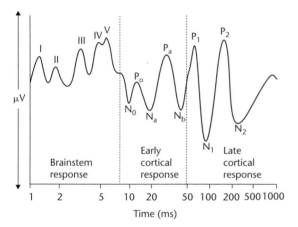

Figure 26.4 AEPs. An auditory stimulus or 'click' is repeated at regular intervals and signal averaging over several cycles used to extract the AEP from background EEG activity. Short-latency (<10 ms) brainstem auditory evoked responses (BAERs) reflect neural activity between the cochlear nucleus (I) and the inferior colliculus (V). BAERs unaffected by anaesthesia but are temperature sensitive making them useful for monitoring the effects of cooling and rewarming. Mid-latency (10–100 ms) AEPs represent cortical processing, which are necessary for awareness and recall of auditory events. Analysis of early cortical AEPs forms the basis of 'depth of anaesthesia' monitors such as the bispectral index (BIS) monitor.

Transcranial doppler

Although the intact adult skull is impervious to the transmission of conventional ultrasound (5–10 MHz), insonation of the basal cerebral arteries is possible using low-frequency ultrasound (2 MHz) directed through regions of the skull where bone is the thinnest (the temporal bones) or absent (the orbit and foramen magnum) (Figure 26.5). Thus, pulsed wave transcranial Doppler (TCD) provides a non-invasive means of

Table 26.2 Clinical applications of TCD

- Detection of cerebral embolism during carotid endarterectomy and cardiac surgery
- Detection of endoaortic balloon clamp migration during port access cardiac surgery
- Diagnosis of circulatory arrest in raised ICP
- Assessment of cerebral autoregulation
- Assessment of CBFV in migraine
- Detection and monitoring of post-subarachnoid haemorrhage vasospasm
- Haemodynamic assessment of vessels feeding arteriovenous malformations
- Assessment of vertebrobasilar insufficiency

measuring cerebral artery blood flow velocity (CBFV), an indirect measure of CBF (Figure 26.6).

Calculation of CBF velocity (CBFV) using the modified Doppler equation is as follows:

$$\text{CBFV} = \frac{c(F_S - F_T)}{2 F_T \cos \theta} \quad \begin{array}{c}\text{Gosling}\\ \text{index}\end{array} = \frac{V_{Sys} - V_{Dias}}{V_{Mean}}$$

where c is the speed of sound in human tissue $\approx$ 1540 m s^{-1}; F_S is the frequency of reflected sound;

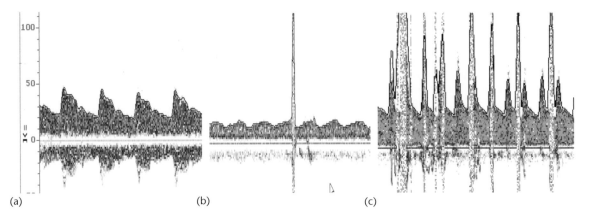

Figure 26.6 TCD examination of the MCA during CABG surgery; before (a), during (b) and immediately after (c) CPB. The high-amplitude signals (b and c) represent cerebral microemboli.

F_T, the frequency of transmitted sound – typically 2 MHz and θ, the angle of incidence or insonation angle. In the absence of vasospasm or vessel stenosis, the pulsatility or Gosling index is a reflection of cerebrovascular resistance, in which V_{Sys} is the systolic flow velocity; V_{Dias}, the diastolic flow velocity and V_{Mean}, the weighted mean flow velocity.

Near infrared spectroscopy

Cerebral near infrared spectroscopy (NIRS) provides a non-invasive means of estimating regional cortical cerebral oxygenation. The physical principles underlying NIRS are given as follows:

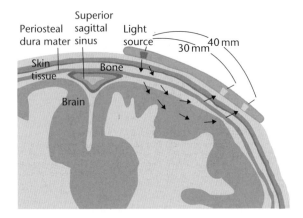

Figure 26.7 Cerebral NIRS. Courtesy of Somanetics Inc.

- Human tissue is relatively translucent to infrared (650–1100 nm) radiation.
- Light traversing the brain is both scattered and absorbed.
- Absorption of light by coloured substances (chromophores) is concentration dependent.
- Oxy-Hb (HbO$_2$) and deoxy-Hb (Hb) have different absorption spectra. The absorption of infrared light by HbO$_2$ and Hb is similar at 810 nm – the isobestic point:
  - Hb has greater absorption at shorter wavelengths,
  - HbO$_2$ has great absorption at longer wavelengths.

Devices for clinical use typically employ self-adhesive sensors, applied to the skin on the sides of the forehead, away from the midline, and a remote processing and display unit. Between 2 and 4 wavelengths of infrared light are generated by photodiodes, and light emerging from the scalp is detected by sensors known as optodes (Figure 26.7). The use of more than one optode allows a correction for the contribution made by blood in the scalp and skull such that around 85%

of the signal is from the brain. In contrast to conventional pulse oximetry, cerebral NIRS does not rely on the pulsatile component of the signal and can, therefore, be used during CPB and deep hypothermic circulatory arrest (DHCA).

In the setting of cardiac surgery, NIRS has been shown to be predictive of postoperative length of hospital stay and cognitive function test performance. In an animal model, cerebral NIRS appears to provide a monitor of safe DHCA duration.

Jugular venous oximetry

Jugular venous oximetry (S$_{JV}$O$_2$) is an invasive method of estimating the balance between global cerebral metabolism (CMRO$_2$) and cerebral oxygenation. The method is analogous to the use of mixed venous oximetry (S_VO_2) as a measure of whole-body oxygen consumption and the adequacy of the systemic circulation:

$$CMRO_2 \approx CBF \times (S_aO_2 - S_{JV}O_2)$$

Using the Seldinger technique, a retrograde catheter is inserted into the internal jugular vein and advanced cephalad into the jugular bulb at the base of the skull. A lateral radiograph of the neck is required to confirm correct catheter placement. $S_{JV}O_2$ can be measured intermittently by drawing serial blood samples for blood-gas analysis or continuously by using a fibreoptic catheter. The latter is prone to calibration drift. Normal values for $S_{JV}O_2$ are in the range of 60–75%.

Increased cerebral oxygen delivery or decreased $CMRO_2$ causes increased $S_{JV}O_2$, whereas decreased cerebral oxygen delivery or increased $CMRO_2$ decreases $S_{JV}O_2$ (Table 26.3).

In neurosurgical critical care, $S_{JV}O_2$ monitoring has been used to guide the management of raised ICP and cerebral hyperaemia. In the setting of head injury $S_{JV}O_2 < 50\%$ has been shown to be associated with a doubling of mortality.

In cardiac surgery, $S_{JV}O_2$ measurement may be particularly useful during CPB when systemic hypotension, cerebral hypoperfusion and anaemia may have a significant impact on cerebral oxygenation. Excessive and/or rapid rewarming may produce cerebral hyperthermia and reduced $S_{JV}O_2$. The magnitude of cerebral arteriovenous oxygen difference ($D_{AV}O_2$) during rewarming has been shown to correlate with cognitive dysfunction.

Multimodal monitoring

Although single-modality monitoring may produce useful information, it is possible that potentially adverse events may not be detected. Furthermore, observed changes may lead to a misinterpretation of events. By reducing the impact of the technical limitations and disadvantages of each individual monitor, multimodal monitoring offers improved detection of cerebral ischaemia permitting targeted intervention to reduce

Table 26.3 Common causes of changes in cerebral oxygen delivery and consumption ($CMRO_2$)

	O₂ Delivery	O₂ Consumption
↑	Hypercapnia	Hyperthermia
	Hypertension	Pain
	Gross hypoxia	Light anaesthesia
	Vasodilators	Seizures
	(e.g. isoflurane)	
↓	Hypocapnia	
	(<3.5 kPa)	
	Vasospasm	Drugs (e.g. thiopental)
	Hypotension	Stroke
	Low CO	Coma
	Hypoxia	Hypothermia
	Anaemia	Brain stem death

↑, increased; ↓ decreased.

Table 26.4 Multimodal neuromonitoring algorithm. Suggested responses to EEG slowing

Time	Temperature	MAP	CBFV	rCVOS	Problem (intervention)
Any	NC	NC	NC	↑	Anaesthesia-induced EEG depression (decreased depth anaesthetic)
Pre-CPB	NC	NC	↓ V_{Sys}	↓	Reposition aortic cannula
	NC	NC	↓ V_{Dias}	↓	Reposition venous cannula
Onset CPB	NC	NC	NC	↓	Acute haemodilution (no intervention)
On CPB	NC	NC	Emboli	↓	Neuroprotection protocol
	NC	↓	↓ V_{Mean}	↓	Dysautoregulation (increased MAP)
	↓	NC	↓ V_{Mean}	NC	Normal flow–metabolism coupling
	↑	NC	NC	↓	Flow–metabolism uncoupling (increased depth of anaesthesia)
Post-CPB	NC	NC	↓ V_{Dias}	↓	Cerebral oedema, obstructed cerebral microcirculation (neuroprotection protocol)

Adapted from Edmonds *et al.* (1996) and Austin *et al.* (1997). A neuroprotection protocol may include administration of thiopental, phenytoin, corticosteroids or a free-radical scavenger. rCVOS, regional cerebral oxygen saturation; NC, no change. VSys, systolic velocity; VDias, diastolic velocity; VMean, mean velocity.

neurological injury. A typical monitoring scheme will include both routine (i.e. MAP, CVP, temperature) and specialized (e.g. EEG, NIRS and TCD) measures.

With the exception of profound hypothermia, EEG slowing is the principle manifestation of cerebral ischaemia. For this reason EEG slowing is considered as a precondition for most intervention algorithms (Table 26.4).

Key points

- The risk of neurological injury is reduced by early detection and intervention.
- At normothermia, the EEG is a sensitive measure of cerebral ischaemia.
- TCD measures CBF velocity, not absolute CBF rate.

- NIRS monitoring during CABG surgery has been shown to be predictive of adverse outcome.
- Multimodal neuromonitoring has been shown to improve clinical outcome.

Further reading

Arrowsmith JE, Grocott HP, Newman MF. Neurologic risk assessment, monitoring and outcome in cardiac surgery. *J Cardiothorac Vasc Anesth* 1999; **13(6)**: 736–743.

Austin EH 3rd, Edmonds HL Jr., Auden SM, Seremet V, Niznik G, Sehic A *et al*. Benefit of neurophysiologic monitoring for pediatric cardiac surgery. *J Thorac Cardiovasc Surg* 1997; **114(5)**: 707–715.

Edmonds HL Jr. Advances in neuromonitoring for cardiothoracic and vascular surgery. *J Cardiothorac Vasc Anesth* 2001; **15(2)**: 241–250.

ROUTINE CORONARY HEART SURGERY

27 PREMEDICATION, INDUCTION AND MAINTENANCE

A.I. Gardner & P.R. Joshi

The aims of anaesthesia for cardiac surgery are: prevention of perioperative cardiac ischaemia, tight haemodynamic control, early extubation and avoidance of non-cardiac complications. The following description is only applicable to the low-risk, elective CABG surgery patient.

Preoperative visit

Preoperative assessment in the setting of a pre-admission clinic, allows the early identification of potential problems, alerts the transfusion service of likely demand and significantly reduces the likelihood of late cancellation. The principal objective of anaesthetic assessment is to gauge the patient's ability to withstand the intended surgical procedure. It also provides an opportunity to explain anaesthetic procedures, to obtain consent for specific interventions and to offer reassurance. The presence of previously documented symptoms and signs (see Chapter 15) should be verified, the results of preoperative investigations reviewed and any undiagnosed or new, intercurrent illness excluded. A more detailed discussion of the objective assessment of operative risk can be found in Chapter 18. The main determinants of risk are summarized below:

- Patient age
- Gender
- LV function
- Urgency of surgery
- Previous cardiac surgery
- Combined procedures
- Coronary arterial anatomy
- Valvular pathology

In addition to a routine preoperative history and examination, specific areas of interest include:

- *Intended conduit harvest sites* may restrict placement of monitors and cannulae.
- *Recent history of anticoagulant use* e.g. aspirin, clopidogrel, heparin and warfarin.
- *Permanent pacemaker (PPM)/implantable cardiodefibrillator (ICD)* may need reprogramming before induction of anaesthesia.
- *Presence of oesophageal pathology* contraindicates TOE.

Preoperatively the patient's regular anti-anginal, anti-hypertensive and anti-cardiac failure medications should be continued (Table 27.1). Ideally antiplatelet medications, which act irreversibly on platelets should be discontinued at such time before surgery to allow a return to normal or near normal platelet function.

Premedication

Sedative premedication reduces anxiety, may induce a degree of amnesia and probably reduces the risk of ischaemia (secondary to hypertension and tachycardia)

Table 27.1 A guide to which regular medications should be taken until the morning of surgery

Continue	Controversial	Discontinue
β-blockers	ACE inhibitors	Diuretics
Nitrates		Oral hypoglycaemics
Calcium antagonists		Aspirin
K$^+$-channel openers		NSAIDs
Corticosteroids		MAO inhibitors
Antidysrhythmics		Antiplatelet medications
Bronchodilators		

In some units, for simplicity, all cardiac medications are continued until the time of surgery. MAO, monoamine oxidase.

Table 27.2 Examples of premedication for adult cardiac surgical patients

Intramuscular
Morphine sulphate 0.2–0.3 mg kg^{-1}
Hyoscine hydrobromide 200–400 µg   45–60 min before induction of anaesthesia

Oral
Lorazepam 2–4 mg   90–120 min before induction of anaesthesia

during induction. Although opioids, benzodiazepines and antihistamines are commonly prescribed, the precise choice of agent(s) is subject to institutional variability. The use of longer acting drugs, such as morphine and lorazepam, has remained popular. As respiratory depression is a common sequel of sedative premedication, supplemental oxygen should be prescribed with other premedicant drugs and administered until induction of anaesthesia (Table 27.2).

Preparation

Drugs, which should be immediately available, include: inotropes, antidysrhythmics, calcium, potassium, magnesium, heparin and protamine.

Equipment
- Anaesthetic machine
- Monitoring (transducers, TOE)
- Infusion pumps and transfusion apparatus
- Laryngoscopes and intubation aids
- Suction apparatus
- Arterial and venous cannulae
- Defibrillator

Drugs to be drawn up
Anaesthetic
- Local anaesthetic (lidocaine)
- Analgesic (fentanyl, remifentanil, sufentanil)
- Muscle relaxant (pancuronium, rocuronium)
- Induction agent (etomidate, propofol, midazolam)

Cardiac
- Vagolytic (atropine)
- Vasopressor (metaraminol, phenylephrine)
- Vasodilator (GTN, SNP)

Other
- IV fluids
- Prophylactic antibiotics
- Anticoagulant (heparin)
- Antifibrinolytic (tranexamic acid)/aprotinin

Anaesthetic/operating room

On arrival the patient's identity should be verified and consent for surgery confirmed. The availability of cross-matched blood should be checked. The operative site should be clearly marked if appropriate (e.g. thoracotomy, radial artery harvest site). Non-invasive monitoring (ECG, NIBP and pulse oximetry) is then commenced.

Vascular access and monitoring

Cannulae are sited with local anaesthesia in a forearm vein (14G) and the non-dominant radial artery (20G). In the case of non-dominant radial artery harvest, either the dominant radial artery or femoral artery should be cannulated. An IV infusion is commenced, and arterial pressure transduced. Femoral arterial pressure monitoring is used when both radial arteries are required for conduits. Insertion of central (i.e. internal jugular or subclavian) venous catheters may then be undertaken, however, in many centres this is left until after induction of anaesthesia. The use of a PAFC in low-risk cases adds little to management.

Induction

In many centres, induction of anaesthesia takes place in a separate anaesthetic room. The benefits of a quiet environment and reduced 'turnover' time have to be balanced against the risk of cardiovascular collapse requiring urgent CPB.

Many techniques have been described for the induction and maintenance of anaesthesia for cardiac surgery. There is no ideal single agent and there is no place for a 'mono-agent' technique.

Ideal cardiac anaesthetic agent should have:

- unaltered haemodynamics,
- lack of myocardial depression,
- lack of coronary vasoconstriction,
- no coronary steal,
- residual analgesia,
- easy to titrate to effect,
- rapid onset and offset.

Following a period of preoxygenation, balanced anaesthesia is induced with a combination of an induction agent, an opioid and a neuromuscular blocker. Contrary to traditional teaching, the muscle relaxant should

Table 27.3 Drugs for induction of anaesthesia

	Most commonly used	Alternatives
Induction agents	Etomidate 0.15–0.30 mg kg^{-1}	Thiopental 3–4 mg kg^{-1} Midazolam 0.05–0.10 mg kg^{-1} Propofol 1.0–1.5 mg kg^{-1}
Opioids	Fentanyl 5–10 μg kg^{-1}	Sufentanil 0.5–1.0 μg kg^{-1} Remifentanil 0.5–1.0 μg kg^{-1}
Neuromuscular blockers	Pancuronium 0.10–0.15 mg kg^{-1}	Vecuronium 0.1 mg kg^{-1}

Table 27.4 Procedures following anaesthetic induction

Tracheal intubation	Securing tube on left side of mouth allows easier insertion of TOE probe.
Mechanical ventilation	Tidal volume ~7–10 ml kg^{-1}.
F$_I$O$_2$ of 0.6 in air	Although theoretically possible to use N$_2$O in early pre-CPB period, failure to switch to air could increase risk of air embolus. Most anaesthetists avoid N$_2$O.
Maintain anaesthesia	Volatile or IV agent(s).
Secure additional vascular access	Central venous – if not undertaken prior to induction. Use short internal jugular lines ~10–12 cm or do not insert >12 cm into patient.
Urinary catheterization	A suprapubic catheter may be inserted at end of case and before transfer to ICU if transurethral catheterization is not possible.
Antibiotics prophylaxis	Dictated by local protocols.
Patient protection	Eyes closed and taped. Heels padded. Knees slightly flexed. Protect ulnar and radial nerve pressure points.
Temperature monitor	Nasopharyngeal/rectal/bladder.
TOE probe	Easier to insert before the patient is prepared and draped for surgery.
Gastric tube	NG/orogastric tube used in some centres to reduce PONV.
Confirm patency of peripheral lines	Peripheral and central venous lines should run freely. Arterial line should aspirate easily.

be given early to prevent opioid-induced coughing or chest wall rigidity. Drugs for induction of anaesthesia and the procedures following induction are given in Tables 27.3 and 27.4.

Transfer to operating room

When an anaesthetic room has been used for induction it is necessary to transfer the patient to the operating room. Although this procedure has the potential for complications (e.g. accidental removal of vascular lines and even the ETT), observing simple precautions can minimize them.

On arrival in the operating room, the patient should first be re-connected to the ventilator, the capnograph, pulse oximeter and ECG. A temperature probe should be inserted. Monitoring transducers are then re-connected and re-zeroed. Venous lines are checked for patency and access to three-way taps confirmed *before* the patient is prepared and draped for surgery. To avoid inadvertent intra-arterial drug administration, it is essential that arterial and venous injection ports are physically separated and clearly labelled. In many centres the arterial port is placed to the left of the patient's head and venous ports to the right.

Drug infusion lines should be checked and correct functioning of infusion pumps should be confirmed. The IV agents are commonly used to maintain anaesthesia but take time to achieve a steady-state concentration. Some anaesthetists find it convenient to use a volatile agent (0.5–1.0 MAC) and delay starting an infusion until arrival in the operating room.

Anaesthetic check list prior to start of surgery

Ventilation
Zero monitoring lines
The Five 'A's
  Access
  Anaesthesia
  Arterial gas
  ACT
  Antibiotics
Check cross-matched blood

Surgical stimulation	
High	**Low**
Laryngoscopy	Post intubation
Tracheal intubation	Preparing and draping
Skin incision	Surgical 'delays'
Sternotomy	Internal mammary artery harvesting
Sternal retraction	
Sternal elevation	

Anaesthetic management needs to take into account the wide variation in surgical stimuli in the pre-CPB period.

Before treating hypertension with vasodilators (e.g. GTN, SNP, phentolamine, K^+ and Mg^{2+}), adequate depth of anaesthesia should be ensured. A supplemental dose of opioid is frequently administered a few minutes before sternotomy. The harvest of bypass graft conduits may result in significant concealed haemorrhage; therefore blood volume status should be assessed before treating hypotension with a vasoconstrictor. When transducers are fixed to the operating table, the influence of lateral table tilt (i.e. the height of the transducers in relation to the patient's RA) must be taken into account before acting on changes in MAP or CVP.

The ECG, and TOE if present, should be monitored closely for evidence of myocardial ischaemia. The use of surgical retractors and retrocardiac swabs may make ECG interpretation difficult. The surgeon should be alerted if there is doubt about the presence of ischaemic changes. Attempts may be made to treat these changes pharmacologically with systemic administration of GTN or a β-blocker. CPB should be instituted if ischaemic changes persist or circulatory collapse ensues. Completion of conduit harvesting then takes place during 'non-ischaemic' CPB – i.e. prior to AXC placement.

Following pericardotomy, the anaesthetist should observe the heart to gain an appreciation of its size, filling and contractility. Elevation of the legs during skin preparation may significantly increase preload. This may be beneficial in the hypovolaemic patient or detrimental when LV function is already on the 'flat' part of the Frank–Starling curve. Fluid administration is guided by MAP, CVP and TOE findings. There appears to be little to choose between crystalloid and colloid solutions, although glucose-containing solutions are best avoided. Cardio-vascular collapse due to severe colloid allergy, which is likely to be indistinguishable from other causes of hypotension, is fortunately rare.

Key points

- The goals of cardiac anaesthesia are tight haemodynamic control and avoidance of perioperative cardiac ischaemia.
- Supplemental oxygen should be administered to the patient when sedative premedication is used.
- Good communication between anaesthetist, surgeon and perfusionist is vital for safe transition to and separation from CPB.

S.J. Gray & D. Gifford

Preparation

The CPB system is assembled, primed and tested before the patient is anaesthetized. Disposable CPB systems are supplied 'closed' (i.e. with arterial and venous lines in continuity) to preserve sterility, and to allow circulation of prime before connection to the patient. During closed circulation, the prime is filtered, to remove bubbles and particulate matter, and warmed to 37°C. An adult CPB system typically requires a 1400–2000 ml prime, consisting of crystalloid, colloid and/or blood, in addition to heparin, calcium and mannitol. The precise 'recipe' varies from institution to institution and is, in part, patient dependent.

It is essential for the perfusionist to note the patient's height, weight and haematocrit. This allows the calculation of 'safe' pump flows based on body surface area and the potential requirement for packed red cells based on the predicted initial haematocrit on CPB.

Clear and unambiguous communication between perfusionist, anaesthetist and surgeon is of paramount importance in the safe conduct of CPB.

Anticoagulation

Adequate systemic anticoagulation, usually with unfractionated heparin, is an absolute requirement for CPB. Anticoagulation usually precedes or accompanies cannulation of the patient, but the precise timing is subject to considerable variation. The advantages of early heparinization (i.e. salvage of blood lost during mammary artery harvesting and readiness for urgent CPB) have to be balanced against the disadvantages (i.e. increased haemorrhage from all operating sites). A heparin dose of 300 units kg^{-1} (3 mg kg^{-1}) is usually sufficient. An objective measure of the adequacy of anticoagulation must be achieved before the onset of cardiotomy suction or CPB. For this reason, a point-of-care anticoagulation monitor, such as a Hemochron-activated clotting time monitor, is mandatory. A normal celite-ACT is in the order of 100–130 s. An ACT >300 s is required for use of cardiotomy suckers

and >400 s for institution of CPB. Heparin resistance and heparin alternatives are discussed elsewhere.

In many centres, a lysine analogue (e.g. tranexamic acid) or aprotinin is used to reduce perioperative blood loss and transfusion requirements. It is recommended that lysine analogues be administered *after* heparinization. As aprotinin prolongs the celite-ACT, a heparin dose of 500 units kg^{-1} and a celite-ACT >700 is recommended for CPB.

If nitrous oxide has been used, it should be discontinued prior to the onset of CPB. Due to the risk of air embolism during cannulation and the first few minutes of CPB, some anaesthetists routinely switch to 100% oxygen following heparinization.

Connection

Cannulation of the ascending aorta, or occasionally a femoral artery, is almost always performed first. Excessive hypertension (MAP >80 mmHg) should be avoided during this procedure to reduce the risk of localized arterial dissection. The connection between the arterial and venous lines is then cut and the former attached to the arterial cannula in such a way as to exclude air. Correct positioning of the cannula is confirmed by the presence of a pulsatile blood–prime interface in the cannula and by reference to the arterial line pressure monitor.

RA cannulation may be accompanied by haemodynamic instability secondary to atrial dysrhythmia, impeded venous return and/or haemorrhage. For this reason, and because of the relative ease of fluid administration via the arterial cannula, venous cannulation invariably follows arterial cannulation.

Onset

Gradually releasing the venous line clamp – diverting venous blood into the venous reservoir – initiates CPB. The speed of the pump is gradually increased to achieve a flow rate of 2.2–2.4 $1 min^{-1} m^{-2}$. Ventilation of the lungs is discontinued when full CPB has been established.

Table 28.1 'AVID' – key considerations at the onset of CPB

A Arterial inflow	
Arterial blood oxygenated?	Colour/oximetry
Arterial cannula malposition?	Unilateral facial oedema and anisocoria
	High arterial line pressure
Evidence of aortic dissection?	High arterial line pressure
	↓ Reservoir level
	↑ or ↓ radial artery pressure
	Inability to arrest heart with antegrade cardioplegia
V Venous inflow	
Venous drainage good?	Reservoir level maintained
	Right atrium not distended and ↓ CVP
Evidence of SVC obstruction?	Heart rotated about base for surgical access, ↑ CVP
	Facial engorgement or conjunctival oedema
I Incomplete bypass	
Evidence of incomplete CPB?	Pulsatile arterial and PA pressures
	↓ Venous drainage
	Aortic insufficiency
	Considerable bronchial venous flow
	Target pump flow not reached
D Drugs	Reduce or discontinue vasoactive drug administration
	Discontinue ventilation

Acute haemodilution produces an abrupt fall in blood viscosity and SVR. Consequently, transient hypotension (MAP: 30–40 mmHg) at the onset of CPB is common and usually responds to vasoconstrictors. The mnemonic 'AVID' addresses some of the key issues to be considered upon initiation of CPB (Table 28.1).

Perfusion

Despite considerable research, the characteristics of optimal CPB are yet to be defined. Areas of controversy – including flow rate, perfusion pressure, flow pulsatility, acid–base management and temperature – are discussed in Chapter 49. As oxygen consumption decreases exponentially (~7% per °C), pump flow is usually reduced during hypothermic CPB. The most commonly used indices (Table 28.2) of the adequacy of CPB are SvO_2 and ABGs (PO_2, PCO_2 and pH). Arterial

Table 28.2 Physiological considerations during CPB

Mean arterial pressure	50–70 mmHg
Central venous pressure	0–5 mmHg
Arterial blood gases	Alpha stat preferred
Mixed venous O_2 saturation	>65%
Haematocrit	>20–25%

blood is drawn every 30 min for blood gas analysis and measurement of K^+, haematocrit and glucose.

Anaesthesia

At the onset of CPB – when circulating drugs are subject to haemodilution, altered protein binding and sequestration – there is a risk of inadequate anaesthesia, or even awareness. In practice, however, drugs administered prior to sternotomy and sternal retraction, coupled with an inevitable degree of hypothermia (~35°C), make this unlikely.

Where anaesthesia is maintained by continuous infusion (e.g. propofol $4 \, mg \, kg^{-1} hr^{-1}$), the rate of administration is typically left unaltered. The exclusion of the lungs from the circulation requires that the responsibility for inhalational agent administration be transferred to the perfusionist during CPB. Failure to maintain inhalational anaesthesia during and after CPB may lead to inadequate anaesthesia.

Cardioplegia

Depending on institutional practice, either the perfusionist or the anaesthetist may be responsible for the delivery of cardioplegic solutions. Crystalloid cardioplegia can be prepared before the onset of CPB. In contrast, blood cardioplegia cannot be prepared until after the onset of CPB because it requires the addition of heparinized blood to a crystalloid base solution. Cardioplegic solutions must be free of air and particulate matter. The principles underlying cardioplegia are discussed in Chapter 20.

Rewarming

Restoration of normothermia is achieved by the heat exchanger, which warms blood returning to the patient. Rewarming should be a gradual process to avoid excessive thermal gradients, incomplete thermal equilibration and neurological injury. Excessively rapid blood rewarming denatures plasma proteins and may induce bubble formation. Despite its accuracy, nasopharyngeal temperature monitoring may underestimate cerebral venous temperature by up to 3.4°C when rewarming is very rapid. As little as 0.5°C hyperthermia may exacerbate ischaemic CNS injury. Conversely, inadequate rewarming combined with further heat loss during chest closure, results in shivering, vasoconstriction, increased oxygen consumption (VO_2) and coagulopathy. In practice the difference between arterial inflow and nasopharyngeal temperature should be <4.0°C, and venous SO_2 should be >65% during rewarming.

De-airing

Removal of intracardiac air following CABG surgery is usually only necessary when an open-heart (e.g. LV aneurysmectomy or valve surgery) procedure has been performed concurrently. Air is typically expelled via a ventriculotomy or proximal aortotomy. In both cases the lungs are ventilated, to expel air from the pulmonary circulation, and the patient positioned to ensure that the venting site is superior. Transventricular de-airing is performed in the Trendelenberg position, whereas de-airing via the ascending aorta is performed in the supine position. Confirmation of the adequacy of deairing is greatly assisted by TOE.

Defibrillation

VF frequently accompanies rewarming and coronary reperfusion following removal of the AXC. Prolonged VF with LV distension must be avoided as the increase in myocardial oxygen consumption may cause subendocardial ischaemia. Defibrillation is usually achieved with a 10–20 J monophasic (or 4–10 J biphasic) shock delivered by internal 'paddles'.

Cardiac pacing

Temporary pacing is established by suturing-coated steel wires onto the epicardium, which are tunnelled through the chest wall and connected by reusable cables to either a single or dual-chamber pacemaker device. The small risk of cardiac damage during insertion, and haemorrhage following removal have to be balanced against the potential therapeutic benefit. The perception of this balance is subject to considerable inter-surgeon variation, with some using atrial and ventricular wires in all cases, and others reserving them for high-risk cases. Generally speaking, the placement of pacing wires may be omitted in low-risk cases (i.e. uncomplicated CABG with HR >70 that responds to atropine). Atrial wires may be considered redundant in patients with chronic AF.

In the operating theatre environment, fixed-rate, dual-chamber pacing (i.e. 'DOO', rate 80–100, AV delay 120–150 ms) is the mode of choice as it is insensitive to diathermy radiofrequency interference. The atrial and ventricular pacing voltages should be high enough to ensure reliable capture. An excessively high atrial pacing voltage may produce simultaneous ventricular activation and impeded diastolic filling (*cv*-waves on CVP trace and arterial hypotension). Similarly, incorrect connection of the pacing cable to the pacemaker may also have unexpected and unwanted effects.

Offset

Before weaning the patient from CPB, the operating table should be levelled and all pressure transducers re-zeroed. Upon restarting mechanical ventilation the venous return to the pump is gradually occluded and optimal cardiac filling achieved by gentle transfusion from the reservoir. The mnemonic TRAVVEL provides a useful checklist prior to terminating CPB (Table 28.3).

Decannulation

Following termination of CPB, the venous cannula and vents are removed. Before giving protamine, any residual pericardial or pleural blood is returned to the venous reservoir and cardiotomy suction discontinued thereafter. After alerting the perfusionist, a test-dose of protamine (10–20 mg) is then given and the patient observed for 1–2 min. If no major adverse haemodynamic instability occurs, the remainder of the dose (~1.0 mg for each 100 units of heparin given) is then administered over 2–5 min. Mild protamine-induced hypotension is common and generally responds to transfusing blood from the venous reservoir via the

Table 28.3 The TRAVVEL checklist for termination of CPB

T	Temperature	Nasopharyngeal 36–37°C
R	Rate	Stable cardiac rate and rhythm
		Epicardial pacing may be required
A	Air	Techniques to remove intracardiac air
		TOE may be used to confirm adequacy
V	Venting	Venting lines either clamped or removed before coming off bypass
V	Ventilation	Mechanical ventilation restarted
		Left lower lobe expansion visually confirmed (if pleura open)
E	Electrolytes	Normalize metabolic indices
		Base excess $< -5\,mmol\,l^{-1}$, $Po_2 > 10\,kPa$, $Pco_2 \sim 5\,kPa$
		Haematocrit $> 20\%$, $K^+ > 4.5\,mmol\,l^{-1}$
L	Level	Operating table

aortic cannula. Following removal of the aortic cannula, the anaesthetist assumes sole responsibility for fluid administration. In some centres, where the aortic cannula is removed shortly after administration of the protamine test-dose, the anaesthetist must be prepared to respond rapidly to profound hypotension. In many centres any blood remaining in the CPB system is drained and returned to the patient. Both the anaesthetist and surgeon must agree to this, as subsequent reinstitution of CPB is made more difficult.

Haemostasis

The adequacy of heparin reversal should be confirmed by ACT measurement. Further arterial blood analysis is undertaken to assess oxygenation, ventilation, haematocrit and K^+. Closure of the pericardium or sternum may be accompanied by haemodynamic instability. Chest reopening may be required if 'tamponade' or graft kinking occurs.

As surgery draws to an end, preparations for transfer to the ICU should be made. The airway, vascular lines, pacing wires, catheters and surgical drains should be protected when moving the patient from the operating table. As hypotension and dysrhythmias may occur, the patient should be monitored throughout transfer. Occasionally a coronary air embolus may induce severe

hypotension or VF. Deferring transfer should be considered when MAP $<60\,mmHg$. An additional supply of oxygen, ventilation apparatus, IV fluids and emergency drugs should be immediately available.

Key points

- Clear and unambiguous communication between anaesthetist, perfusionist and surgeon are essential to safe CPB conduct.
- Excessive hypertension should be avoided during aortic cannulation.
- Confirmation of adequate anticoagulation must be obtained before the use of cardiotomy suction.
- Pump flows are based on patient's body surface area and temperature.

Further reading

Cook DJ, Orszulak TA, Daly RC, Buda DA. Cerebral hyperthermia during cardiopulmonary bypass in adults. *J Thorac Cardiovasc Surg* 1996; **111**(1): 268–269.

Grocott HP, Newman MF, Croughwell ND, White WD, Lowry E, Reves JG. Continuous jugular venous versus nasopharyngeal temperature monitoring during hypothermic cardiopulmonary bypass for cardiac surgery. *J Clin Anesth* 1997; **9**(4): 312–316.

ROUTINE EARLY POSTOPERATIVE CARE 29

M. Screaton

The high volume and repetitive nature of cardiothoracic surgical critical care has meant that in many centres nursing staff have taken over much of the routine postoperative care previously undertaken by medical staff. The use of *critical care pathways* and protocols allows senior nurses to manage uncomplicated cases relatively independently with medical staff only being consulted when patient progress deviates from a clearly defined pathway. Since new members of the medical staff may not be accustomed to this style of patient care, it is essential that they read and *understand* the protocols, appreciate the indications for medical referral and be aware of management steps prior to referral. Medical staff without previous cardiothoracic ICU experience should be guided through several straightforward cases in order to understand the key principles.

ICU admission

ICU should ideally be located adjacent to and on the same floor level as the operating theatre. Invasive monitoring should be continued throughout transfer from the operating theatre to the ICU.

Priorities on arrival are:
Capnography
Invasive monitoring
Oximetry
ECG
Pacing

It is essential that all relevant patient, anaesthetic and intraoperative details are clearly conveyed to the admitting nurse:

- *Patient details*
  - Name, age and preoperative risk factors.
  - Allergies/drug sensitivities.
- *Surgical*
  - Planned and actual surgical procedure performed.
  - Complications and other significant events.
  - Ease of weaning from CPB.
  - Optimal cardiac filling pressures in theatre.
  - Haemodynamic support – vasoactive drugs, pacing and IABP.
- *Anaesthetic*
  - Vascular line types and insertion sites.

- Laryngoscopy grade – if difficult intubation.
- Current drug infusions and administration rates.
- Blood products used (and ordered for later administration).
- Fluids administered, use of haemofiltration and urine output.
- Post-CPB blood gases, ACT, glucose, K^+ and haematocrit.
- Pending laboratory investigations.
- *Patient-specific ICU goals*
  - Acceptable ranges for MAP, CVP, (LAP, PAWP and CO).
  - Expected duration of sedation and mechanical ventilation.
- *Investigations*
  - A baseline CXR is routinely undertaken in some centres to check lines and ETT positions.

Sedation and ventilation

Although it may be possible to extubate patients in theatre, most consider that the risks of bleeding, haemodynamic instability and hypothermia outweigh any potential benefits. Simple volume controlled ventilation is adequate for the majority of patients using 10 breaths per minute, a tidal volume of 7–$10\,ml\,kg^{-1}$ and 60% oxygen. ABG analysis is used to guide changes in ventilator settings to maintain $Po_2 > 10\,kPa$ and $Pco_2 \sim 5\,kPa$. Sedation and mechanical ventilation are usually continued for 2–4 h in order to allow rewarming and exclude significant bleeding.

Criteria for patient extubation by nurse:	
Airway	Ability to protect airway; easy intubation
Breathing	Adequate ventilation and oxygenation
Circulation	Haemodynamic stability
Metabolic	Base deficit $<5\,mmol\,l^{-1}$
CNS	Appropriate

Analgesia

Median sternotomy is associated with moderate to severe postoperative pain. Effective postoperative analgesia reduces pain on movement and deep inspiration, facilitating early weaning from mechanical ventilation. In most centres IV morphine is the analgesic of choice. Although NSAIDs are effective, they should be used with caution in patients with a coagulopathy or impaired renal function. The use of epidural analgesia is discussed in Chapter 60.

Haemodynamic goals

The maintenance of adequate systemic perfusion is vital to the preservation of cerebral, myocardial and visceral function.

HR	Usually 60–100 bpm
Rhythm	Preserve sinus rhythm
MAP	60–80 mmHg
CVP	6–10 mmHg (on IPPV)
Perfusion	Good peripheral perfusion
Urine output	$>0.5\,ml\,kg^{-1}h^{-1}$

Common early postoperative haemodynamic problems include: hypertension, hypotension, tachycardia and bradycardia.

Hypertension

Pain, hypoventilation and intolerance of ETT may all cause hypertension. Treatment should be directed at the underlying cause. If hypertension persists despite good analgesia, adequately ventilation, resedation or extubation, a vasodilator for example, SNP or GTN should be used.

Hypotension

Reductions in preload, contractility and afterload may contribute to hypotension. Most commonly hypotension is caused by hypovolaemia secondary to urinary loss, haemorrhage and peripheral vasodilation. Hypotension that does not respond to a colloid challenge (200–400 ml) is an indication for additional support. Temporary pacing should be optimized before instituting inotropic therapy. If possible, haemodynamically unstable tachydysrhythmias should be converted pharmacologically or electrically. Further investigation with a chest radiograph (to exclude covert haemorrhage), a PAFC or TOE is indicated in patients with refractory hypotension.

Tachycardia

Possible causes include pain, hypovolaemia, inotropic/chronotropic therapy and tamponade. The diagnosis of tamponade is discussed in more detail in Chapter 52.

Bradycardia

Epicardial pacing wires allow rapid treatment of bradycardias. In the absence of AF, atrial (AAI) pacing is

preferable to ventricular (VVI) pacing because of the contribution of atrial systole to CO. Dual chamber (DDD) pacing is required if A-V conduction is impaired.

Communication

The day of surgery is understandably very stressful for relatives. It is courteous and good practice for medical or nursing staff to contact relatives by telephone within the first hour of ICU admission to give a brief report. Relatives should be encouraged to telephone or visit thereafter.

Haemorrhage

Bleeding is an inevitable consequence of cardiac surgery. Excessive postoperative bleeding, however, is associated with increased morbidity and mortality. Bleeding, which may be overt or covert, is frequently described as being 'surgical' (i.e. from a blood vessel), 'anaesthetic' (i.e. coagulopathic) or both! Overt blood loss through mediastinal and pleural drains is relatively easy to diagnose, whereas a diagnosis of covert haemorrhage requires a high degree of clinical suspicion.

Time (h)	Acceptable blood loss $(ml\,kg^{-1}h^{-1})$
1	3
2–4	2
5–12	1

In an effort to identify patients requiring surgical re-exploration earlier, some units use a blood loss nomogram. This method allows better visualization of bleeding trends and a comparison with other patients operated on at the same institution. Re-exploration must be considered if haemorrhage exceeds the 95th centile for two successive hours (Figure 29.1).

The development of algorithms for the investigation and management of excessive postoperative bleeding can help decision-making.

Fluid balance

Fluid intake (crystalloid and colloid), urine output and chest tube drainage are recorded hourly. Following CPB, most patients are in positive crystalloid balance. Total crystalloid intake (oral and IV is restricted to $750\,ml\,m^2$ in the first 24h and $1000\,ml\,m^2\,day^{-1}$ thereafter. Colloid (e.g. hydroxyethyl starch, succinylated gelatin and blood) is given when the patient has low MAP with low CVP or oliguria.

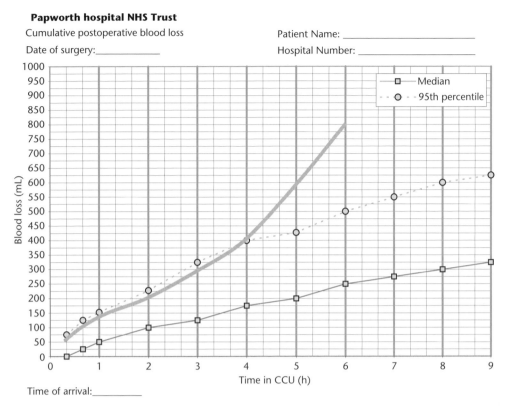

Figure 29.1 The Papworth critical care unit (CCU) postoperative blood loss chart. The median and 95th percentile ICU blood loss is plotted against time. In the example shown, an abrupt increase in the expected rate of bleeding for two consecutive hours should prompt surgical re-exploration. (Courtesy of C Gerrard and A Vuylsteke, ICU, Papworth hospital).

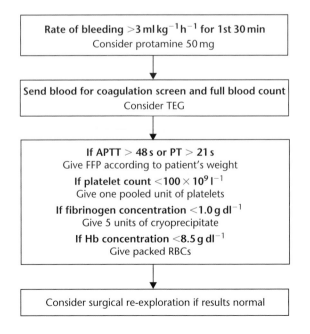

Serum potassium concentration should be maintained between 4.5 and 5.5 mmol l^{-1}. Hypokalaemia is common for several reasons – preoperative diuretic therapy, haemodilution, the humoral response to surgery, catecholamine use and significant post-CPB diuresis. Hypokalaemia is associated with dysrhythmias and must be aggressively corrected. If [K$^+$] < 4.5 mmol l^{-1}, 10 mmol KCl is given via the central venous line over 10 min, whereas if [K$^+$] < 4.0 mmol l^{-1}, 20 mmol KCl is given over 20 min.

Hyperkalaemia is less common in the early postoperative period. No action is required if [K$^+$] < 6.5 mmol l^{-1}. In the absence of cardiac dysfunction a [K$^+$] > 6.5 mmol l^{-1} may be treated with a loop diuretic (e.g. frusemide 20 mg) or a dextrose (25 g) and insulin (15 units) infusion. Intravenous calcium (CaCl$_2$: 10 mmol) may be considered in the presence of cardiac dysfunction.

Oliguria

Oliguria is defined as a urine output <0.5 ml $kg^{-1}h^{-1}$ for two consecutive hours and may have a pre-renal, renal or post-renal cause. Anuria is unusual and may indicate a blocked urinary catheter. Before intervening the patient's chart should be reviewed to establish the normal preoperative BP and to exclude reduced renal perfusion pressure (i.e. MAP–CVP). An incorrectly positioned IABP may cause renal artery occlusion.

Fluid challenge
250 ml over 10 min
Repeated if rise in CVP not sustained after 30 min

Diuretic
e.g. frusemide 20 mg or mannitol 0.25 g kg^{-1}

Increase MAP/CO
Consider pacing
Inotrope e.g. dopamine 2–5 μg kg^{-1} min^{-1}

Metabolic acidosis

Mild metabolic acidosis is common following cardiac surgery. In the absence of significant renal impairment, a persistent acidosis may indicate inadequate CO and visceral ischaemia. Since the base deficit is a useful 'barometer' of the effectiveness of treatment, bicarbonate should not be administered unless there is evidence of end-organ dysfunction (i.e. myocardial depression).

Gastrointestinal problems

Abdominal distension with absent bowel sounds, nausea and vomiting are relatively common. Although NG tubes are used routinely in some centres, their use may increase the risk of nosocomial respiratory tract infection. The presence of a gastric bubble on a CXR should prompt insertion of a NG tube. Nausea and vomiting may be treated with phenothiazines (e.g. prochlorperazine), or serotonin antagonists (e.g. ondansetron).

Failed extubation

Failure to maintain adequate ventilation and/or gas exchange after tracheal extubation is rare. Reintubation and reinstitution of ventilation should be considered in the presence of significant bleeding, neurological impairment or worsening haemodynamic instability. Although a review of the anaesthetic record may predict an easy reintubation, it should be remembered that vocal cord or glottic oedema might make intubation more difficult. In most cases early, elective intervention is preferable to an emergency reintubation following cardiorespiratory collapse.

The essential requirements for reintubation are:

Skilled assistance
Full haemodynamic monitoring
Laryngoscopes, ETTs
Intubation aids
Suction apparatus
Functioning capnograph
Induction agent and muscle relaxant
Vasopressor and other emergency drugs
Colloid solution
Sedative drug infusion(s)

First postoperative day

Timing of chest drain removal is a surgical decision. The drains are usually removed when there is no air leak and residual drainage is <25 ml h^{-1} for two consecutive hours.

The arterial line is removed before the patient is transferred to the ward, although it may be retained if the patient is being transferred to a stepdown or high-dependency area.

Epicardial pacing wires are usually left *in situ* even if the drains are taken out. They are normally removed on the 5th or 6th postoperative day.

The central venous line is retained and any lumen not in use should be flushed with heparinized saline and capped. It is usually removed on the 3rd or 4th postoperative day. The pharmacological treatment of tachydysrhythmias (e.g. AF) is greatly facilitated if the line is not removed too early.

The urinary catheter is retained for at least 2 days. Accurate fluid balance is essential as oliguria frequently precedes postoperative complications.

Key points

- Problems in the early postoperative period are common – most can be effectively managed by the application of locally developed protocols.
- Demand (rather than fixed-rate) pacing should be used to reduce the risk of VF.
- Maintain a high index of suspicion for covert bleeding and tamponade.
- Good communication between anaesthetists, intensivists, surgeons and nursing staff is fundamental.

I.M. Davies & A.T. Lovell

History

Initial attempts at coronary artery surgery involved intricate surgery on a moving heart in a bloody operative field. The introduction of CPB and cardioplegic arrest effectively relegated beating-heart surgery to centres unable to afford the costs associated with CPB. In time, the suspicion that many of the complications of cardiac surgery were secondary to CPB led to the 'rediscovery' of beating-heart CABG surgery. Re-evaluation of the technique and the development of cardiac stabilization devices, retractors and intracoronary shunts have facilitated widespread uptake of off-pump coronary artery bypass (OPCAB). In essence cardiac surgical practice has come full circle (Figure 30.1).

Initially OPCAB was practised only by enthusiasts and restricted to low-risk patients requiring one or two bypass grafts on the anterior cardiac surface. The demonstration that OPCAB is both safe and efficacious in high-risk patients with multi-vessel disease has led to a broadening of indications. The uptake of OPCAB surgery varies widely between centres and

individual surgeons. In some centres, >90% of isolated revascularization procedures are performed off pump (Figure 30.2).

Rationale

Interest in OPCAB has been driven by a desire to avoid the perceived ill effects of CPB, develop less invasive surgical approaches and reduce costs. To some extent commercial pressures and the wide availability of information about OPCAB have contributed to both cardiologist and patient demand for the technique. Objective evidence that OPCAB surgery has achieved these aspirations is tantalizingly close, yet incomplete (Table 30.1).

Surgical approach

The majority of OPCAB procedures are performed through a conventional median sternotomy. Not only does this approach provide excellent access to the heart

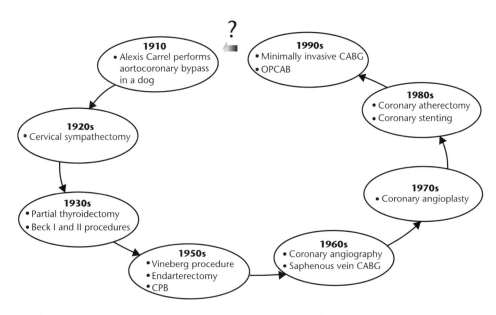

Figure 30.1 The management of coronary artery disease – a century of evolution.

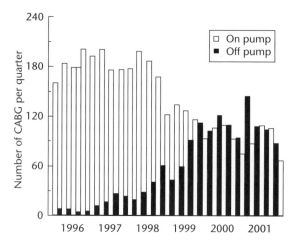

Figure 30.2 The transition to OPCAB in one UK cardiac centre.

and the internal mammary arteries, but also it facilitates the rapid institution of CPB, if required.

In the small number of patients with single-vessel LAD disease, who are not suitable for percutaneous intervention, a limited anterior short thoracotomy (LAST) may provide sufficient surgical access for minimally invasive direct coronary artery bypass (MIDCAB). Proponents of MIDCAB cite reductions in length of hospital stay, postoperative infection rates and postoperative analgesic requirements to support their continued use. Those opposed to MIDCAB cite, the not insignificant 'conversion' rate, limited resuscitation access and *increased* postoperative analgesic requirements as reasons *not* to pursue the technique.

Multi-vessel coronary revascularization via a median sternotomy will necessitate displacement of the heart from its natural position. The uptake of OPCAB has been greatly assisted by the introduction of single-use and reusable mechanical stabilization devices

Table 30.1 The rationale for OPCAB surgery – putative benefits and areas of controversy

	Advantages	Disadvantages
General	Avoids air and particulate emboli from extracorporeal circuit Avoids risk of cannulation site injury (i.e. aortic dissection) Avoids median sternotomy for single vessel disease	Labour-intensive anaesthesia Technically challenging Cannot be extended to deal with incidental intracardiac pathology (e.g. MR) Anterior thoracotomy may be more painful than median sternotomy
Myocardial	No requirement for cardioplegia Transient interruption to normal coronary blood flow ↓ Release of markers of myocardial injury (i.e. troponins, creatine kinase) ↓ Incidence of perioperative infarction ↓ Myocardial reperfusion injury	Potential for incomplete revascularization Quality of coronary anastamoses uncertain Long-term graft patency uncertain Impact on postoperative AF unclear
Neurological	No requirement for aortic cannulation ↓ Cerebral microemboli – ↓↓ if all aortic instrumentation avoided ↓ Incidence of stroke – in large retrospective studies	↓ Cognitive dysfunction unproven
Renal	↓ Risk of dialysis-dependent renal failure in patients with pre-existing renal dysfunction	↓↓ CO during posterior (e.g. circumflex) grafting
Pulmonary	Ventilation and pulmonary circulation maintained throughout procedure	No significant improvement in lung function despite ↓ Inflammatory response
Haematological	Full heparinization may be avoided ↓ Haemorrhage and blood product requirements	Claims for significant ↓ transfusion requirements unblinded and may be biased
Immunological	↓ Systemic inflammatory response Avoids increases in vascular permeability and total body water associated with CPB	
Cost	↓ Duration of intensive care and length of hospital stay ↓ Disposable costs (i.e. CPB equipment) ↓ Use of blood and blood products	Perfusionist and CPB system required to be available on 'stand-by'

and double- or triple-limb intracoronary shunts. The Medtronic Octopus™ has the advantage of attaching to the surface of the heart via suction cups and reduces the degree of cardiac chamber compression caused by other devices (Figure 30.3).

Anaesthetic management

Patients scheduled for OPCAB surgery should undergo the same preoperative assessment and management as those scheduled for conventional surgery with CPB. Similarly, the goals of anaesthetic management – prevention of perioperative cardiac ischaemia, tight haemodynamic control, minimizing cardiovascular depression and avoidance of non-cardiac complications while providing adequate depth of anaesthesia – are identical. The requirement for a double-lumen

endotracheal tube and lung isolation to improve surgical access via a LAST incision should be discussed with the surgeon before induction of anaesthesia.

Since the recovery following OPCAB is often more rapid than that following conventional surgery, anaesthetic techniques have evolved to facilitate early extubation. As might be expected, no single anaesthetic technique has been shown to be superior (Table 30.2).

Monitoring

Surgical retraction, elevation and rotation of the heart may impede venous return and ventricular outflow. It follows that the haemodynamic impact is typically greatest when the heart is positioned for circumflex and posterior descending artery grafting, and that the rationale for advanced intraoperative monitoring is the early detection of a fall in CO (Table 30.3).

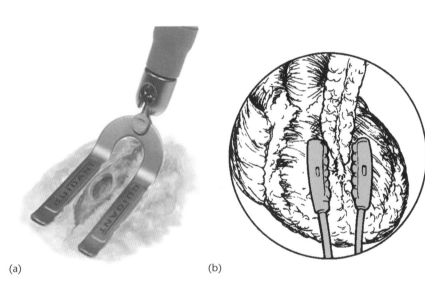

(a)   (b)

Figure 30.3 (a) The Guidant stabilization device (courtesy of Guidant Corporation) and (b) the Octopus™ suction stabilization device (courtesy of Medtronic Inc.).

Table 30.2 Anaesthetic drugs for OPCAB surgery

Premedication	Short-acting benzodiazepines, avoid lorazepam
Induction agents	Similar to 'on pump'
Opioids	Remifentanil use may expedite earlier extubation
Muscle relaxants	Pancuronium considered acceptable by many; shorter-acting agents may be preferred by those aiming for early or 'on-table' extubation
Maintenance	TIVA techniques using propofol are popular; volatile techniques

TIVA, total intravenous anaesthesia.

Table 30.3 Causes of haemodynamic instability during OPCAB surgery

- Reduction of venous return
- RV and LV compression
- Ventricular septal displacement secondary to chamber compression
- Valve distortion and regurgitation (particularly the MV)
- Partial aortic clamping (side-biting clamp for proximal anastamoses)
- Conduction system ischaemia leading to heart block (particularly during RCA grafting)

RCA, right coronary artery.

Table 30.4 Intraoperative monitoring for OPCAB surgery

Basic monitoring
Multilead ECG with ST analysis
Haemodynamic: MAP, CVP
Airway: F_IO_2, $F_{ET}CO_2$, S_pO_2
Temperature, urine output, arterial blood gases

Advanced monitoring
CO measurement: PAFC (intermittent or continuous);
ODM; Pulse-contour monitoring
Regional wall motion: TOE
Neurological: TCD, EEG, NIRS.

Table 30.5 Heat conservation during OPCAB surgery

Maintenance of high ambient temperature (~25°C)
Use of heated mattress
Use of sterile lower body forced air blanket (after
  saphenous vein harvest)
Use of IV fluid warming device
Use of insulating material to reduce cranial heat loss

Despite the theoretical advantage of truly continuous monitors of CO (e.g. oesophageal Doppler monitoring, ODM), there is little evidence to suggest that intermittent, PAFC-based monitoring results in poorer clinical outcomes (Table 30.4). In the setting of OPCAB, some anaesthetists argue that arterial pressure monitoring and capnography provide a rapid and reliable means of detecting a fall in CO!

More subtle changes in regional ventricular wall function can only be effectively detected with TOE. As discussed in Chapter 25, myocardial ischaemia reduces systolic thickening and inward motion long before changes in the surface ECG become apparent. During cardiac elevation, reliance must be placed on the mid-oesophageal views, as the transgastric views may be unobtainable.

In a small number of centres, advanced neurological monitoring is used to detect critical reductions in global and regional cerebral blood flow. As with all neurophysiological monitoring during surgery, the relationship between observed changes and clinical outcome is inconsistent and unreliable. At present there is no objective evidence that using transcranial Doppler (TCD), near infrared cerebral spectroscopy (NIRS) or EEG – either alone or in combination – has any impact on clinical outcome in the setting of OPCAB surgery.

Heat conservation

In anticipation of rapid recovery and early postoperative extubation, intraoperative heat loss should be minimized and active warming measures employed. Convective and radiant losses from prolonged exposure of thoracic contents present a considerable challenge and, unlike conventional CABG, there is no rewarming period. Various methods have been advocated to minimize the incidence and severity of hypothermia (Table 30.5).

Haemodynamic management

The options to ameliorate the cardiovascular disturbances that may occur during OPCAB surgery are physical, pharmacological and electrical. In the early days of beating-heart surgery, a pharmacologically induced bradycardia (<40 bpm) was favoured by many surgeons. Improvements in cardiac stabilization, recognition of the importance of maintaining vital organ perfusion and growing operator confidence have reduced the importance of HR control. To maintain CO and avoid the risks of ventricular distension, some surgeons prefer to operate on a heart paced at 80–90 bpm (Table 30.6).

Table 30.6 Haemodynamic management during OPCAB surgery

Physical
Fluid administration: avoidance of hypovolaemia
Maintenance of cerebral perfusion: avoidance of gross
  CVP elevation
Posture: use of Trendelenburg position and lateral tilt
Opening right pleural cavity to reduce the impact of
  cardiac rotation
IABP in high-risk cases

Pharmacological
↓ HR: esmolol (IV diltiazem in USA)
↑ Contractility: inotrope
Vasoactive drugs: GTN, SNP, α_1-agonists
Anti-dysrhythmics: K^+, Mg^{2+}

Electrical
↑ HR: fixed rate, epicardial atrial pacing (AOO)

Anticoagulation

Interruption and manipulation of vascular endothelium necessitates some degree of anticoagulation. In the vast majority of cases the drug of choice is unfractionated heparin because of its predictable pharmacology. Opinion is divided as to the dose of heparin that should be used. While some surgeons favour full anticoagulation (i.e. 300 units kg^{-1} and ACT >400 s), the majority prefer partial anticoagulation (i.e. 100–150 units kg^{-1}). Full anticoagulation facilitates the rapid institution of CPB but may increase bleeding. Reversal of anticoagulation is also subject to considerable variation. Practices include complete reversal, partial reversal and no reversal.

Institution of bypass

In some cases conversion to 'on-pump' surgery is required, although the indications and thresholds for conversion vary considerably. Indications for CPB include inadequate surgical access, gross haemodynamic instability, refractory dysrhythmia and the diagnosis of new valvular pathology requiring surgical correction. Full anticoagulation is required for CPB.

Postoperative management

Although the goals of postoperative management are similar to 'on-pump' CABG, it is important to appreciate subtle differences in analgesic requirements, fluid management and temperature control.

Postoperative analgesic requirements are dependent on the type of surgical incision, the type and dose of intraoperative opioid and the use of local or regional anaesthetic techniques. The pain associated with median sternotomy is largely unaltered by the use of CPB and it should be borne in mind that patients undergoing OPCAB might have received substantially less intraoperative analgesia. For patients with a LAST incision, intrapleural analgesia, intercostal blockade and paravertebral blockade can produce excellent analgesia, without the risk of a peri-spinal haematoma that is inherent with central neuraxial techniques. Suboptimal analgesia should not, however, be the price paid by the patient for early extubation.

Patients undergoing OPCAB are not subjected to the considerable fluid load associated with CPB and administration of cardioplegic solutions. For this reason their postoperative fluid requirements are greater.

The use of adequate intraoperative measures to prevent heat loss and maintain body temperature should render the OPCAB patient relatively immune from the so-called 'after-drop' phenomenon commonly seen after hypothermic CPB. While intraoperative measures should be continued into the early postoperative period, hyperthermia should be avoided.

Complications

The complications of OPCAB surgery are similar to those of conventional CABG surgery. Although the reported rates of complications following OPCAB are lower, it should be borne in mind that study populations may not be comparable. In most of the large, 'off-pump' versus 'on-pump' series reported to date, there was no randomization and patients in 'off-pump' groups had fewer bypass grafts. This observation has led some to raise the issue of incomplete revascularization.

The future

The uptake of OPCAB surgery is likely to increase if large, randomized studies conclusively demonstrate lower complication rates and equivalent graft patency rates. Recognition of the importance of aortic atheroma in the genesis of neurological injury has led to a reduction or avoidance of instrumentation of the proximal aorta. New devices, capable of forming a proximal anastomosis without aortic clamping, are currently undergoing investigation.

Key points

- OPCAB is increasingly being performed.
- Displacement of the heart from its natural position is frequently associated with hypotension and a reduced CO.
- The use of OPCAB *may* reduce the incidence and severity of major complications.

Further reading

Ascione R, Reeves BC, Chamberlain MH, Ghosh AK, Lim KHH, Angelini GD. Predictors of stroke in the modern era of coronary artery bypass grafting: a case control study. Ann Thorac Surg 2002; **74(2)**: 474–480.

Mehta Y, Juneja R. Off-pump coronary artery bypass grafting: new developments but a better outcome? *Curr Opin Anaesthesiol* 2002; **15(1)**: 9–18.

Stamou SC, Jablonski KA, Pfister AJ, Hill PC, Dullum MK, Bafi AS et al. Stroke after conventional versus minimally invasive coronary artery bypass. *Ann Thorac Surg* 2002; **74(2)**: 394–399.

Watters MPR, Ascione R, Ryder IG, Ciulli F, Pitsis AA, Angelini GD. Haemodynamic changes during beating heart coronary surgery with the 'Bristol technique'. *Eur J Cardiothorac Surg* 2001; **19(1)**: 34–40.

ANAESTHETIC MANAGEMENT OF SPECIFIC DISORDERS

J.H. Mackay & J.E. Arrowsmith

The aortic valve (AV) comprises the left (posterior), right (anterior) and non-coronary semilunar cusps (Figure 31.1). The main functions of the AV are to permit unimpeded LV systolic ejection and to prevent regurgitation of the stroke volume (SV) during diastole. The normal AV orifice area is 2–4 cm^2.

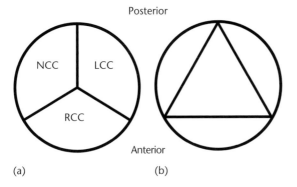

(a)   (b)

Figure 31.1 The AV (as seen on TOE) during: (a) diastole, and (b) systole, NCC, non-coronary cusp; RCC, right coronary cusp; LCC, left coronary cusp.

Aortic stenosis

Aortic stenosis (AS) is defined as a fixed obstruction to systolic LV outflow:

Severity	Valve area (cm^2)	Mean pressure gradient (mmHg)
Mild	1.5–2.0	<25
Moderate	1.0–1.5	25–50
Severe	<1.0	>50

Clinical features

Patients may be asymptomatic for many years, though normally present with one or more of the classic triad of symptoms, namely angina, syncope or breathlessness. Less fortunate patients may present with sudden death.

Presenting symptom	50% Survival rate (years)
Angina	5
Syncope	3
Breathlessness	2

Pathology

In most cases, AS is an acquired disease. Degenerative calcification causes thickening and stiffness of the leaflets. It is associated with advanced age (>70 years) and is often associated with mitral valve (MV) annular calcification. Chronic rheumatic aortic disease causes commissural fusion and aortic regurgitation (AR) is more common.

With a prevalence of 2%, bicuspid AV, is one of the most common congenital heart lesions. Patients with bicuspid AV have a shorter latency period to symptom onset due to earlier AV degeneration and calcification.

More rarely, stenosis may be at a supra- or sub-valvular level. Similar principles of anaesthetic management apply.

Pathophysiology

The fixed obstruction to LV ejection causes chronic LV pressure overload and increased wall tension (Figure 31.2). This increase in wall tension is offset

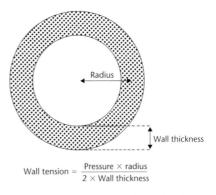

$$\text{Wall tension} = \frac{\text{Pressure} \times \text{radius}}{2 \times \text{Wall thickness}}$$

Figure 31.2 Laplace's law. The relationship between wall tension or stress, intracavity pressure, radius of curvature and wall thickness.

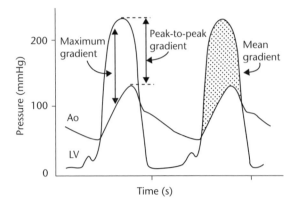

Figure 31.3 Pressure curves obtained simultaneously from the LV cavity and the aortic root in AS. The *peak-to-peak* gradient is measured in the catheter laboratory and is the difference between the peak systolic pressures in the LV cavity and aortic root. (*Note* that peak aortic root pressure is reached later than peak ventricular pressure.) The maximum or *instantaneous* gradient is measured by the Doppler ultrasound. Reproduced with permission from Otto CM, 2000.

by the development of concentric LVH at the price of diastolic dysfunction secondary to impaired relaxation and reduced compliance, manifest as elevated LVEDP (Figure 31.3). LV end-diastolic dimensions are usually preserved in early AS.

Angina pectoris

An imbalance between myocardial oxygen supply and demand. Angina may occur even in the absence of significant coronary artery disease (CAD). The combination of LVH and increased wall tension increases systolic myocardial oxygen demand, while a reduction in coronary perfusion pressure decreases oxygen supply (Figure 31.4).

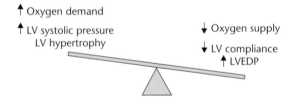

Figure 31.4 The imbalance between myocardial oxygen supply and demand in AS.

Syncope

Syncope typically occurs on exertion. SV is limited in moderate or severe AS giving a 'fixed' CO. Although inability to compensate for exercised induced peripheral arterial vasodilatation is the most common explanation for syncope, a ventricular dysrhythmia is another potential cause.

Breathlessness

Breathlessness is the most sinister of the triad of symptoms and may herald the onset of LV decompensation/dilatation. Increased LVEDP necessitates higher left-sided filling pressures, which lead to pulmonary congestion (Figure 31.5). Decompensation arises when the LV wall tension can no longer be maintained by systolic wall thickening and the LV dilates. LV dilatation is associated with increased wall tension (Laplace's law).

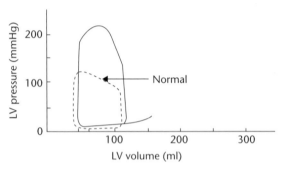

Figure 31.5 LV pressure–volume loop in AS. Note elevated end-diastolic pressure, elevated systolic pressure and preservation of SV.

Investigations

- *Electrocardiogram (ECG)*   Increased R- and S-wave amplitude, T-wave inversion (strain pattern) in anterior chest leads.
- *Two-dimensional (2D) echo*   AV anatomy and function, LV function, aortic root size.
- *Doppler*   Peak AV gradient = $4 \times$ peak velocity^2.
- *Coronary angiography*   To exclude coronary disease; mandatory in males >40 years or females >50 years.
- *Ventriculography*   LV function, peak-to-peak AV gradient (Figure 31.3).

Anaesthetic goals

Sinus rhythm and the 'atrial kick' are very important in these poorly compliant hearts. Atrial contraction can account for 30–40% diastolic filling in these patients (*cf.* 15–20% in normal patients). AF and nodal rhythm result in failure to maintain preload and are poorly tolerated.

TOE provides a better direct objective measure of LV filling (i.e. LVEDA) than the PAFC (i.e. PAWP) but the former is not available during the critical induction period.

Tachycardia may cause myocardial ischaemia by reducing diastolic filling time and should be avoided. Bradycardia should also be avoided due to the 'fixed' CO. Systolic function is usually well preserved in the early stages of AS. Maintaining contractility is usually only a problem in end-stage AS associated with LV decompensation. Attempts to improve SV by reducing afterload are misguided and dangerous in AS, as afterload is effectively fixed at the AV level. It is a fundamental requirement that SVR must be maintained during anaesthesia for AS.

Preload	Better full than empty
HR	60–80 is ideal
Rhythm	Preserve sinus rhythm
Contractility	Maintain (but most tolerate mild depression)
SVR	Maintain (or slightly increase) to maintain coronary perfusion pressure

Treatment of hypotension

Hypotension is common following induction and must be anticipated. Initial treatment is usually IV fluid and a vasoconstrictor to maintain preload and afterload, respectively. Early intervention is required to prevent an inexorable downward spiral of hypotension leading to myocardial ischaemia and cardiac arrest. If cardiac arrest does occur, external cardiac massage is generally ineffective. Survival after prolonged arrest is unusual without the facility for rapid institution of CPB.

Aortic regurgitation

Aortic regurgitation (AR) is defined as diastolic leakage across the aortic valve which causes volume overload of the left ventricle.

Clinical features

Presenting features are highly dependent on whether aetiology is acute or chronic.

- *Chronic AR* Compensatory LV changes allow many patients with chronic AR to be asymptomatic for over 20 years. Symptoms, typically exertional dyspnoea, accompany LV decompensation. Angina is less common in AR than AS because the increase in myocardial oxygen demand with volume overload is smaller than that with pressure overload.
- *Acute AR* Typically presents with pulmonary oedema, tachycardia and poor peripheral perfusion.

Pathology

AR may be secondary to aortic root dilatation, abnormalities of the leaflets or both.

Both aortic dissection (discussed in Chapter 34) and infectious endocarditis cause acute AR. Endocarditis may cause leaflet perforation and vegetations may impede diastolic leaflet closure.

Pathophysiology

Factors affecting severity of AR (Figure 31.6) include:

- regurgitant orifice area,
- diastolic pressure gradient across the AV,
- length of diastole (inversely related to HR).

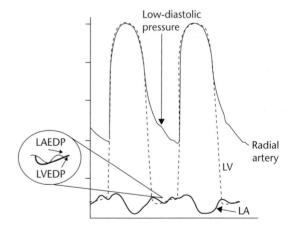

Figure 31.6 Pressure curves for AR. A fall in diastolic pressure leads to a widening of pulse pressure.

Aortic root dilatation	Congenital	Marfan's syndrome.
	Acquired	Long-standing hypertension, aortic dissection, atheromatous aortic disease, syphilitic aortitis, connective tissue disorders.
Leaflet abnormality or damage	Congenital	Bicuspid AV (frequently become incompetent after fourth decade and have well recognized association with coarctation of aorta).
	Acquired	Aortic dissection, chronic rheumatic heart disease, infective endocarditis; connective tissue disease (e.g. systemic lupus erythematosus, rheumatoid arthritis, ankylosing spondylitis); balloon valvuloplasty.

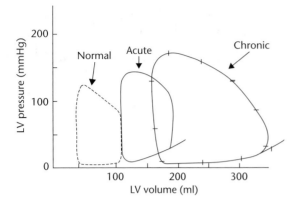

Figure 31.7 Pressure–volume loops for acute and chronic AR. In chronic AR, LVEDV and SV are greatly increased. In acute AR, where there has been no adaptive increase in LV compliance, the increases in LVEDV and SV are smaller.

In both chronic and acute AR, the primary problem is LV volume overload. In chronic AR, the increase in diastolic filling volume induces adaptive changes in the LV. Muscle elongation results in an increased LV radius and eccentric LVH. Unlike MR, where the LV offloads into the LA during the early part of ejection, there is no reduction in LV pressure during systole. LV wall thickness increases to match the increased radius and reduce wall tension (Laplace's law). True compliance is changed only slightly but the ventricle operates much further to the right on the pressure–volume curve (Figure 31.7).

Hearts in chronic AR, the so-called 'bovine' hearts, can develop the largest LV end-diastolic volume (LVEDV) of all the valvular heart lesions. Systolic SV is increased (LVEDV increases by more than LV end-systolic volume (LVESV)) in order to compensate for diastolic regurgitant volume and maintain an 'effective' SV. Although Starling mechanisms initially maintain LV systolic function, increasing LVEDV eventually leads to decompensation evidenced by a decrease in the slope of end-systolic pressure–volume relationship (ESPVR). The rise in LVESV is accompanied by a fall in LV ejection fraction (LVEF).

Acute AR causes diastolic volume–pressure overload in a normal-sized, non-compliant LV. The acute rise in LVEDP reduces coronary perfusion pressure, causes early closure of the MV and necessitates higher LA filling pressures.

Investigations

- *2D echo*   AV leaflet pathology, aortic root dimensions, LV function. LV end-systolic dimension

>5.5 cm and LVEF <50% are signs of systolic dysfunction and are indications for surgery.
- *Colour flow Doppler*   To assess the width of regurgitant jet at origin in relationship to width of LVOT. Diastolic flow reversal in the descending aorta suggests severe AR. The presence and severity of associated MR needs to be established (Figure 31.8).
- *Continuous wave Doppler*   Calculation of regurgitant valve orifice size using the pressure half-time method. Diastolic regurgitant blood flow velocity decreases more rapidly in severe AR .
- *Coronary angiography*   To exclude coronary disease.

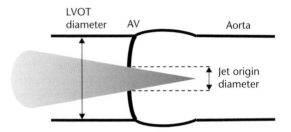

Figure 31.8 Echocardiographic assessment of the severity AR using the ratio of jet origin diameter to LVOT diameter (<0.3 = mild, 0.3–0.6 = moderate, >0.6 = severe).

Anaesthetic goals

	Acute AR	Chronic AR
Preload	Increase	Increase
HR	Fast	Medium to fast
Rhythm	Sinus	Sinus
Contractility	Support	Maintain
SVR	Low – maintain	Low

Preload   needs to be higher in acute AR to overcome higher LVEDP. A modest tachycardia shortens diastole and reduces regurgitant flow. It also reduces the time for anterograde filling through the MV, which reduces LV distention, lowers LVEDP and improves coronary perfusion. In acute AR and the latter stages of chronic AR, sinus rhythm is particularly beneficial because it facilitates anterograde LV filling.

Contractility   must be maintained and inotropic support is often required in acute AR.

Afterload reduction lowers the diastolic AV gradient and, therefore, the regurgitant volume. Vasodilator therapy is commonly used to delay the development of systolic dysfunction. Afterload reduction may not be tolerated in the presence of a low aortic diastolic pressure, particularly in the emergency scenario.

Treatment of hypotension

Strategies are based on inotropes and vasodilators. The IABP is contraindicated due to its tendency to worsen regurgitation and cause LV dilatation.

Key points

- Aortic stenosis (AS) produces both systolic and diastolic LV dysfunction.
- Tachycardia, *severe* bradycardia and vasodilatation are poorly tolerated in AS.

- Hypotension should be treated early in AS to prevent haemodynamic collapse.
- Volume overload in chronic aortic regurgitation (AR) results in the largest left ventricular end-diastolic volume (LVEDV) of all the valvular heart lesions.

Further reading

Otto CM, Textbook of Clinical Echocardiography. 2nd edition. Philadelphia: Saunders, 2000.

J.H. Mackay & F.C. Wells

The recent trend towards repair, rather than replacement of the MV, together with increased use of perioperative TOE, have stimulated cardiac anaesthetists to gain a greater understanding of MV anatomy.

Normal MV area is 4–6 cm². Unlike other heart valves, the MV consists of two asymmetric leaflets. The *anterior* leaflet makes up 65% of valve area but only 35% of the circumference. The *posterior* leaflet consists of three main scallops. The leaflets are joined at the anterolateral and posteromedial commissures (Figure 32.1). The anterior MV leaflet shares the same fibrous attachment as the non-coronary cusp of the AV.

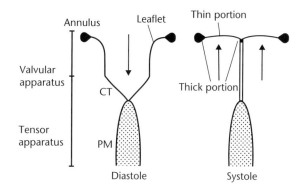

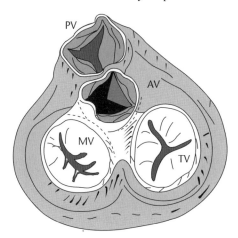

Figure 32.1 Anatomy of the cardiac valves (viewed from above).

Figure 32.2 illustrates the valvular and tensor apparatus during diastole and systole. The leaflets and annulus make up the valvular apparatus:

- During diastole, leaflet opening should permit unimpeded flow from LA to LV.
- During systole, co-aptation of the leaflets protects the pulmonary circulation from high LV pressures.

The tensor apparatus consisting of chordae tendinae and papillary muscles make significant contributions to LV function and ejection fraction.

MV surgery is usually undertaken through a sternotomy though right or left thoracotomy may be used particularly for redo or minimally invasive mitral surgery.

Figure 32.2 Mitral leaflet opening during diastole and co-aptation and apposition during systole. CT, chordae tendinae; PM, papillary muscle. From Oka Y, Goldiner PL. *Transesophageal Echocardiography*. Philadelphia JB Lippincott 1992.

Mitral stenosis

MS is defined as area <2 cm² and classified as severe or critical when valve area is <1 cm².

The vast majority of cases are secondary to rheumatic fever, though a history of acute febrile illness is often absent. Leaflet thickening and commissural fusion occurs secondary to the inflammatory process. Other valve disease, particularly involving AV and TV are common. Pure MS is less common than mixed stenosis and regurgitation.

Clinical features

Breathlessness on exertion is the commonest presentation and onset is usually insidious. Other presentations include haemoptysis, AF, or peripheral embolic events.

Pathophysiology

Fixed obstruction to blood flow, between LA and LV creates a pressure gradient across the MV. Left atrial pressure (LAP) increases to maintain CO.

$$\text{Pressure gradient} = \left[\frac{\text{Flow rate}}{K} \times \text{Valve area} \right]^2$$

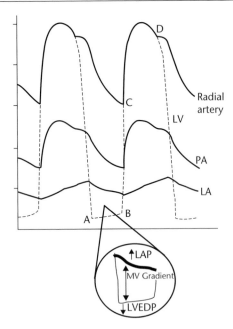

Figure 32.3 Pressure curves for MS.

where K is the hydraulic constant. Elevated LAP and the presence of low LV end-diastolic pressure (LVEDP) result in an increased MV gradient (see Figure 32.3).

Impact of elevated LAP includes:

• LA dilatation
• AF
• reduced pulmonary compliance
• pulmonary hypertension.

AF reduces LV filling particularly when associated with fast ventricular rates. Pulmonary hypertension is initially reversible but becomes irreversible following sustained chronic elevation of PVR.

The LV pressure–volume loop in MS is small and shifted to the left due to a reduction in LV pressure and volume loading (Figure 32.4).

LV systolic function may be depressed due to myocardial fibrosis and chronic underloading. Figure 32.5 illustrates that effect of reducing valve orifice area on the relationship between transmitral flow rate and pressure gradient. Decreasing valve area has a dramatic effect on the flow rate required to generate the diastolic pressure gradient at which pulmonary oedema develops.

Investigations

• *Two-dimensional (2D) echo* Leaflets thickened, possibly calcified, doming and reduced opening.

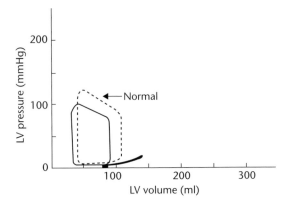

Figure 32.4 LV pressure–volume loop in MS.

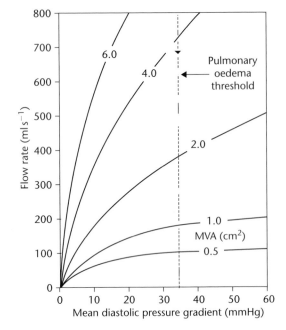

Figure 32.5 Rate of transmitral diastolic blood flow versus mean diastolic MV gradient for normal (4–6 cm^2) and stenotic MVs (0.5–2 cm^2).

• *Doppler gradient (pressure half-time, PH–T)* MV inflow is quantified with PWD or CWD. The rate of fall of blood flow velocity of the E-(early diastolic filling) wave is attenuated in MS. The PH–T method uses the slope of E-wave deceleration to calculate MV orifice area (MVA) (Figure 32.6):

$$\text{MV Orifice Area} = \left[\frac{220}{\text{PH-T}} \right]$$

Calculation of MVA by the PH–T method is unreliable in the presence of an incompetent AV. AR contributes

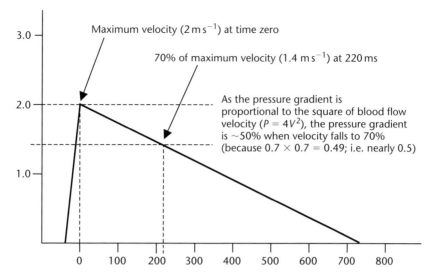

Figure 32.6 Estimation of MVA using diastolic transmitral blood flow velocity to calculate the PH-T. The PH-T is defined as the time required for the magnitude of the instantaneous transmitral pressure gradient to fall by half. From the modified Bernouilli equation $P = 4 \times V^2$ (where P is pressure and V is velocity) it can be deduced that for pressure to halve, velocity must fall by 30%. In the example above, the PH-T is 220 ms, which gives an MVA of $220/220 = 1.0 \, cm^2$.

to LV diastolic filling causing transmitral blood flow velocity to decline more rapidly. The net result is that in the presence of AR, the PH–T method will underestimate the severity of MS.

Anaesthetic goals

Preload	High
HR	Avoid tachycardia
Rhythm	Sinus rhythm better than AF
SVR	Maintain
Contractility	Maintain
PVR	Avoid increase

High LAP is required to overcome the resistance to LV filling. Excessive preload may cause LA distention and AF. Control of HR is paramount. Tachycardia does not allow time for LV filling and results in reduced LVEDV. Bradycardia is poorly tolerated due to relatively fixed SV. Loss of sinus rhythm can decrease CO by 20%. Consider synchronized direct current (DC) shock in acute onset AF – if no LA thrombus present.

SVR needs to be maintained particularly in patients with tight stenosis and an active sympathetic nervous system. LV contractility is rarely a problem in pure MS where greater emphasis should be placed on protecting the RV from increases in PVR and pulmonary hypertension.

Treatment of hypotension

Hypotension is usually associated with tachycardia. Consider DC cardioversion if tachycardia is due to acute onset AF. Sinus tachycardia is generally best treated initially with volume and phenylephrine. Esmolol is useful if these measures fail to improve haemodynamics.

External chest compressions are unlikely to be successful in patients with severe MS. In the event of full-blown cardiac arrest, the emphasis should be on institution of internal cardiac massage and emergency CPB.

Surgery

Percutaneous transeptal balloon valvotomy is an alternative to surgery in patients with favourable valve morphology (non–calcified, pliable valves and absence of commissural calcification) in the absence of significant MR or LA thrombus. Valvotomy is a palliative procedure and recurrence is common. Patients with valvular calcification, thickened fibrotic leaflets and subvalvular calcification, who have a greater incidence of complications and recurrence, fair better with open surgery.

Mitral regurgitation

Mild MR is a common finding in patients with ischaemic heart disease undergoing cardiac surgery. Most of these patients do not require surgical intervention to the valve. Lesions typically amenable to repair include myxomatous degeneration, posterior leaflet prolapse and chordal rupture. Cardiac anaesthetists can assist the surgical decision-making process using TOE by providing information on aetiology, severity and likely natural history of the regurgitant lesion.

Pathology

Acute MR is usually caused by rupture or ischaemia of papillary muscles or rupture of chordae tendinae. Posterior papillary dysfunction is more common than anterior papillary dysfunction. (The posterior papillary muscle has a single coronary artery supply whereas the anterior papillary muscle is supplied by two coronary arteries.)

1 *Myxomatous degeneration of valve leaflets* Most commonly affects MV, posterior > anterior, chordae thin and prone to rupture. Leaflets appear redundant and thickened. Size disproportion between mitral leaflets and LV cavity causes prolapse.
2 *Chronic rheumatic heart disease* Leads to scarring and contraction of chordae and leaflets, which become thickened and often calcified.
3 *Ischaemic MR* Papillary muscle dysfunction with reduced contractility and consequent prolapse, mitral annular dilatation, papillary muscle rupture.
4 *Endocarditis* Leaflet perforation, chordal rupture, vegetations, abscess formation or scarring may interfere with co-aptation.

Clinical features

Breathlessness on exertion and easy fatigability are the commonest presentations for chronic MR. Symptoms frequently deteriorate with the onset of AF. Patients with acute MR do not have time to develop LA enlargement and may present with acute LV failure and pulmonary oedema.

Pathophysiology

The effect of systolic ejection of blood into the low-pressure LA is largely dependent on whether the onset of MR is acute or chronic.

- *Acute MR* results in a sudden increase in LAP. The LA and LV are not accustomed to increased volume load. Increased LVEDP and LAP result in acute pulmonary oedema. SVR increases to maintain BP. The balance between myocardial oxygen supply and demand is adversely affected by reduced CO and increased HR. There is a particularly high

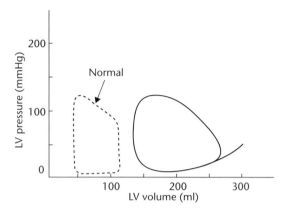

Figure 32.7 LV pressure–volume loop in chronic MR.

risk of ischaemia when acute MR is secondary to ischaemic papillary muscle dysfunction or rupture.
- *Chronic MR* results in LV volume overload and LV dilatation and a shift of the curve to the right (Figure 32.7). Increased LVEDV occurs without any increase in LVEDP in the early stages of the disease process.

Anaesthetic goals

Acute MR	
Preload	Maintain
HR	Maintain
Rhythm	Sinus preferable
SVR	Main coronary perfusion
Contractility	Support
PVR	Maintain
Chronic MR	
Preload	Maintain
HR	Control ventricular rate
Rhythm	Generally in AF
SVR	Slight decrease tolerated
Contractility	Maintain
PVR	Maintain

Patients with chronic MR are not infrequently in AF. Sinus rhythm is useful, but less critical than for other valve lesions, as much of the blood entering the LV in late diastole is immediately returned to the LA in early systole.

Reduced afterload is generally desirable because of improved forward flow. Patients with non-ischaemic MR tolerate a lower MAP than patients with AR because coronary perfusion pressure (i.e. aortic root pressure) is maintained during diastole.

Treatment of hypotension

Risk of downward spiralling hypotension, as resistant to medical treatment is less than that in stenotic valvular lesions. *Hypotension therefore rarely interferes with the important and interesting task of acquiring good TOE images of the valve.* Nevertheless, profound hypotension may occur, particularly in MR secondary to acute ischaemia. Patients with a competent AV usually respond to small dose of phenylephrine, otherwise inotropes are the first-line treatment for systemic hypotension.

Investigations

The LA provides an excellent acoustic window for examination of the MV. TOE is superior to transthoracic echocardiography (TTE) for examining posterior cardiac structures. MV repair and endocarditis surgery are both Category I indications for TOE (see Table 24.3).

Transoesophageal echo

The surgeon needs information about the aetiology and functional severity of MR.

Two dimensional

A thorough 2D examination using oesophageal and transgastric views provides the cornerstone of MV evaluation. Figure 32.8 illustrates the scanning planes

through the MV for mid-oesophageal (ME) views at 0°, 60°, 90° and 150°.

Features to look for on 2D echo:

Leaflets	Structure: Are the leaflets thin and pliable?
	Movement: Do the leaflets open well?
	Co-aptation: Is the point where the leaflets meet below annulus?
	Apposition: Are both leaflets at same height relative to annulus at the end of systole?
Annulus	Size: Is the annulus dilated?
Sub-valve	Structure: Is there chordal lengthening, thickening or rupture?
LV	Structure: Is there LV dilatation?
	Function: Is a regional wall motion abnormality affecting papillary muscle function?

The diagrammatic representation of the classification of MR (the Carpentier classification) is given in Figure 32.9.

Colour flow doppler

MR jets appear red or yellow on colour flow doppler as flow is going towards the transducer. Doppler studies of MR are highly dependent on loading conditions.

As the Doppler shift is a function of the cosine of the angle of incidence, the severity of MR may be

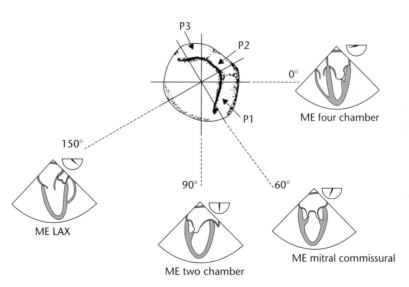

Figure 32.8 ME TOE scanning planes perpendicular to the MV demonstrating the effect of ultrasound plane rotation. P1, anterior scallop of posterior leaflet; P2, middle scallop of posterior leaflet and P3, posterior scallop of posterior leaflet. All three scallops of the posterior leaflet can usually be visualized with the ME 60° (commissural) and 150° views.

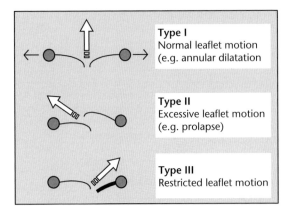

Figure 32.9 Diagrammatic representation of the Carpentier classification of mitral regurgitation. The direction of the regurgitant jet (open arrow) often aids determination of the aetiology. A central jet is usually due to annular dilatation (type I, normal leaflet motion), whereas an eccentric jet may indicate leaflet prolapse (type II, excessive leaflet motion) or restriction (type III, restricted leaflet motion). The jet is directed 'away' from a prolapsing leaflet, and 'towards' a restricted leaflet.

underestimated in the presence of an eccentric regurgitant jet. For the same reason, if the jet is angled away from the ultrasound plane – the so called *third dimension effect* measurements of the velocity of the regurgitant jet will tend to be underestimated (see Table 24.2)

The apparent severity may be significantly influenced by the haemodynamic state of the anaesthetized patient. Relative hypovolaemia and reduced SVR may lead to an underestimation of severity. Pharmacological intervention may be required to reproduce near-normal resting conditions (Table 32.1).

Surgery

In comparison to MV replacement, MV repair is associated with better preservation of LV function, less risk of bacterial endocarditis, reduced need for postoperative anticoagulation, lower operative mortality and better long-term survival. Virtually all type I, and the majority of type II lesions are repairable. Common problems and their surgical solutions are discussed below (Table 32.2).

Table 32.1 Assessment of severity of mitral regurgitation

Size of regurgitant jet is proportional to
- Size of orifice, pressure gradient, compliance of LA and LV

Classification of jets
- Orientation (central or eccentric), Size of jet (volume of LA filled)

Assessment of severity of MR
- Colour flow Doppler (CFD) in several planes: measure proportion of LA filled by colour
- Blunting or reversal of systolic pulmonary venous flow
- Calculation of regurgitation fraction (i.e. difference in forward flow through MV versus second site such as AV)
  - Aortic valve must be competent
- Radius of proximal isovelocity surface area (PISA).
  - The velocity of blood converging on the MV increases as it nears the regurgitant valve during systole
  - When the velocity exceeds the Nyquist limit, aliasing occurs
  - Interface between aliasing velocities forms a semicircular line
  - Radius of curvature of this line (distance between mitral orifice and semicircular line) is proportional to the severity of MR

Pitfalls of CFD
- Gain settings on echo machine, direction of regurgitant jet, influence of cardiac rhythm, atrial preload, afterload

---

Table 32.2 Aetiology of mitral regurgitation and surgical solutions

Carpentier type	Mechanism	Solution
Type I	Annular dilatation	Annuloplasty ring
	Leaflet perforation	Pericardial patch
Type II	Posterior leaflet prolapse (cord rupture/elongation)	Quadrangular resection + simple/sliding annuloplasty
	Anterior leaflet prolapse	Posterior leaflet flip over; Gortex® cords; edge to edge (Alfieri) apposition
	Commissural prolapse	Resection/plicaton; edge to edge; partial homograft

Emergency surgery in the setting of acute MR carries greater morbidity and mortality. LA enlargement, which typically accompanies chronic lesions and facilitates surgical access, is normally absent in MR of acute onset.

Surgical repair of rheumatic and ischaemic (type III) lesions is challenging. Extensive rheumatic leaflet calcification often leaves little pliable leaflet tissue remaining. Partial or complete homograft replacement or the use of pericardial extension has yet to demonstrate long-term stability and durability.

Myocardial ischaemia may result in type I (annular dilatation), type II (papillary muscle rupture), or type III (fibrosis of sub-valve apparatus) lesions. The mechanisms of MR are often complex – having more to do with LV function than a structural valve abnormality. Type III lesions caused by fibrotic distortion of the ventricular wall following infarction are particularly difficult to repair. In contrast, ischaemic rupture of the head of a papillary muscle is usually simple to repair. Patients with mild MR will often improve with coronary revascularization alone. More severe regurgitation may be better treated with valve replacement with preservation of the sub-valve apparatus.

The mechanical complications of MV repair include persistent regurgitation, iatrogenic stenosis and LVOT obstruction. (Table 32.3)

High-velocity regurgitant jets may produce severe haemolysis. Anaemia and haematuria may necessitate repeat surgery. Obstruction of the LVOT secondary to SAM is a rare complication, ranging from severe (failure to wean from CPB) to mild/transient (exertional symptoms). The aetiology of SAM is now recognized as being due to the following: (Table 32.4)

Table 32.3 Mechanical complications of mitral valve repair

Problem	Mechanism	Discussion
Regurgitation	Leaflet distortion	Badly positioned or ill-sized annuloplasty ring
	Paravalvular leak	Gaps between the sutures or annuloplasty sutures cutting out through the annulus creating a hole between the ventricle and the LA
Stenosis	Severe reduction of MV orifice	May be trivial, all degrees possible Repeat surgery may be indicated
LVOT obstruction	Systolic anterior motion (SAM) of anterior MV leaflet	Anterior leaflet moves into LVOT during systole

Table 32.4 Aetiology of Systolic Anterior Motion (SAM)

Aetiology	Mechanism	Prevention/Treatment
Excessive height of the posterior leaflet	Pushes anterior leaflet into LVOT in early systole. As systole progresses the leaflet is carried further and further into the LVOT producing potentially complete obstruction	Ensure that the posterior leaflet is not left too tall when being reconstructed
Small/rigid annuloplasty ring		Use of appropriate ring size
Septal hypertrophy	Reduces LVOT diameter	
LV cavity size	Reduces LVOT diameter	Avoidance of hypovolaemia Cautious use of inotropes

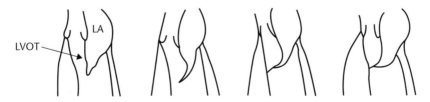

Figure 32.10 The mechanism of LVOT obstruction due to SAM of the anterior mitral leaflet.

Postoperative management specific to the MV repair patient includes anticoagulation, treatment of dysrhythmias and prevention of secondary infection:

- *Anticoagulation*
  If in sinus rhythm after surgery:
  – long-term anticoagulation not necessary,
  – evidence for use of antiplatelet therapy not strong.
  If in AF after surgery:
  – anticoagulation indicated at the level determined by AF as the primary indication.
- *Dysrhythmias*
  – AF is the most common dysrhythmia, particularly in the elderly.
  – Onset often accompanied by hypokalaemia/hypomagnesaemia.
  – Amiodarone has largely replaced digoxin as first-line therapy.
  – Amiodarone continued until at least first outpatient clinic visit.
- *Infection*
  – The risk of bacterial endocarditis is lower following MV repair than MV replacement.

– In practice, most patient are given antibiotic prophylaxis before dental, genitourinary and gastrointestinal surgery.
– Consult local or national formulary for latest details.

Up to 50% of patients in AF before surgery will revert to sinus rhythm when the atrial stretching effect of MR has been corrected. The likelihood and durability of reversion to sinus rhythm is largely determined by the duration of AF prior to surgery.

Key points

- Mitral sub-valvular apparatus makes a significant contribution to LV function.
- Tachycardia and *severe* bradycardia are poorly tolerated in MS.
- The assessment of LV function is difficult in severe MR.
- Relative hypovolaemia and reduced SVR during anaesthesia may lead to underestimation of severity of MR.

J. Graham

Redo surgery

Redo surgery has greater risk compared with first operations. It is essential to be prepared for the increased likelihood of haemodynamic instability and haemorrhage in the pre-CPB period.

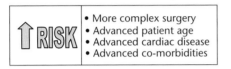

⬆ RISK	• More complex surgery • Advanced patient age • Advanced cardiac disease • Advanced co-morbidities

Anaesthetic preparation

- Avoid cannulation of intended conduits (e.g. radial artery).
- Substantial venous access.
- External defibrillator/pacing electrodes placed before induction.
- Cross-matched blood must be checked before sternotomy.
- Heparin drawn up and immediately available before sternotomy.
- Consider TOE (Category 2 indication).

Management of haemorrhage

Extensive adhesions following first time surgery may cause cardiac structures (e.g. the RV) and major vessels (e.g. aorta, innominate vein, coronary bypass grafts) to be attached to the undersurface of the sternum making them vulnerable to injury during resternotomy. Catastrophic haemorrhage resulting from laceration of these structures during resternotomy has an estimated mortality of 20%.

During cardiac reoperations division of adhesions may significantly prolong the procedure and increase blood loss and transfusion requirements. In the event of catastrophic haemorrhage, bleeding should be controlled with local compression and CPB instituted immediately (Tables 33.1 and 33.2).

Dysrhythmias

Surgical manipulation of the heart and damage to existing bypass grafts may provoke haemodynamically significant dysrhythmias during sternotomy and dissection. These dysrhythmias may occur before adequate exposure has been achieved to allow use of internal defibrillator paddles. For this reason, external defibrillator pads or paddles *must* be placed on the patient before induction of anaesthesia.

Myocardial protection

Effective myocardial protection is more difficult in redo CABG. Antegrade cardioplegia will not reach myocardium supplied by a patent mammary arterial

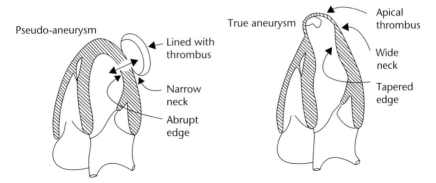

Figure 33.1 False and true aneurysm of the LV (from Otto CM, 2000 with permission).

Table 33.1 Strategies to reduce bleeding and transfusion requirements

Preoperative
- Consider erythropoietin and autologous blood donation
- Consider abstinence from aspirin and other antiplatelet drugs
- Correct existing coagulopathy
- Alter surgical approach to avoid sternotomy (e.g. thoracotomy)

Before sternotomy
- Consider use of aprotinin or lysine analogue
- Consider normovolaemic haemodilution
- Perfusionist must be in the operating room
- Groins prepared to allow access to femoral vessels for CPB
- Consider full anticoagulation and femoro-femoral CPB

Sternotomy
- Use of oscillating saw to reduce likelihood of soft tissue damage
- Ventilation of lungs usually continued in this circumstance

Intraoperative
- Intraoperative cell salvage

Postoperative
- Salvage of shed mediastinal blood

Table 33.2 Surgical Access for CPB following catastrophic haemorrhage

Stage of procedure	Cannulae *in situ*	Surgical strategies
Immediately following sternotomy	No femoral vessel cannulation	Cannulation of femoral vessels Femoro-femoral CPB
	With femoral artery cannulated	Cardiotomy sucker – femoral artery CPB
Later in dissection	No aortic or femoral artery cannulation	Cannulation of femoral artery Cardiotomy sucker – femoral artery CPB
		Cannulation of aorta Cardiotomy sucker – aorta CPB
		Cannulation of aorta and RA Conventional CPB
	With aortic or femoral artery cannulation	Cardiotomy sucker – aorta CPB, or Cardiotomy sucker – femoral artery CPB

graft. Administration of antegrade cardioplegia through existing vein grafts may be associated with distal atheroembolism. Although the use of retrograde cardioplegia, administered via the coronary sinus, avoids these two problems RV protection may be inadequate.

Ventricular aneurysm

It is important to distinguish between false and true LV anaeurysms. A *false* or pseudo-aneurysm is a free wall rupture of the ventricular contained by the surrounding pericardium (Figure 33.1). Ventricular rupture has a peak incidence 5–10 days after an MI. As the likelihood of further rupture and tamponade is high,

surgical repair is indicated. Ventricular pseudo-aneurysm may also occur following MV and AV surgery and after congenital heart surgery.

A *true* ventricular aneurysm is an area of the ventricle where thin stretched scar tissue has replaced muscle. During diastole, the aneurysm appears as a protruding segment of ventricular wall beyond the expected outline of the ventricular cavity. During systole, the segment appears either akinetic or dyskinetic (Figure 33.2):

- The overwhelming majority of LV aneurysms are secondary to coronary artery disease.
- >80% of LV aneurysms involve the anterior wall or apex and are associated with occlusion or high-grade stenosis of the LAD.

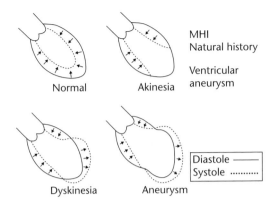

Figure 33.2 The natural history of a true LV aneurysm (from Grondin P, Kretz JG, Bical O, *et al.* Natural history of saccular aneurysms of the LV. *J Thorac Cardiovasc Surg* 1979; **77**: 57–64 with permission from Elsevier).

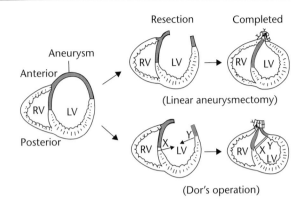

Figure 33.3 Surgical approaches to LV aneurysmectomy – the linear repair and the Dor procedure (from Ohara K. Current surgical strategy for post-infarction LV aneurysm: from linear aneurysmectomy to Dor's operation. *Ann Thorac Cardiovasc Surg* 2000; **6**: 289–294).

- An LV aneurysm may be evident on ventriculography within 2 weeks of transmural MI.

Approximately 8% of patients with coronary artery disease referred for coronary angiography have an LV aneurysm. Associated MR may occur.

Ventricular dysrhythmias and LV failure are the commonest causes of death. Although the overall risk of thromboembolic events is small, patients with mural thrombus or low LV ejection fraction (LVEF) (i.e. <25%) should be anticoagulated.

Indications for surgery

Patients with LV aneurysm who are asymptomatic have a good prognosis without surgical intervention. In patients with triple vessel disease, surgery reduces symptom severity *and* improves survival. LV aneurysm repair is often performed together with coronary revascularization.

There is currently a trend towards more aggressive management of LV aneurysm – a more detailed discussion about the decision to plicate, resect or ignore the LV aneurysm is beyond the scope of this chapter. The generic term 'Laplace operations' has been applied to these procedures which all reduce ventricular size and, thus, wall stress.

The traditional operation for LV aneurysm is the *linear repair*, in which the aneurysm is resected and the defect closed. This inevitably results in some distortion of LV geometry and that part of the aneurysm involving the ventricular septum is not repaired.

More recently, complete resection of the aneurysm, including any septal component, with placement of a patch at the base of the aneurysm and a tight suture around its apex, has been advocated. Whether outcome

from patch repair techniques are superior to those following linear repair, is controversial (Figure 33.3).

Sternal wound debridement

Mediastinal infection following cardiac surgery occurs in 1–2% patients and carries an overall mortality of 5%. Risk factors for both superficial and deep mediastinal infections include:

- diabetes mellitus,
- re-sternotomy for haemorrhage,
- bilateral mammary artery harvesting,
- obesity,
- renal failure.

Patients with mediastinal infection who require surgical re-exploration and debridement are invariably systemically unwell. In addition to fever and general malaise there may be signs of pericardial tamponade or constriction, as well as cardiac, respiratory and renal dysfunction. Patients with apparently superficial infection may be found to have much more extensive infection at operation. The prudent anaesthetist will arrange for postoperative admission to the ICU and prepare for the worst-case scenario!

Further reading

Cohn LH, Edmunds LH. *Cardiac Surgery in the Adult*. New York: McGraw-Hill, 2003.

Machiraju VR. How to avoid problems in redo coronary artery bypass. *J Card Surg* 2002; **17**(1): 20–25.

Yeo TC, Malouf JF, Oh JK, Seward JB. Clinical profile and outcome in 52 patients with cardiac pseudoaneurysm. *Ann Intern Med* 1998; **128**(4): 299–305.

AORTIC DISSECTION

34

A.C. Knowles & J.D. Kneeshaw

Acute aortic dissection is one of the most common cardiothoracic surgical emergencies. An understanding of pathophysiology and aims of surgical management is essential.

Definition

Aortic dissection occurs when the intima and media of the aortic wall become separated resulting in the production of true and false lumens.

Pathogenesis

Aortic dissection is usually associated with a tear in the aortic intima secondary to shear stress, although it may occur in the absence of a demonstrable tear. Rupture of the vasa vasorum in the medial layer may lead to intramural haematoma formation and subsequent intimal rupture. Conditions predisposing to the condition are shown in Table 34.1.

Table 34.1 Causes of aortic dissection
Acquired
• Arterial hypertension, atherosclerosis, pregnancy
• Trauma, cocaine abuse
• Iatrogenic (e.g. IABP, aortic cannulation, cardiac catheterization)
Congenital
• Marfan's syndrome, Ehler's–Danlos syndrome, male gender

The velocity and pressure of cardiac ejection are the driving forces that cause propagation of a dissection. Distal propagation – typically in a spiral fashion – is common, although proximal extension towards the coronary ostia and aortic valve may occur.

Classification

The Stanford and DeBakey classifications are the most commonly used to describe aortic dissection (Figure 34.1).

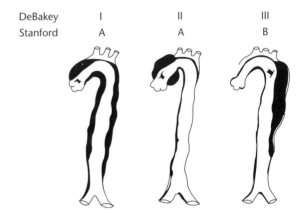

Figure 34.1 Classification of aortic dissection. In DeBakey type I, the intimal tear occurs in the ascending aorta with propagation of the dissection to the arch and DTA. In type II, a tear in the ascending aorta does not propagate beyond the innominate artery. In type III, the tear is beyond the origin of the left subclavian artery. The Stanford classification simply divides dissections into either type A or B. Type A involves the ascending aorta regardless of the extent of the dissection. Type B lesions involve the DTA distal to the origin of the left subclavian artery.

A new classification has been proposed as a subdivision of the Stanford and DeBakey classifications to include aetiology (Table 34.2).

Clinical presentation

The symptoms and signs of aortic dissection are diverse (Table 34.3). As diagnosis may not be easy, a high index of suspicion is required. The differential diagnosis includes: acute coronary syndrome, aortic regurgitation (AR) or aneurysm, acute pericarditis, pulmonary embolism, pleurisy, musculoskeletal pain and cholecystitis.

Diagnosis

The aim is to rapidly confirm the diagnosis, localize the initial tear, establish the extent of propagation and the presence of complications (aortic root dilatation, AR,

Table 34.2 New classification of aortic dissection based on aetiology

Class 1	Classical aortic dissection with intimal flap between true and false lumens
Class 2	Medial disruption with intramural haematoma/haemorrhage formation
Class 3	Discrete/subtle dissection without haematoma, eccentric bulge at tear site
Class 4	Plaque rupture leading to aortic ulceration, penetrating aortic atherosclerotic ulcer with surrounding haematoma, usually subadventitial
Class 5	Iatrogenic and traumatic dissection

Svennson *et al.* 1999.

Table 34.3 Symptoms and signs of acute aortic dissection

Pain
- Sharp, tearing or ripping – maximal intensity at time of onset
- Retrosternal in proximal dissection
- Interscapular/back in descending dissections

Syncope
- Severe pain, cardiac tamponade or obstruction of cerebral vessels
- Up to 20% have syncope without typical pain or neurological findings

Dyspnoea
- Severe aortic regurgitation
- Extrinsic bronchial constriction
- MI following coronary artery involvement

Stroke
- Vessel involvement in dissection

Shock
- Tachycardia, hypotension, diaphoresis, oliguria, cyanosis

Pulse deficits
- Unequal upper limb BPs
- 'White arm' – subclavian occlusion

Murmur
- Aortic regurgitation – new early diastolic murmur
- Heart sounds may be soft in the presence of pericardial effusion

Stroke
- Vessel involvement in dissection

Other
- *Haemoptysis*: bronchial compression/rupture
- *Hoarseness*: recurrent laryngeal nerve compression
- *Abdominal pain*: mesenteric ischaemia
- *CXR*: widened mediastinum, pleural effusion
- *ECG*: hyperacute changes of infarction, low amplitude

MI and tamponade). The various diagnostic tests include:

- *CXR* Mediastinal widening may suggest the diagnosis but is not specific.
- *CT ± contrast* This is the most commonly used non-invasive imaging technique. It has high sensitivity (>90%) and specificity (>85%) and can be performed rapidly. It can detect intramural haematoma and the extent of dissection.
- *MRI* This produces higher-quality images than CT and has the highest sensitivity and specificity. It allows functional assessment of the AV and LV, and can differentiate peri-aortic haematoma from false aneurysm thrombosis. The specialized equipment required for monitoring the critically ill patient during imaging limits the use of this modality.
- *Aortography* This is time-consuming and invasive procedure associated with both complications and death. It allows localization of the intimal tear, determines the extent of dissection and involvement of major aortic branches, and permits coronary angiography. It is now less frequently performed due to introduction of less-invasive imaging techniques.
- *TOE* This allows minimally invasive, real-time structural and haemodynamic evaluation of the majority of thoracic aorta. In particular, it allows detailed examination of AV, aortic root, proximal ascending aorta, distal arch and descending thoracic aorta (DTA). To minimize the haemodynamic changes that may occur with TOE, general anaesthesia is recommended.

A comparison of the diagnostic value is given in Table 34.4.

Management

Type B dissections are usually managed conservatively (i.e. medically). The aim of medical treatment is to reduce BP and ejection velocity, as uncontrolled hypertension may lead to further propagation or rupture. Although the majority of type B dissection heals by fibrosis, a small number may ultimately require surgery. Surgery in the acute phase is required in the presence of vital organ (e.g. renal and mesenteric) ischaemia, aortic rupture or continuing pain.

In contrast, type A dissections occur more commonly and have a higher initial mortality compared to type B dissection (60% versus 10%). The risk of death is greatest in the first few hours. Most require surgical

Table 34.4 Comparison of diagnostic value of imaging techniques in aortic dissection

	CT	MRI	Aortography	TOE
Sensitivity	++	+++	++	++
Specificity	++	+++	++	+++
Tear localization	−	++	+	+++
Aortic regurgitation	−	++	++	+++
Pericardial effusion	++	++	−	+++
Brachiocephalic involvement	++	++	+++	+
Coronary artery involvement	−	+	+++	++

treatment, although surgical mortality is appreciable (10–40%). The aim of surgery is to prevent death by proximal propagation. This is achieved by replacing the segment of ascending aorta containing the tear with a synthetic interposition graft. Additional surgical procedures, such as AV replacement or repair, and CABG, may be required.

BP control before surgery is an important facet of management. Reducing the rate of aortic pressure change (i.e. dP/dt) reduces propagation driving force. A combination of drugs may be required to reduce myocardial contractility, HR and SVR (Table 34.5).

Table 34.5

β-blockers
- *Esmolol*: An ideal agent; high β_1 specificity and short duration of action make it easily titratable
- *Labetalol*: Combined α and β-blockade

Vasodilators
- *GTN*: Coronary artery dilatation desirable
- *SNP*: More potent and predictable action; reflex tachycardia may be troublesome

Analgesics
- *Opioids*: Pain control should not be overlooked

Patient transfer

Most patients with aortic dissection are admitted to hospitals without cardiac surgical facilities. Patients with type A dissection must be transferred to a specialist unit for further investigation and treatment. Effective medical therapy must be initiated prior to transfer. Substantial IV access, and invasive arterial and central venous monitoring are mandatory. Medical escorts must have experience in advanced resuscitation and the use of vaso-active drugs. Ideally all medical notes, the results of any investigations and cross-matched blood should accompany the patient.

Anaesthesia

Surgery should be expedited once the diagnosis is confirmed. Whenever possible a brief history should be taken and physical examination performed. At least six units of cross-matched blood must be available.

A rapid sequence induction should be considered in every case. The choice of anaesthetic technique should take into account the need for haemodynamic stability – particularly during laryngoscopy. As the surgical approach is invariably via a sternotomy, a single-lumen ETT tube is used.

Monitoring

In addition to standard monitoring procedures, a left upper limb arterial line is preferred because of the risk of innominate artery involvement. If the arch vessels are to be isolated, a femoral arterial line is required. A large bore (8F) central venous cannula is often used for rapid transfusion. Repair of aortic dissection is a category I indication for TOE, and should be considered in every case (Chapter 24). Nasopharyngeal *and* bladder temperature monitoring should be used if deep hypothermic circulatory arrest (DHCA) is anticipated.

Surgery

The patient is placed in a supine position with the groins exposed and prepared for possible femoral cannulation. Full anticoagulation and femoral artery cannulation are often undertaken prior to median sternotomy to allow sucker-CPB in the event of rupture or to facilitate arch replacement. Where possible, conventional atrial–aortic CPB is then established. If DHCA is required to facilitate aortic arch repair, selective anterograde or retrograde cerebral perfusion may be considered. The use of aprotinin in the setting of aortic dissection repair and DHCA is controversial and is discussed in Chapter 50.

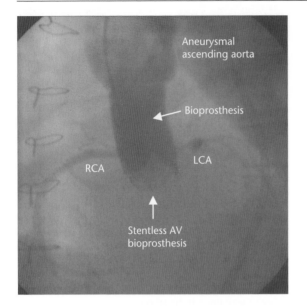

Figure 34.2 Aortic root angiogram following replacement of the aortic root with a Shelhigh stentless valved biosprosthesis. The right and left coronary arteries (RCA and LCA, respectively) have been re-implanted.

Post bypass

In most cases the surgeon will request a degree of arterial hypotension to assist haemostasis. Due to the importance of maintaining CO greater emphasis should be placed on vasodilatation rather than reducing myocardial contractility. The high incidence of coagulopathy contributes to postoperative haemorrhage. Thromboelastography may guide the rational use of blood products.

Postoperative care

A period of sedation and ventilation should follow during which there should be meticulous BP control to reduce stress on the surgical suture lines and aortic wall. During this time the patient's temperature, acid–base status, haematology and biochemistry should be normalized. Assessment of neurological function is important prior to tracheal extubation although in other respects, postoperative management is broadly similar to that for any cardiac surgical patient.

Complications

- *Myocardial dysfunction* Dysrhythmia, impaired contractility.
- *Embolic injury* Thrombus, atheroma, air.
- *Haemorrhage* Coagulopathy, surgical.
- *Neurological dysfunction* Secondary to dissection, embolic stroke, hypoperfusion.
- *Renal impairment* Secondary to dissection, low CO state.
- *Respiratory impairment*

Key points

- Signs and symptoms are highly variable depending on the site of dissection.
- Type A dissection is a surgical emergency with a high mortality.
- Mortality is due to aortic rupture, tamponade or myocardial infarction.
- Tight BP control throughout the perioperative period is mandatory.

Further reading

Erbel R, Alfonso F, Boileau C, Dirsch O, Eber B, Haverich A *et al.* Diagnosis and management of aortic dissection. *Eur Heart J* 2001; **22(18)**: 1642–1681.

Hagan PG, Nienaber CA, Isselbacher EM, Bruckman D, Karavite DJ, Russman PL *et al.* The International Registry of Acute Aortic Dissection (IRAD): new insights into an old disease. *JAMA* 2000; **283(7)**: 897–903.

Kouchoukos NT, Dougenis D. Surgery of the thoracic aorta. *N Engl J Med* 1997; **336(26)**: 1876–1888.

Svensson LG, Labib SB, Eisenhauer AC, Butterly JR. Intimal tear without hematoma: an important variant of aortic dissection that can elude current imaging techniques. *Circulation* 1999; **99(10)**: 1331–1336.

35

A.C. Knowles & J.D. Kneeshaw

The aortic arch is the segment of thoracic aorta lying above the aortic insertion of the fibrous pericardium at the level of the sternal angle. The arch therefore begins *proximal* to the brachiocephalic artery and ends *distal* to the left subclavian artery and ligamentum arterioisus. Conditions affecting the aortic arch include dissection, aneurysmal dilatation and traumatic rupture. Aortic dissection was discussed in the previous chapter.

Traumatic rupture

Indirect or blunt (deceleration) injury to the aorta is much more common than penetrating (e.g. gunshot or stabbing) injury. Road traffic accidents and falls from significant heights account for the majority of non-penetrating injuries. In 95% cases the site of aortic rupture is the isthmus – the site of insertion of the ligamentum arteriosum – where the relatively fixed arch joins the more mobile descending thoracic aorta (DTA). The condition carries a considerable immediate mortality. A patient will only survive until hospital admission when the rupture is confined by the aortic adventitia or surrounding structures. Surgical repair of a tear at the isthmus is undertaken via a left thoracotomy, involving the same principles and practice of those for surgery on the DTA. On rare occasions, delaying surgery may be necessary to avoid the risks of CPB in the presence of other injuries.

Aneurysm

An aneurysm is a permanent, localized aortic dilatation >150% of the normal aortic diameter. The incidence increases with age and has been reported as 6 per 100,000 person-years. Aneurysms of the aortic arch represent only 10% of aneurysms of the thoracic aorta. The risk of rupture is much greater than that for abdominal aortic aneurysm. The aetiology of thoracic aortic aneurysms is shown in Table 35.1.

Symptoms and signs

Aneurysms commonly present as an incidental finding during investigation for other conditions or at necropsy following sudden death. Symptoms are typically absent until enlargement encroaches on surrounding structures Table 35.2.

The sudden onset of severe retrosternal or interscapular pain radiating to the neck or jaw may indicate impending rupture. The presence of haemodynamic collapse and signs of haemothorax or haemopericardium suggest established rupture.

Imaging

The aims of imaging are to confirm the location, extent and operability of the aneurysm.

- *CXR* This is generally poor in detecting arch pathology and may appear 'normal'. It may be difficult to differentiate an aneurysm from other mediastinal masses. Enlargement of the aortic knuckle and tracheal deviation are suggestive of aneurysm,

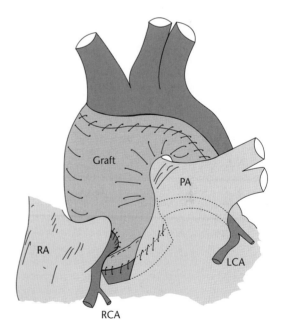

Figure 35.1 Example of a patch graft repair of the ascending aorta and aortic arch. The distal end of the graft is attached to the under surface of the arch. The right and left coronary arteries (RCA and LCA, respectively) have been re-implanted into the proximal end of the graft.

Table 35.1 The aetiology of thoracic aortic aneurysm

Atherosclerosis
- The main cause of thoracic aortic aneurysms
- The principle co-factor is hypertension
- Aortic wall ischaemia and decrease in medial nutrient supply occurs as a result of:
  - Gross intimal thickening with massive fibrosis and calcification
  - An increase in the distance between endothelium and media
  - Adventitial fibrosis and vasa vasorum occlusion

Cystic medial degeneration
- Fragmentation and loss of elastic tissue
- Loss of smooth muscle cells

Congenital
- Marfan's and Ehlers Danlos syndromes
- Presents in younger age group
- Defective synthesis of glycoprotein fibrillin, a component of the elastic tissue of the medial layer

Inflammatory
- Kawasaki's disease, Takayasu's arteritis
- Destroys the medial layer leading to wall weakness

Infective
- Bacterial, fungal, syphilis
- Destroys the medial layer leading to wall weakness

Mechanical
- Post (aortic) stenotic dilatation
- Turbulence distal to a bicuspid AV or aortic coarctation may result in aneurysmal dilatation
- Post-traumatic

Table 35.2 The origins of symptoms associated with thoracic aortic aneurysm

Sympathetic efferents	Jaw, neck and interscapular pain
Recurrent laryngeal nerve	Hoarseness
Trachea	Stridor
Oesophagus	Dysphagia
SVC	Oedema and engorement
Aortic root dilatation	AR, congestive heart failure

whereas mediastinal widening suggests dissection or rupture.
- *Aortography* This was previously considered the gold standard for delineating the aortic arch and its branches. In view of the likely age of the patient, the potential benefits of concurrent coronary angiography must justify the risks associated with the use of contrast media.
- *CT* This is the most widely used non-invasive imaging technique. Image acquisition times with spiral CT are in the order of a few seconds. Contrast enhancement may be required to demonstrate rupture and extravasation.

- *MRI* This can provide clear images of the aorta and its branches without contrast media. Prolonged image acquisition sequences may not, however, be suitable for haemodynamically unstable patients.
- *TOE* This can be performed relatively rapidly at the bedside but incomplete imaging of the aortic arch limits its utility. Ventricular and valvular performance can be readily assessed.

Surgery

Surgical repair of the aortic arch is performed via a median sternotomy in the supine position. The procedure typically involves the replacement of either part or the entire arch with re-implantation of the arch vessels. In many cases an aortic (Carrel) patch is used to anastamose the arch vessels to an aortic graft Figure 35.1. Surgical repair of the distal aortic arch and DTA are discussed in Chapter 36.

Anaesthetic considerations

Preoperative assessment

The goal of preoperative assessment prior to elective surgery is the exclusion of concomitant cardiovascular, respiratory, renal and neurological disease, which are the principle causes of perioperative morbidity and mortality. Assessment of the cardiovascular system should include echocardiography and, if indicated, stress testing and coronary angiography. The patient should be encouraged to abstain from tobacco use for at least 6 weeks before surgery and pulmonary function tested objectively. Intercurrent respiratory tract infection should be treated aggressively and surgery delayed if necessary. Preoperative renal impairment is an independent predictor of postoperative renal dysfunction and renal failure. It should be borne in mind that up to 50% of nephrons may be lost before the serum urea and creatinine concentrations become elevated. Significant carotid artery stenosis (>80%) increases the already high risk of neurological injury associated with aortic arch surgery. Consideration should be given to carotid endarterectomy before arch surgery. The extent of planned surgery together with the methods of cerebral protection to be used must be discussed with the surgical team.

In the emergency situation, the time for preoperative evaluation is limited. In most cases, the role of the anaesthetist is to establish substantial venous access, initiate invasive monitoring and resuscitate the patient.

Induction

The maintenance of haemodynamic stability is paramount. A standard cardiac anaesthetic technique is appropriate for most elective cases. A rapid sequence induction should be considered in emergency cases.

Monitoring

In addition to standard intraoperative monitoring, bladder or rectal temperature monitoring should be used if deep hypothermic circulatory arrest (DHCA) is anticipated. The use of non-invasive cerebral monitoring (e.g. near infrared spectroscopy, NIRS) may assist in detecting and limiting neurological injury.

Cerebral protection

Aortic arch surgery requires the temporary interruption of anterograde cerebral blood flow. The primary method for providing protection against cerebral injury is deep hypothermic circulatory arrest. A period of circulatory arrest for up to 30–40 min at a body temperature of 15–18°C is well tolerated by the majority of patients. More recently two techniques have been developed with the aim of reducing this cerebral morbidity on the basis that some flow is better than no flow.

These are retrograde cerebral perfusion (RCP) and selective anterograde cerebral perfusion (SACP). The intention of these techniques is to ensure some oxygen delivery to the brain while the normal anterograde flow is interrupted. DHCA is discussed in Chapter 50.

Aprotinin

The use of aprotinin in the setting of thoracic aortic surgery and DHCA is the subject of considerable debate and its routine use remains controversial. Although aprotinin use may at first glance appear to be logical, paradoxically increased bleeding, organ thrombosis and renal dysfunction have been reported. Adequate anticoagulation (i.e. heparin 400 units kg^{-1} prior to CPB and 100 units kg^{-1} prior to DHCA) is essential, if aprotinin is to be used.

Temperature

Following the completion of surgery, there must be adequate re-warming. Ongoing blood loss is likely due to anastamotic leaks and coagulation defects secondary to hypothermia, prolonged bypass and previous blood loss. A coagulation screen or thromboelastograph must be performed following protaminization. In the case of significant ongoing losses then a cell-saver should be used.

Intensive care goals

- Normothermia
- Normal acid–base balance
- Correction of coagulopathy
- Assessment of cardiac, respiratory and renal function
- Strict control of hypertension using beta-blockers or vasodilators
- Cessation of sedation to allow cerebral assessment prior to extubation.

Key points

- Haemodynamic control is essential in cases of aneurysm, dissection or trauma which present as emergencies.
- Surgery to the aortic arch is likely to involve circulatory arrest with or without either retrograde cerebral perfusion or selective anterograde cerebral perfusion.
- The use of aprotinin in the setting of thoracic aortic surgery and DHCA is the subject of considerable debate.
- Haemostatic and haemodynamic control are vital in postoperative period.

Further reading

Gravlee GP. Con: Aprotinin should not be used in patients undergoing hypothermic circulatory arrest. *J Cardiothorac Vasc Anesth* 2001; **15(1)**: 126–128.

Kouchoukos NT, Dougenis D. Surgery of the thoracic aorta. *N Engl J Med* 1997; **336(26)**: 1876–1888.

Royston D. Pro: Aprotinin should be used in patients undergoing hypothermic circulatory arrest. *J Cardiothorac Vasc Anesth* 2001; **15(1)**: 121–125.

Westaby S, Katsumata T, Vaccaria G. Arch and descending aortic aneurysms: influence on perfusion technique on neurological outcome. *Eur J Cardiothorac Surg* 1999; **15(2)**: 180–185.

DESCENDING THORACIC AORTA SURGERY 36

E.J.S. Taylor & J.H. Mackay

The descending thoracic aorta (DTA) extends from the distal aortic arch to the diaphragm. Conditions affecting the DTA can be broadly classified into three main groups:

- Aneurysm
- Dissection
- Transection

Aneurysm

The aetiology is multi-factorial, but the vast majority are degenerative and associated with atherosclerosis. Other causes include trauma and infection (mycotic). DTA aneurysm may extend to involve the abdominal aorta. The Crawford classification, types I–IV, depends on the extent of involvement of the thoracoabdominal aorta (Figure 36.1).

Presentation

A chance finding on CXR – 40% patients are asymptomatic. Common presenting symptoms are vague chest, back, flank or abdominal pain, secondary to rupture, or compression and erosion of adjacent structures. Other symptoms and signs include:

- dyspnoea/cough/wheeze;
- haemoptysis – bronchial or pulmonary parenchymal erosion;
- hoarseness – stretching or compression left recurrent laryngeal nerve;
- dysphagia;
- Horner's syndrome – stellate ganglion compression.

The high mortality and morbidity associated with DTA surgery, dictates that all potential candidates undergo thorough preoperative assessment. Absolute indications for *consideration for* surgery include:

- leaking aneurysm,
- increased diameter >5 mm over 6 months in an aneurysm >6 cm,
- persistent pain,
- transection,
- false or mycotic aneurysm.

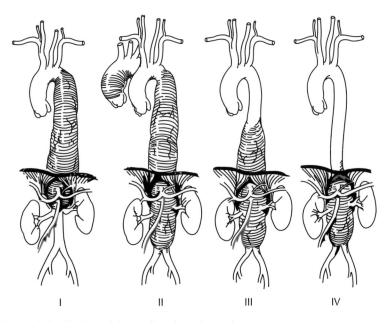

I II III IV

Figure 36.1 The Crawford classification of descending thoracic–aortic aneurysms.

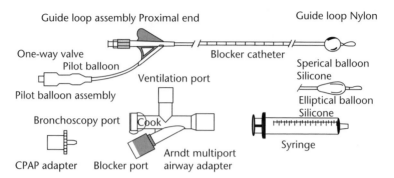

Figure 36.2 The Cook Univent® bronchial blocker. CPAP, continuous positive airway pressure.

Complication of repair

- MI: 7–17%
- Paraplegia: 4–38%
- CVA: 3%
- Respiratory failure: 8–33%
- Renal failure: 5–15%

Anaesthetic management

The anaesthetic management of these patients is extremely challenging for the following reasons:

- Co-existing coronary artery disease is common and accounts for half of early deaths.
- Aortic cross clamp (AXC) induces significant haemodynamic changes and is associated with spinal cord, renal and mesenteric injury.
- The potential for coagulopathy and massive blood loss.
- One-lung ventilation for left thoracotomy – maximally invasive surgery.

Specific considerations

Surgical strategy and intended spinal cord protection techniques should be discussed and agreed in advance.

One-lung anaesthesia

One-lung ventilation provides improved access to and visualization of the operative site, reducing the likelihood of retraction trauma to the left lung and cardiac compression. Various strategies can be used to collapse the left lung.

- *Right double-lumen tube*   Avoids left main bronchus instrumentation. Displacement may obstruct right upper lobe ventilation.
- *Left double-lumen tube*   Eliminates concern about right upper lobe ventilation. Anatomic displacement by the aneurysm may make placement difficult and risks aneurysm rupture.

- *Right endobronchial tube*   Gordon Green (carinal hook) – provides stability and a large bronchial lumen, but precludes suction from left lung.
- *Single-lumen tube with bronchial blocker*   Univent® tube with blocker placed in left main bronchus (Figure 36.2). Useful if either double-lumen tube placement is not possible or the right upper lobe bronchus has a very proximal/tracheal origin. Drawbacks include lack of stability and limited facility for suctioning.

Monitoring and vascular access

The risks of major haemorrhage, hypoxaemia and cardiovascular instability mandate significant venous access and the use of invasive monitoring. Proximal and distal aortic pressures should be transduced throughout:

- *Arterial access*
  - Proximal: Right radial artery.
    The left radial artery is avoided as intraoperative AXC placement may occlude the left subclavian artery.
  - Distal: Right common femoral artery or right dorsalis pedis artery. The left common femoral artery is commonly used for partial bypass.
- *Venous access*   Large bore (⩾14G) peripheral and (8F) central venous introducer connected to rapid infusion/warming system.

Patient positioning

Right lateral decubitus position with an axillary roll and left arm splint. The duration of surgery necessitates scrupulous attention to protecting pressure points, neurovascular bundles and the eyes.

Other considerations

Subarachnoid CSF drainage via a catheter at L3/4 may improve spinal cord perfusion.

Table 36.1 Physiological effects of application and removal of aortic cross clamp

Clamp application	Clamp removal
↑SVR – sudden impedance to aortic outflow	↓SVR – 'declamping shock'/reactive hyperaemia
↑LVEDP (preload) – blood volume redistribution	Pulmonary hypertension
↑Contractility and coronary blood flow (CBF)	Sequestration of blood in capacitance vessels
↑Catecholamines, renin and angiotensin	Ischaemic metabolite actions
↑Intraspinal (CSF) pressures	Alteration of liver, kidney and gut integrity

Epidural catheter – potential difficulty with the differential diagnosis of neurological injury has to be balanced against the benefits of postoperative analgesia.

Somatosensory and/or motor evoked potential (SSEP and MEP, respectively) monitoring.

Surgical considerations

Aortic cross clamp

Placed either distal to the left subclavian or between the left subclavian and left common carotid artery. AXC may cause severe proximal arterial hypertension. Other physiological effects caused by application and removal of the AXC include those given in Table 36.1.

The net effects of AXC application are elevation of proximal aortic pressure, LVEDP, PAWP, PAP and CVP, and a reduction in distal aortic pressure, spinal cord perfusion pressure and renal blood flow. The magnitude of these effects is dependent on AXC application site, extent of collateral blood flow, LV function, diastolic filling pressures, vasodilator use and distal perfusion techniques. Hypertension proximal to the AXC may be managed with SNP, GTN, isoflurane, esmolol, phentolamine or diazoxide.

Surgical approaches

Surgical access is achieved via a maximally invasive, left thoracoposterolateral thoracoabdominal incision. Exposure of the proximal DTA and arch is obtained through an incision in the fifth intercostal space and excision of the sixth rib. More distal exposure requires a left paramedian abdominal incision. Five of the commonly employed techniques are described in Figures 36.3–36.7.

Endovascular techniques

The high morbidity and mortality associated with surgical repair has prompted the development of endovascular techniques. Unfortunately it is only

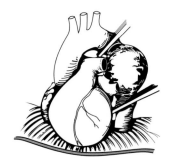

Figure 36.3 DTA repair with proximal and distal AXC. *Advantages*: Simplest method. *Disadvantages*: Highly dependent on short cross-clamp time, distal organ ischaemia, proximal arterial hypertension, metabolic acidosis.

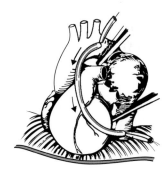

Figure 36.4 DTA repair with proximal and distal AXC and simple shunt. *Advantages*: Controls proximal hypertension primarily by reduced LV afterload, decreased myocardial wall stress, increased splanchnic and renal perfusion, prevention of metabolic acidosis, heparin-coated conduit, therefore systemic anticoagulation not required.

applicable to specific aneurysm anatomy and morphology. Potential benefits include:

- applicable in patients deemed unfit for conventional repair,
- obviates thoracotomy and extensive dissection,
- decreased incidence of paraplegia – AXC avoidance,
- decreased blood loss,
- decreased systemic inflammatory response,
- decreased ICU and hospital stay.

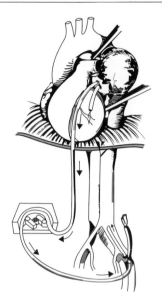

Figure 36.5 DTA repair with left heart (atriofemoral) bypass. *Advantages*: Improved spinal cord/renal perfusion, ability for rapid infusion of warm fluids, supplementary extracorporeal oxygenation. *Disadvantages*: Requires full anticoagulation, risk of vascular injury, air/particulate embolism – stroke, interference with the operative field, increased operative time and increased risk of major haemorrhage.

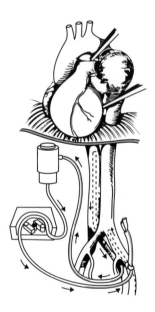

Figure 36.6 DTA repair with femoro-femoral bypass. *Advantages*: No clutter of operative field, supplementary oxygen is provided, circuit can be used for full CPB if required, distal perfusion is independent of patient cardiac output. *Disadvantages*: Systemic heparinization, requires venous reservoir, oxygenator and roller pump.

Acute renal failure

The incidence of ARF is up to 15%. The primary mechanism is reduced renal blood flow associated with the AXC. Alterations in renal haemodynamics induced by changes in the renin–angiotensin and prostaglandin pathways may also contribute to proximal tubular cell damage and reperfusion injury. Despite the lack of evidence to demonstrate efficacy, a number of reno–protective strategies are routinely used, including:

- maintenance of intravascular volume;
- minimizing aortic cross clamp time;
- avoidance of distal hypoperfusion;
- use of partial (left heart) bypass;
- pharmacological – dopamine, mannitol, frusemide.

Spinal cord injury

Postoperative paraplegia occurs in 4–38% cases and remains the most devastating and unpredictable complication of DTA surgery (Figure 36.8). Spinal cord injury is most commonly apparent immediately after surgery, although its onset may be delayed by up to 3 weeks. Although many causes have been suggested, it is difficult to predict which patient will develop paraplegia (Table 36.2).

The arterial supply of the spinal cord is derived from the anterior and posterior spinal arteries (Figure 36.9). The anterior spinal artery is a midline structure formed from branches of each vertebral artery. It supplies the whole of the cord anterior to the posterior grey columns. The smaller posterior spinal arteries are derived from the inferior cerebellar arteries. In its rostral course, spinal branches of the vertebral, deep cervical, intercostal, lumbar, iliolumbar and lateral sacral arteries support the spinal arteries. The anterior radicular arteries, which vary in size and number, tend to be larger in the T4–T9 region, the largest of these is known as the artery of Adamkiewicz. It has a characteristic hairpin bend that perfuses the spinal cord distal to its junction with the anterior spinal

Temp 15 °C
MAP < 20 mmHg

Figure 36.7 DTA repair with full CPB and deep hypothermic circulatory arrest. *Advantages*: Minimal aortic dissection, no proximal AXC, bloodless surgical field. *Disadvantages*: Increased blood loss.

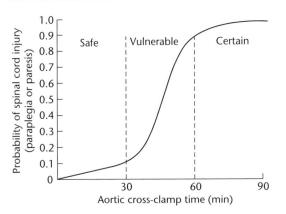

Figure 36.8 Probability of spinal cord injury as a function of AXC duration without distal perfusion. The likelihood of injury is <10% below 30 min, and >90% above 60 min.

artery. It is this portion of the spinal cord, where collateral blood supply is minimal, that is at the greatest risk of ischaemia from prolonged cross clamping or sustained hypotension. Although the artery may arise anywhere from T5 to L1, the origin lies between T5 and T9 in 15% patients, and between T9 and T12 in 60% patients (i.e. above T12 in 75% patients). The 25% patients, in whom it arises below T12, are at increased risk of intraoperative spinal ischaemia.

Strategies to reduce the incidence and severity of spinal cord injury include physical measures, neurophysiological monitoring and pharmacological neuroprotection:

- Physical
  - Increased spinal cord perfusion pressure ±CSF drainage
  - Distal perfusion techniques

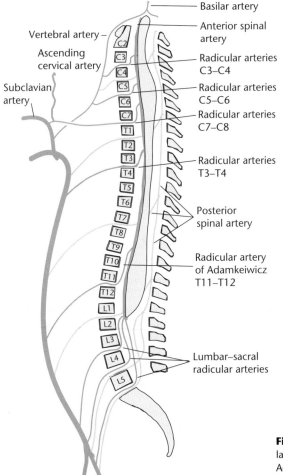

(a)

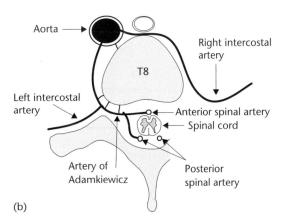

(b)

Table 36.2 Spinal cord injury: patient and perioperative factors

Patient factors	Perioperative factors
Spinal cord blood supply	Duration of AXC
Patient age	Degree/duration
Aortic dissection/rupture	of hypotension
Aneurysm location and	Reperfusion injury
extent	CSF pressure
	Loss of intercostal/
	lumbar arteries
	Hyperglycaemia

Figure 36.9 The arterial supply of the spinal cord. (a) The largest of the anterior radicular arteries in the artery of Adamkeiwicz has a variable origin between T5 and L1. (b) Ligation of intercostal arteries may cause bleeding and reversal of distal blood flow, resulting in spinal ischaemia. Reproduced with permission from Arrowsmith, 2002.

- Reattachment of intercostal and lumbar arteries
- Hypothermia (systemic, epidural, intrathecal)
- Monitoring
  - *SSEP monitoring*
    Slow response time and provides no information about anterior horn cell function
  - *MEP monitoring*
    Readings affected by volatile agents and neuro-muscular blockade
- Pharmacological unlicensed indications
  - *Systemic agents*
    Corticosteroids, barbiturates, naloxone, calcium antagonists, glutamate antagonists, free radical scavengers
  - *Intrathecal agents*
    Papaverine, magnesium

Dissection

Dissections of the DTA are usually managed medically (see Chapter 34). Indications for surgery in DeBakey type B dissection include rupture, continued pain, continued expansion and organ ischaemia.

Transection

Aortic rupture may follow sudden deceleration or blunt or penetrating chest trauma. Of these, deceleration is the most common mechanism, with severity ranging from incomplete laceration to complete transection. Eighty per cent of ruptures occur just distal to the origin of the left subclavian (near the attachment of the ligamentum arteriosum) – a point of aortic fixation where shearing stresses are maximal. Regardless of cause, the prognosis is poor.

The diagnostic triad of increased upper extremity arterial pressure, decreased lower extremity arterial pressure and mediastinal widening is present in more than 50% patients. Other symptoms and signs include:

- Symptoms
  - Dyspnoea
  - Retrosternal/interscapular pain
  - Hoarseness and dysphagia
- Signs
  - Penetrating wound/rib or sternal fractures
  - Upper extremity BP $\gg$ lower extremity BP
  - Left pleural effusion
  - Systolic flow murmur over precordium or medial to left scapula
- Radiological features
  - Mediastinal widening
  - Left-sided pleural collection
  - Associated rib, clavicular or sternal fractures

Management depends on the anatomy of the tear, the condition of the aorta, the degree of haemodynamic instability and the presence of additional injuries. Surgical repair consists of excision with end-to-end anastomosis, patching or interposition grafting. In most cases a 'clamp and sew' technique is used, although shunting or partial CPB may be considered.

Coarctation

Coarctation may present in adulthood with upper extremity hypertension, radio-femoral delay and weak or absent pulses in the lower extremities. CXR may show rib-notching secondary to the development of large collaterals. Repair of coarctation is undertaken via a left thoracotomy. Many of the anaesthetic challenges are similar to DTA aneurysm surgery; namely one lung anaesthesia, AXC-induced haemodynamic changes and postoperative analgesia. Concomitant coronary artery disease is rare and cross-clamp times are shorter. Surgical management of coarctation in neonates is discussed in Chapter 43.

Key points

- Surgery for DTA has a substantial morbidity and mortality.
- As a significant number of patients have co-existing cardiorespiratory disease, careful preoperative assessment is mandatory.
- Preoperative discussion of surgical approach, distal perfusion and neuroprotective strategies is essential.
- Paraplegia following DTA surgery may occur despite all precautions.

Further reading

Arrowsmith JE, Simpson J. Problems in Anesthesia: *Cardiothoracic Surgery*. London. Martin Dunitz Ltd. 2002.

Fann JI. Descending thoracic and thoracoabdominal aortic aneurysms. *Coron Artery Dis* 2002; **13(2)**: 93–102.

O'Connor CJ, Rothenberg DM. Anesthetic considerations for descending thoracic aortic surgery: Part 1. *J Cardiothorac Vasc Anesth* 1995; **9(5)**: 581–588.

O'Connor CJ, Rothenberg DM. Anesthetic considerations for descending thoracic aortic surgery: part II. *J Cardiothorac Vasc Anesth* 1995; **9(6)**: 734–747.

Shenaq SA, Svensson LG. Paraplegia following aortic surgery. *J Cardiothorac Vasc Anesth* 1993; **7(1)**: 81–94.

Wan IY, Angelini GD, Bryan AJ, Ryder I, Underwood MJ. Prevention of spinal cord ischaemia during descending thoracic and thoracoabdominal aortic surgery. *Eur J Cardiothorac Surg* 2001; **19(2)**: 203–213.

Webb TH, Williams GM. Thoracoabdominal aneurysm repair. *Cardiovasc Surg* 1999; **7(6)**: 573–585.

J.A. Chandler & J.H. Mackay

Widening indications for implantation have increased the prevalence of permanent pacemakers (PPMs) and implantable cardioverter defibrillators (ICDs). As these devices have become more complex, the potential for perioperative interference and reprogramming has grown. Patients with these devices are at increased risk of perioperative morbidity and mortality during cardiac surgery.

Permanent pacemakers

Conditions for which there is evidence or general agreement that implantation is beneficial, useful and effective (i.e. Class 1 indications) are summarized in Table 37.1.

Device classification provides a concise means of communicating chamber or chambers paced, chamber or chambers in which native depolarizations are sensed and how sensing affects pacing pattern. The original three-position code (1974) has evolved to the five-position North American Society of Pacing and Electrophysiology/British Pacing and Electrophysiology Group (NASPE/BPEG) generic pacemaker code (Table 37.2).

The original fixed-rate VOO ventricular pacemakers were superseded by VVI systems, which sense

Table 37.1 Class 1 indications for permanent pacemaker implantation

Acquired AV block (in adults)	3rd degree AV block with symptomatic bradycardia or documented asystole, neuromuscular disorders following AV node ablation
Chronic bifascicular and trifascicular block	Intermittent 2nd degree (Mobitz type II) AV block; intermittent 3rd degree AV block
AV block following acute MI	Persistent 2nd degree AV block; transient 3rd degree AV block; need not be symptomatic
Sinus node dysfunction	Documented symptomatic bradycardia; frequent sinus pauses
Prevention of tachycardia	Sustained, pause-dependent VT in which efficacy of pacing has been documented
Carotid sinus hypersensitivity	Recurrent syncope due to carotid sinus stimulation
Specific conditions	Hypertrophic cardiomyopathy; idiopathic dilated cardiomyopathy; cardiac transplantation – persistent bradycardia

From the *ACC/AHA/NASPE Guideline Update* (2002). Indications for pacing in children, adolescents and patients with congenital heart disease (CHD) (not shown) are broadly similar.

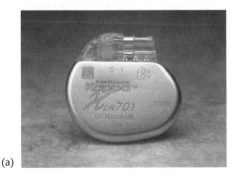
(a)

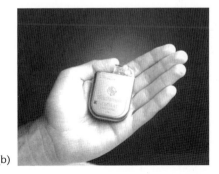
(b)

Figure 37.1 Examples of implantable pacemaker (a) and ICD (b) The ICD weighs <80 g and displaces ~40 cm³. Courtesy of Medtronic, Inc.

Table 37.2 The NASPE/BPEG five-position generic pacemaker code

Position	I	II	III	IV	V
Category	Chamber(s) paced	Chamber(s) sensed	Response to sensing	Rate modulation	Anti-tachycardia functions
Code letters	O	O	O		O
	A	A	T	O	P
	V	V	I	R	S
	D	D	D		D

O, none; A, atrium; V, ventricle; D, dual (A + V); T, triggered; I, inhibited; R, rate modulation; P, anti-tachycardia; S, shock.

Table 37.3 Examples of common permanent pacemaker modes

Code	Indication	Function
AAI	Sinus node disease, normal AV conduction	Demand atrial pacing
VVI	Bradycardia without need for preserved AV conduction, e.g. AF	Demand ventricular pacing
DDD	Bradycardia, impaired AV conduction	Maintains AV concordance
DDDR	Bradycardia, impaired AV conduction	Maintains AV concordance, exercise response

Fixed-rate pacing (AOO, VOO and DOO) is rarely used in PPM.

spontaneous ventricular depolarization and inhibit the delivery of unnecessary ventricular stimuli. VVI pacemakers have a ventricular escape interval, defined as the time after a paced or sensed beat that a pacemaker waits before delivering a pacing stimulus. VVI pacing is appropriate for chronic AF with slow ventricular rate. Most currently implanted PPMs are dual-chamber devices (DDD) capable of pacing and sensing both atria and ventricles. These versatile devices are more haemodynamically efficient than ventricular pacing. Rate-adaptive DDDR devices, which enable HR and CO to increase during exercise, are more physiological. Additional programmable features of DDDR devices include maximal upper rate, minimal lower rate, activity threshold, rate response, and acceleration and deceleration times. Mechanisms of rate adaptation vary. Piezoelectric crystals can detect vibration and body movement. Other sensors detect acceleration, ECG events (QT interval), myocardial contractility, minute volume, and central venous blood temperature or oxygen saturation (Table 37.3).

Implantable cardioverter defibrillators

National Institute for Clinical Excellence (NICE) Guidelines have reinforced the increasing role of these devices in the prevention of 'sudden cardiac death'.

ICDs can be programmed to function as biphasic defibrillators or overdrive pacing units. Modern devices are also capable of sophisticated pacing functions. Battery life is highly dependent on the number of shocks delivered.

Device implantation

Most PPMs are now inserted under local anaesthesia. The device is usually placed in a left pre-pectoral pocket and the endocardial leads inserted via the subclavian vein and positioned with fluoroscopic guidance. General anaesthesia may be required where difficulties are anticipated.

Implantation of ICDs is more complex – both because of the nature of the devices and the population of patients. Introduction of smaller devices has allowed electrophysiologists to implant them without surgical assistance. Conscious sedation is preferred to general anaesthesia in many centres. Invasive arterial monitoring should be considered in all cases. Device testing requires induction of VF and measurement of the minimally effective defibrillation energy threshold (DFT). Most ICDs deliver a biphasic waveform of up to 30 J, which provides a considerable margin of safety over the usual DFT of ~10–15 J. Standard inhalational anaesthetic techniques increase DFT by ~4 J, whereas techniques using subcutaneous lidocaine and intermittent boluses have minimal impact on DFT (Table 37.4).

Table 37.4 Complications of pacemaker and defibrillator insertion

Early complications

Venous access	Pneumothorax, haemothorax, air embolus
Lead related	Perforation, malposition, dislodgement
Pocket	Haematoma, infection

Delayed complications

Lead	Thrombosis, infection, insulation failure
Generator	Erosion, migration, external damage

Device function issues

Pacing/sensing	Oversensing, undersensing, crosstalk
ICD-specific	Failure to deliver shock, ineffective, inappropriate

Table 37.5 Perioperative considerations for patients with pacemakers and ICDs

Original indications for implantation	Medical history and pre-pacemaker symptoms*
Current mode of function?	Pacemaker book/card should be reviewed
Is device functioning properly?	Recent pacemaker checks?
	Recurrence of symptoms* – particularly during exercise
	CXR – location, type and continuity of leads
Is patient pacemaker dependent?	ECG – evidence of pacing spikes and capture?
Is reprogramming necessary before surgery?	PPM usually reprogrammed to fixed-rate pacing prior to induction of anaesthesia for cardiac surgery
What are likely effects of anaesthesia and surgery on device?	Electromagnetic interference
	Diathermy may cause reprogramming to VVI or VOO
	Drugs, electrolytes, defibrillation
What are likely effects of device on anaesthesia and surgery?	Bipolar diathermy where possible, smallest possible currents, avoid unnecessary cautery <5 cm from device

* pre-pacemaker symptoms.

Pacemakers and cardiac surgery

Perioperative considerations for patients with pacemakers and ICDs are shown in Table 37.5.

Unfortunately, because programmers are manufacturer-specific and use different telemetry frequencies and software, technicians may be unable to interrogate all devices. Magnets used to be applied to older PPMs to convert from demand to fixed-rate pacing. Magnet application *and removal* has unpredictable effects on modern PPM devices and is no longer recommended. Most devices will switch to high-rate asynchronous pacing, but some switch to low rate, and others to fixed programmed rates. Cardiac technicians can *usually* check pacemaker function, disable rate-adaptive functions and reprogramme the device to an asynchronous or triggered mode before induction of anaesthesia. It is important to consult cardiac technicians *before* the patient arrives in the operating room.

Induction

Due to its propensity to induce fasiculations, suxamethonium is generally avoided in patients with PPM.

Central and peripheral venous cannulations are generally undertaken on the contralateral side to the pacing system. PAFC is usually not utilized due to the risk of pacing lead dislodgement particularly in recently implanted systems. Diathermy ground plate should be placed so that current pathway is at right angles to the pacemaker leads. In practice, the plate is usually applied to the buttock.

Intraoperative considerations

Surgery is usually undertaken with fixed-rate pacing at $\sim80\,min^{-1}$, though rate can be modified depending on individual cardiac pathophysiology. Hypokalaemia, metabolic disturbances and hypercapnia may alter pacing thresholds and should be avoided. Diathermy may reprogramme or inhibit the device even in fixed-rate modes. Back up pacing via transcutaneous pads should be immediately available. Postoperative shivering is theoretically undesirable. If hypothermic CPB is utilized, adequate rewarming must be undertaken before separating from CPB. Insertion of epicardial pacing wires is rarely necessary in patients with PPM.

Table 37.6 Common perioperative temporary pacing problems

Problem	ECG	Cause	Action
Failure to pace	No A or V pacing spikes	Connection problem, lead problem, pacing box	Check each in turn
Failure to capture	Pacing spikes present	High-pacing threshold	Increase output? Reposition leads
Failure to sense	Asynchronous pacing	Sensitivity too low (*voltage too high*)	*Reduce* voltage on dial to increase sensitivity
Oversensing	Inappropriate output suppression	Artefacts or T-waves may be mistaken for R-waves	*Increase* voltage on dial to reduce sensitivity
Crosstalk	May inhibit V output	High A output, V sensitivity too high	Reduce A output, reduce V sensitivity

Postoperative considerations

The PPM must be checked and reprogrammed on the ICU *before* the patient returns to the ward. If electromechanical dissociation (EMD) arrest (loss of output with an apparently satisfactory paced electrical rhythm) occurs, always consider the possibility of underlying VF. Infection and septicaemia are particularly problematical in PPM patients. Complete device removal with transvenous lead extraction may become necessary. The decision to remove an infected lead is never easy and the explantation procedure is rarely straightforward. CPB standby may be required.

ICDs and cardiac surgery

All the preceding precautions for PPM apply to patients with an ICD. Use of magnets is liable to upset both the device and the electrophysiologist. Since diathermy could be misinterpreted as VF and trigger the delivery of a shock, defibrillation and anti-tachycardia functions must be disabled close to the time of anaesthetic induction. Adhesive patches are applied to the right upper chest and left lower chest *before* disabling the ICD defibrillation function. In the event of external fibrillation, the current is perpendicular to the ICD leads, which minimizes the risk of damaging the device. The internal defibrillation mechanism is reactivated when the patient is stable on the ICU.

Pacing problems

Temporary epicardial pacing via wires attached to the RA and RV may cause problems (Table 37.6). Fixed-rate pacing should almost invariably be converted to demand mode during ICU. Anaesthetists need to become familiar with both the single-chamber and dual-chamber boxes (pulse generators) used in their institution. Atrial wires are brought out through the right chest and ventricular wires through the left chest wall. Patients with long-standing chronic AF usually have ventricular epicardial wires only.

In the event of a possible pacing problem, check that the connections are secure, and that atrial and ventricular outputs are connected to the correct epicardial wires! Atrial wire dislodgement is a common cause of loss of atrial pacing.

Key points

- When patients with PPM or ICD are scheduled for cardiac surgery, cardiac technicians should be informed at an early stage.
- Magnet application has unpredictable effects on modern pacemakers.
- ICDs should be deactivated before surgery.
- Facilities for external defibrillation should be immediately available for the duration that ICD is disabled.
- Devices need to be checked and reprogrammed after surgery.

Further reading

National Institute of Clinical Excellence. *Guidelines on the Use of Implantable Cardioverter Defibrillators for Arrhythmias.* National Institute for Clinical Excellence Technology Appraisal Guidance, No. 11. London: NICE, September 2000.

Senthuran S, Toff WD, Vuylsteke A, Solesbury PM, Menon DK. Implanted cardiac pacemakers and defibrillators in anaesthetic practice. *Br J Anaesth* 2002; **88(5)**: 627–631.

D.W. Wheeler

Abnormal cardiac action potential (AP) production or conduction may be the manifestation of ischaemia, LV dysfunction or structural heart lesions. The classification of cardiac dysrhythmias is given in Table 38.1.

Patients with electrophysiological disorders have an increased risk of perioperative morbidity and mortality. Dysrhythmias may be triggered or worsened during anaesthesia and surgery, leading to myocardial ischaemia and hypoperfusion of vital organs. Patients undergoing investigation or treatment of electrophysiological disorders may require a general anaesthetic. Such procedures include direct current (DC) cardioversion, abnormal conduction pathway ablation, implantable cardioverter defibrillator (ICD) implantation and major cardiac surgery.

Preoperative assessment, intraoperative monitoring and postoperative care should reflect the fact that many patients have severe heart disease. Whenever possible,

a dysrhythmia should be corrected, or the physiological impact minimized, before surgery. Operative manoeuvres and drugs that trigger or worsen dysrhythmias should be avoided, and there should be a treatment plan if a dysrhythmia should arise.

Pathophysiology

Atrial fibrillation

In AF, abnormal AP wavelets are conducted through by atrial myocytes in a self-sustaining fashion, producing uncoordinated atrial contraction (Table 38.2 and Figure 38.1). The atrioventricular (A-V) node is bombarded with atrial APs that are irregularly conducted to produce a rapid and irregular ventricular response. Loss of atrial contraction and a shortened diastolic filling time to reduce SV and CO.

The treatment of AF includes identification and treatment of any underlying cause, electrical or chemical cardioversion (to NSR), control of ventricular rate and prevention of thromboembolic complications.

Table 38.1 Classification of cardiac dysrhythmias

Impulse generation

Supraventricular
- Sinus dysrhythmia, tachycardias, bradycardia
- SVT
- AF, atrial ectopic beats, atrial flutter

Junctional
- Nodal

Ventricular
- Ventricular ectopics, tachycardia, fibrillation

Impulse conduction

Delayed/absent
- Heart block

Abnormal pathways
- Pre-excitation syndromes
- Wolff–Parkinson–White (WPW) syndrome
- Lown–Ganong–Levine (LGL) syndrome
- Mahaim-type pre-excitation

Disordered action potential

Long QT Syndromes
- Inherited: Romano-Ward syndrome, Jervell Lange–Nielsen syndrome
- Acquired: $\downarrow\downarrow Ca^{2+}$, $\downarrow\downarrow K^{+}$, $\downarrow\downarrow Mg^{2+}$, drugs

Table 38.2 Causes of atrial fibrillation

Ischaemic heart disease
Atrial enlargement (e.g. mitral valve disease)
Hyperthyroidism
Idiopathic
Pulmonary embolism
Cardiomyopathy
Other – fever, infection, stroke, trauma

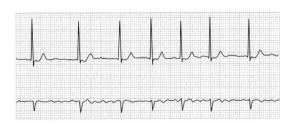

Figure 38.1 Atrial fibrillation.

Atrial flutter

An atrial ectopic beat can initiate a re-entrant atrial 'loop' which discharges at ~300 beats per minute. The ventricular response rate is dependent on A-V nodal conduction, which typically varies between 150 (2:1 block) and 60 min^{-1} (5:1 block). Flutter waves can be difficult to distinguish among QRS complexes if ventricular response is rapid. However, a narrow complex tachycardia of ~150 should be considered to be atrial flutter until proven otherwise. Manoeuvres that increase A-V block (e.g. carotid sinus massage or adenosine) may be diagnostic and therapeutic. In difficult cases, for example flutter with aberrant

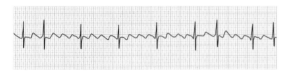

Figure 38.2 Atrial flutter with variable A-V conduction.

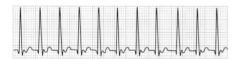

Figure 38.3 Supraventricular tachycardia.

conduction shown in Figure 38.2, an atrial ECG may be helpful. This can be recorded via an oesophageal lead, a transvenous temporary pacing electrode, temporary epicardial atrial pacing wires or by interrogating certain implanted pacemakers or defibrillators.

Supraventricular tachycardia

SVT is a paroxysmal tachycardia and is caused by a rapidly firing ectopic focus in the SA node, atria or A-V node. It may occur in the absence of organic disease or in association with hyperthyroidism, alcohol or caffeine intoxication and pre-excitation syndromes. The ventricular rate ranges from 140 to 240 min^{-1}, with narrow QRS complexes in the absence of bundle branch block (Figure 38.3).

Cardioversion may be achieved with vagal manoeuvres, DC shock, drugs (e.g. adenosine, esmolol and amiodarone) or overdrive pacing. Digoxin and verapamil should not be used unless it is certain the patient does not have Wolff–Parkinson–White (WPW) syndrome.

Pre-excitation syndromes

Disordered cardiogenesis can result in accessory conducting pathways that bypass the A-V node and the annulus fibrosis, which normally electrically insulates the atria from the ventricles (Table 38.3). The majority

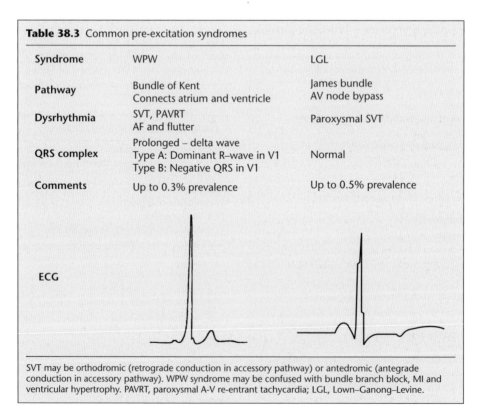

Table 38.3 Common pre-excitation syndromes

Syndrome	WPW	LGL
Pathway	Bundle of Kent Connects atrium and ventricle	James bundle AV node bypass
Dysrhythmia	SVT, PAVRT AF and flutter	Paroxysmal SVT
QRS complex	Prolonged – delta wave Type A: Dominant R–wave in V1 Type B: Negative QRS in V1	Normal
Comments	Up to 0.3% prevalence	Up to 0.5% prevalence
ECG		

SVT may be orthodromic (retrograde conduction in accessory pathway) or antedromic (antegrade conduction in accessory pathway). WPW syndrome may be confused with bundle branch block, MI and ventricular hypertrophy. PAVRT, paroxysmal A-V re-entrant tachycardia; LGL, Lown–Ganong–Levine.

of affected patients are young and have no evidence of other cardiac abnormality. The speed and direction of conduction via these pathways is highly variable, and dependant on their relative refractory periods. If conduction is predominantly via the A–V node, then the PR interval is normal. If conduction occurs via a faster accessory pathway, then the PR interval is shortened (<0.12 s). The morphology of the QRS complex depends on the level at which the accessory pathway joins the His–Purkinje system (Figure 38.4).

The treatment of WPW and SVT represents a particular challenge as many of the drugs commonly used to treat SVT may cause life-threatening dysrhythmias in WPW. Vagal manoeuvres or adenosine may terminate re-entrant tachycardia, but precipitate AF, which may progress to VF and sudden cardiac death. The drugs of choice are class Ic (e.g. propafenone or flecainide) or class III (e.g. sotalol or amiodarone) anti-dysrhythmics. Procainamide (class Ia) may be used to treat refractory dysrhythmics.

The termination of pre-excited AF in WPW syndrome warrants particular care. Digoxin, verapamil and other drugs that normally slow A–V conduction can paradoxically accelerate ventricular response and are contraindicated. If there is haemodynamic compromise, synchronized DC cardioversion is indicated; otherwise amiodarone or procainamide may be used (Figure 38.5).

In the long term, patients with symptomatic pre-excitation syndromes should undergo electrophysiological assessment. Ablation the accessory pathway is effective in most cases and has few complications.

Heart block

A-V (heart) block commonly indicates the presence of ischaemic or structural heart disease. It is important to identify patients with block that may progress to complete heart block (CHB) and cardiovascular collapse (e.g. bifascicular block or LBBB with first-degree heart block). Although these patients are at high risk of developing bradydysrhythmias with haemodynamic compromise, progression to CHB is independent of whether first-degree block is present and not as common as previously thought. Historically transvenous pacing was considered necessary before

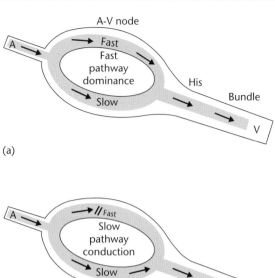

(a)

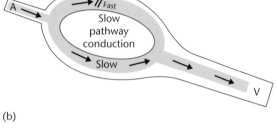

(b)

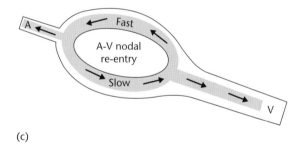

(c)

Figure 38.4 In WPW syndrome the accessory pathway may conduct APs retrogradely from the His–Purkinje system to the RA (orthodromic conduction) (a, *normal sinus impulse*). If an atrial extrasystole reaches the A-V node and accessory pathway when the accessory pathway is still in its refractory period, then the AP is conducted to the His–Purkinje system via the A-V node (b, *premature atrial impulse*). If the accessory pathway is no longer refractory when the impulse reaches the His–Purkinje system, it can be conducted retrogradely into the atria triggering a self-sustaining re-entrant loop that results in tachycardia (c, *A-V nodal re-entrant tachycardia*).

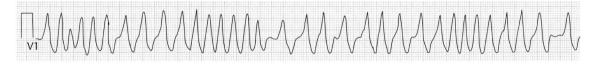

Figure 38.5 Pre-excited AF in WPW syndrome. The irregular rate and widened QRS morphology may be mistaken for VT.

anaesthesia. Nowadays it is recommended that brady-dysrhythmias be treated with chronotropic drugs, with facilities for temporary pacing on 'standby'.

Ventricular dysrhythmias

Ventricular extrasystoles are relatively common and usually benign. They may be a normal variant or secondary to ischaemic heart disease (IHD), hypoxaemia, hypercapnoea, electrolyte imbalance or drugs (e.g. halothane and anti-dysrhythmics). The presence of two or more ectopic foci (i.e. multifocal extrasystoles) is of more concern. They rarely require treatment unless the R wave coincides with the previous T wave (the 'R on T phenomenon'), when other dysrhythmias may be triggered (Figure 38.6).

A run of three or more consecutive ventricular extrasystoles constitutes VT or torsades des pointes (Figure 38.7). The rhythm is sustained by a rapidly

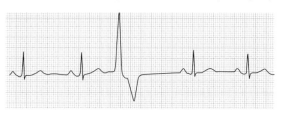

(a)

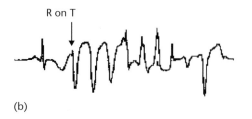

(b)

Figure 38.6 (a) Ventricular extrasystole. (b) R on T phenomenon triggering torsades des pointes.

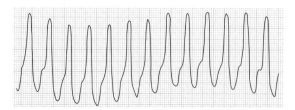

Figure 38.7 Ventricular tachycardia.

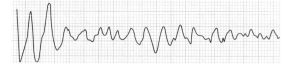

Figure 38.8 Degeneration of VT into coarse VF.

discharging ventricular focus. If there is no CO, immediate DC cardioversion is indicated. If the patient remains conscious, however, DC cardioversion should be undertaken under general anaesthesia. In the relatively asymptomatic patient, overdrive pacing, lidocaine or amiodarone may be considered.

Degeneration of the rhythm to VF (Figure 38.8) is an indication for immediate DC cardioversion. No anaesthetic is required!

Long QT syndromes

Prolongation of the QT interval >440 ms increases the risk of the R on T phenomenon, particularly if the corrected QT interval (QTc = QT interval/$\sqrt{RR}$ interval) is very variable (Figure 38.9).

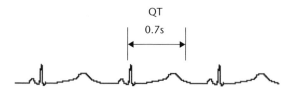

Figure 38.9 Prolonged QT interval.

Long QT syndrome (LQTS) may be acquired or secondary to inherited disorders of cardiac ion channels. Although the majority of patients are asymptomatic, LQTS may present as stress-induced syncope, cardiac arrest or 'seizures'. In addition, there may be a family history of LQTS or unexplained sudden cardiac death. A large number of drugs may prolong the QT interval (Table 38.4).

Table 38.4 Causes of QT interval prolongation

Inherited
Romano Ward syndrome (autosomal dominant)
Jervell and Lange–Nielsen syndrome (autosomal recessive)

Acquired
MI, CHB, cardiomyopathy, rheumatic fever
Hypokalaemia, hypcalcaemia, hypomagnesaemia

Drug induced
- Class Ia and Ic anti-dysrhythmics: procainamide, flecainide
- Class III anti-dysrhythmics: amiodarone, sotalol
- Antipsychotics: droperidol, thioridazine, risperidone
- Antidepressants: fluoxetine, sertraline
- Antimicrobials: erythromycin, clarithromycin, halofantrine
- Prokinetics: cisapride
- Antihistamines: terfenadine

Anaesthetic considerations

Patients with known dysrhythmias may require anaesthesia for electrophysiological studies, ablation therapy, dysrhythmia surgery or unrelated surgical procedures. Occasionally, a dysrhythmia may be diagnosed during elective surgery (e.g. the asymptomatic child who is found to have delta waves on the ECG monitor during the course of minor surgery).

A far more common scenario is the elderly patient with a supraventricular dysrhythmia (e.g. AF) or intermittent heart block who requires anaesthesia non-dysrhythmia surgery. Management goals include identification and treatment of any precipitating causes (Table 38.2), correction of hypovolaemia and electrolyte disturbances, ventricular rate control and avoidance of exacerbating factors in the perioperative period. As patients with long-standing AF and atrial enlargement are unlikely to respond to cardioversion, ventricular rate control and anticoagulation assume precedence. A small number of patients with bradydysrhythmias will require permanent preoperative pacing on prognostic and symptomatic grounds (Table 38.5).

Additional considerations apply when patients undergo procedures designed to characterize or treat a dysrhythmia. These include:

- DC cardioversion
- electrophysiological testing and aberrant pathway ablation
- ICD implantation
- the maze procedure.

Cardioversion

Elective, synchronized DC cardioversion is probably the most common anti-dysrhythmic procedure conducted under general anaesthesia. Although normally safe and uneventful, cardioversion may occasionally result in cardiovascular collapse or pulmonary aspiration. For these reasons, elective cardioversion should be carried out in an anaesthetic room or the ICU. Patients must be fasted, adequately anticoagulated (i.e. INR >2) and normokalaemic ($K^+ >4.0\,mmol\,l^{-1}$). Premedication is rarely necessary. Non-invasive monitoring and preoxygenation should precede induction of anaesthesia. In most cases a short-acting IV agent (e.g. propofol) is used rather than a combination of drugs. Inhalational agents are rarely necessary. Patients should be transferred to a designated recovery area for post-anaesthetic care.

Mapping and ablation

The characterization (mapping) and treatment (ablation) of paroxysmal tachydysrhythmias may require the deliberate triggering of the dysrhythmia. Although often performed under 'conscious sedation', general anaesthesia may be required for lengthy procedures, children and profoundly symptomatic patients. Tracheal intubation and intermittent positive pressure volume (IPPV) reduces the risk of hypoxia, hypercapnoea and aspiration. Invasive arterial monitoring should be considered if not undertaken by the electrophysiologist. Total IV anaesthesia (TIVA) avoids the adverse influence that inhalational agents (e.g. isoflurane) may have on the refractory period of an accessory pathway.

ICD implantation

Recurrent life-threatening ventricular dysrhythmias are increasingly being treated with ICDs. In most cases, implantation and testing is performed under local anaesthesia and monitored conscious sedation. The indications for ICD implantation and the perioperative management of patients with ICDs are discussed in Chapter 37.

Table 38.5 Consideration for patient undergoing general anaesthesia for the investigation and treatment of dysrhythmias

Isolated site
The cardiac catheterization laboratory or coronary care unit may be isolated from the operating theatres, recovery room and ICU

Hostile environment
Crowded room; limited access to patient; ionizing radiation – risk to patient, operators and anaesthetist

Skilled assistance
Staff may be unfamiliar with the anaesthetic equipment and procedures (e.g. preoperative fasting, administration of regular cardiac medication)

Co-morbidity
Dysrhythmias may indicate severe cardiovascular disease

Maze procedure

Chronic symptomatic AF that cannot be controlled pharmacologically may be amenable to surgical intervention, particularly if CABG or MV surgery is being contemplated. Although a number of procedures have been described, they all result in interruption of the atrial conduction routes by the creation of insulating scar tissue and an electrical 'maze' or 'labyrinth'. Surgical incision of the atria during CPB is gradually being superseded by radio frequency, microwave and cryo-ablation techniques. These latter techniques have permitted the introduction of minimally invasive, off-pump and percutaneous procedures.

The potential complications associated with open CPB procedures include bleeding, atrial standstill and persisting AF. A significant number of patients may require permanent pacing.

Key points

- A broad-complex tachycardia may indicate SVT with aberrant conduction.

- Digoxin and verapamil should not be used to treat SVT unless WPW syndrome has been excluded.
- Perioperative progression of chronic bifascicular block or LBBB to CHB is rare. Routine prophylactic insertion of a temporary pacemaker is rarely indicated.
- An undiagnosed conduction abnormality may become apparent during the course of general anaesthesia for a non-cardiac surgical procedure.

Further reading

Booker PD, Whyte SD, Ladusans EJ. Long QT syndrome and anaesthesia. *Br J Anaesth* 2003; **90(3)**: 349–366.

Cannom DS. Atrial fibrillation: nonpharmacologic approaches. *Am J Cardiol* 2000; **85(10A)**: 25D–35D.

Esberger D, Jones S, Morris F. ABC of clinical electrocardiography. Junctional tachycardias. *Br Med J* 2002; **324(7338)**: 662–665.

Gauss A, Hubner C, Radermacher P, Georgieff M, Schutz W. Perioperative risk of bradyarrhythmias in patients with asymptomatic chronic bifascicular block or left bundle branch block; does an additional first degree atrioventricular block make a difference? *Anesthesiology* 1998; **88(3)**: 679–687.

CARDIOMYOPATHIES AND CONSTRICTIVE PERICARDITIS

39

J.H. Mackay & F. Falter

Hypertrophic obstructive cardiomyopathy

Hypertrophic obstructive cardiomyopathy (HOCM) is a progressive disease, also referred to as idiopathic hypertrophic subaortic stenosis (IHSS) and aymmetrical septal hypertrophy (ASH). Inheritance is autosomal dominant with heterogeneous phenotypes within families.

Pathology

The predominant lesion is ventricular septal hypertrophy, with narrowing of the LVOT. The LV free wall, in comparison, remains relatively thin.

Clinical features

The most common presentation is sudden death in a previously asymptomatic patient. A small number of patients develop symptoms similar to AS – typically breathlessness, angina and syncope/pre-syncope on exertion. Atrial and ventricular dysrhythmias are also common.

Pathophysiology

HOCM causes dynamic LVOT obstruction, functional AS and dynamic MR. These lead to a secondary increase in left atrial pressure (LAP), reduced CO and hypotension.

Narrowing of the LVOT during systole leads to increased systolic ejection velocity, which draws the anterior mitral leaflet (AMVL) towards the hypertrophied septum by a Venturi effect. Systolic anterior motion (SAM) brings the AMVL into contact with the septum leading to LVOT obstruction in mid-systole to late systole. Distortion of MV results in mid-systolic and late systolic MR. The sequence of events are summarized in Figure 39.1.

Increased muscle mass, decreased LV volume and myocardial fibrosis lead to decreased compliance and diastolic dysfunction. Reduced calcium re-uptake by sarcoplasmic reticulum increases myoplasmic calcium and contributes to impaired relaxation.

Factors influencing the LVOT pressure gradient and obstruction are summarized below:

Factors increasing LVOT obstruction	Factors decreasing LVOT obstruction
↓ Arterial BP	↑ arterial BP
↓ Preload	↑ LV volume
↑ Blood flow velocity inotropes	↑ Blood flow velocity β-blockers/verapamil
↓ SVR	↑ SVR

Investigations

- *2D echo* This determines end-diastolic septal thickness and LVOT diameter, characterizes SAM and identifies the leaflet–septum contact point.
- *Colour Doppler* Characteristic systolic turbulence in LVOT with posteriorly directed jet of MR.
- *CWD* Characteristic 'sharks tooth' velocity contour in LVOT differs from AS (Figure 39.2). Velocity of blood increases during systole due to SAM.
- *PWD* The determination of transmitral and pulmonary venous blood flow velocities allows assessment of impairment of LV relaxation (see Chapter 25).

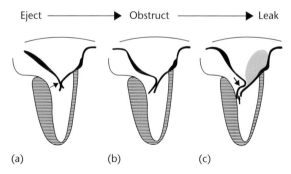

Figure 39.1 SAM of the AMVL, dynamic LVOT obstruction and MR in HOCM. (a) Onset of systole, (b) early systole and (c) mid-systole. Adapted from Journal of the American College of Cardiology **20**: 42–52. Grigg *et al.* © 1992 with permission from the American College of Cardiology Foundation.

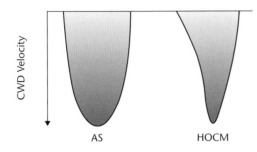

Figure 39.2 CWD in AS and HOCM.

Management

- *Medical* β-blockers and Ca^{2+}-channel blockers of the verapamil type are first-line medical treatment. Implantation of a DDD pacing device improves symptoms in some patients.
- *Surgical* Septal myectomy through the aortic valve is considered in patients with symptoms not controlled by maximal medical treatment and LVOT gradient >50 mmHg.

Anaesthetic goals

Preload	Better full than empty
HR	60–80 is ideal
Rhythm	Preserve sinus rhythm
Contractility	Maintain (but most tolerate mild depression)
SVR	Maintain (or slight ↑) to maintain coronary perfusion pressure

The basic rule is to avoid haemodynamic derangements that worsen the obstruction. If an inhalational technique is used, halothane is said to be superior to isoflurane. Surgery for relief of dynamic LVOT obstruction is considered a Category I indication for perioperative TOE (Chapter 24).

Complications of surgery

These include residual LVOT obstruction, VSD and conduction abnormalities requiring permanent pacing.

Constrictive pericarditis

Constrictive pericarditis is an uncommon cause of diastolic dysfunction.

Pathology

Pericardial inflammation leads to fibrosis and calcification. Ultimately the heart becomes 'encased' in a non-compliant sac, which prevents normal diastolic filling and the transmission of intrathoracic pressure changes to the cardiac chambers.

Idiopathic	? Post-viral
Infection	Tuberculosis
Malignancy	
Ionizing radiation	Radiotherapy
Post-cardiac surgery	
Connective tissue disorders	Rheumatoid arthritis

Pathophysiology

Constriction gives rise to rapid early diastolic filling, which ceases abruptly when the limits of ventricular expansion are reached (Figures 39.3 and 39.4).

Overall cardiac volume is relatively fixed which leads to exaggerated ventricular interdependence. There is

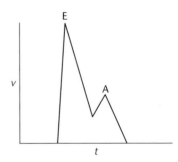

Figure 39.3 Transmitral diastolic flow pattern in constrictive pericarditis. Note the high-velocity E-wave and short deceleration time.

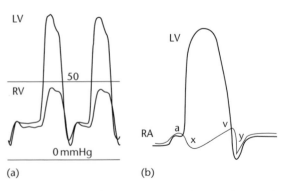

(a)   (b)

Figure 39.4 Typical pressure tracings in constrictive pericarditis. (a) The pathognomonic 'square root sign' can be seen in both the LV and RV pressure traces (b) Rapid, unimpeded early diastolic filling gives rise to a deep y-descent in the RA pressure trace. The short duration of the y-descent is due to abrupt cessation of early diastolic filling.

dissociation between intrathoracic and intracardiac pressures.

During normal spontaneous respiration, inspiration increases venous return to the right heart with a slight shift of the ventricular septum to the left. In contrast, increased pulmonary capacitance (fall in PAWP > fall in LVEDP) reduces venous return to left heart resulting in a fall in arterial pressure by up to 10 mmHg. In constrictive pericarditis, where changes in intrathoracic pressure are not transmitted to the ventricles, this so-called *respiratory paradox* is exaggerated and LV filling can vary by more than 25% during the respiratory cycle (Figure 39.5).

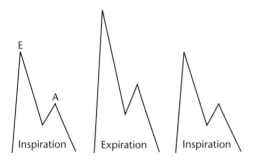

Figure 39.5 The effect of spontaneous respiration on diastolic LV filling in constrictive pericarditis.

Diagnosis

Diagnosis is often difficult and needs high index of suspicion. Patients present with a variety of symptoms and usually show signs of right heart failure. The differential diagnosis from restrictive cardiomyopathy can be difficult but is important, as treatment options are very different (Table 39.1):

- Patients with constrictive pericarditis need surgical pericardectomy.
- Patients with restrictive cardiomyopathy need medical treatment or transplantation.

Anaesthetic goals

Anaesthetic considerations are similar to those for cardiac tamponade. Both the conditions are associated with impaired diastolic filling, increased atrial pressures, tachycardia and reduced SV. In constrictive pericarditis, however, ventricular filling occurs early in diastole, whereas in tamponade, ventricular filling occurs predominantly in late diastole.

Preload	Increased
HR	High
Rhythm	Sinus preferable but limited atrial kick
Contractility	Maintain
SVR	Maintain

Surgical pericardiectomy is associated with significant perioperative mortality because patients are often in poor condition, and are prone to major haemorrhage and haemodynamic instability during dissection. Unlike relief of tamponade, pericardial stripping does not usually result in an instantaneous reversal of pathophysiology.

Unstable cases may need CPB standby and cannulation of the groin is an option. Most surgeons use median sternotomy as cannulation is easier if CPB is required. If anterolateral thoracotomy utilized, patients will require a double-lumen tube. The institution of intermittent positive pressure ventilation may be associated with a significant reduction in LV filling and profound

Table 39.1 Differential diagnosis

	Constrictive pericarditis	Restrictive cardiomyopathy
CXR	Diffuse calcification of pericardium	Normal heart size
CVP	Prominent y- ≫ x-descents	Elevated. Prominent cv-wave in the presence of TR
PA catheter	PA systolic pressure normally <40 mmHg	PA systolic pressure ⩾50 mmHg
LV catheter	'Square root' sign RVEDP = LVEDP RV systolic pressure ⩽50 mmHg	LVEDP − RVEDP >5 mmHg RV systolic pressure ⩾50 mmHg
2D echo	Pericardial thickening and effusion	Normal pericardium
Doppler echo	Restrictive pattern Respiratory swing >25% variation peak mitral velocities during inspiration	Little respiratory swing in velocities
CT and MRI	Pericardial thickness >4 mm	Pericardial thickness <4 mm

hypotension. For this reason positive end-expiratory pressure (PEEP) should not normally be applied.

Restrictive cardiomyopathy

This very rare condition causes severe diastolic dysfunction. Although many of the presenting symptoms and signs are similar to those of constrictive pericarditis, the principles of management are widely different.

Pathology

Conditions characterized by myocardial stiffening (thickening and fibrosis) and endocardial thrombosis. The diagnosis can only be confirmed by myocardial biopsy:

- Primary
  - Idiopathic
- Secondary
  - Amyloidosis
  - Sarcoidosis
  - Haemochromatosis
  - Glycogen storage diseases
  - Eosinophilic (Löefflers) endocarditis
  - Tropical endomyocardial fibrosis.

Clinical features

Patients present with signs and symptoms of biventricular failure. Signs of right heart failure tend to predominate.

Pathophysiology

There are many similarities to constrictive pericarditis. Marked myocardial stiffening and very low ventricular compliance cause the characteristic pattern of rapid but early diastolic filling (see Figure 25.11).

Anaesthetic goals

Preload	High
HR	High
Rhythm	Sinus – preferred, but little dependence on late diastolic filling
Contractility	Maintain – inotropic support invariably needed
SVR	Maintain in the face of 'fixed' CO

Dilated cardiomyopathy

Dilated cardiomyopathy (DCM) is the most common primary cardiomyopathy. Peak incidence in middle-aged males.

Pathology

Characteristically four-chamber cardiac enlargement, cardiomyocyte hypertrophy and a propensity towards formation of intracardiac thrombus. Cardiomyopathy secondary to myocardial ischaemia may be limited to the LV. Endomyocardial biopsy is rarely diagnostic. The characteristics are summarized as:

- Primary
  - Idiopathic
  - Hb-SS disease
  - Muscular dystrophy (Duchenne)
- Secondary
  - Ischaemia
  - Valvular disease
  - Infection (viral, trypanosomal)
  - Toxic (ethanol, adriamycin)
  - Peripartum
  - Myxoedema.

Clinical features

DCM is characterized by progressive left, right or biventricular failure and declining functional status. Ventricular dysrhythmias are common. Patients are at risk of pulmonary or arterial embolism from intracardiac thrombi if inadequately anticoagulated.

Pathophysiology

Impaired systolic *and* diastolic function, low CO and elevated LVEDP. Subsequent atrioventricular valve regurgitation worsens atrial enlargement, increasing the likelihood of AF. Ventricular compliance is reduced. Diastolic transmitral blood flow velocity measurement reveals impaired relaxation early in the process, progressing to 'pseudo-normalization' and ultimately a restrictive filling pattern (see Chapter 25).

Anaesthetic goals

Preload	Increased due to ↑ LVEDP
HR	Avoid tachycardia, if ventricular relaxation impaired
Rhythm	Sinus preferred – little contribution in end-stage disease
Contractility	Inotropic support may be required
Afterload	Increases poorly tolerated

Key point

- The differential diagnosis of constrictive pericarditis and restrictive cardiomyopathy can be difficult.

CARDIAC TRANSPLANTATION

40

F. Falter & J.H. Mackay

Fewer road traffic accidents, improved medical treatment of subarachnoid haemorrhage and better neurosurgical intensive care have reduced the availability of hearts suitable for transplantation over the past decade.

Heart transplantation requires full anticoagulation and hypothermic aorto-caval CPB. Explantation is invariably incomplete in order to facilitate implantation. The remnants are a cuff of LA (incorporating the four pulmonary veins), and a cuff of RA (incorporating the SVC and IVC). Implantation then requires anastomosis of the donor and recipient atria, aorta and PA.

Good coordination is crucial to minimize the cold ischaemic time of the donor heart as duration has a considerable impact on the performance of the donor heart after weaning from CPB. The maximum time from application of the aortic cross-clamp (AXC) at donor hospital to removal of the AXC in the recipient should be <4h.

Patient selection

In practice, most recipients have dilated or ischaemic cardiomyopathy. Rarer indications for heart transplantation include unresectable cardiac tumours,

end-stage valvular disease, hypertrophic obstructive cardiomyopathy (HOCM), sarcoidosis, amyloidosis and active myocarditis.

- Indications
  - Physiological age <60 years
  - Emotional and social stability
  - Compliant with drugs
  - Strong motivation
- Relative contraindications
  - Peripheral vascular disease
  - Severe COPD
  - Diabetes mellitus with end-organ dysfunction
  - Conditions likely to be worsened by immunosuppression
  - Ventilator dependence
- Absolute contraindications
  - Active substance abuse
  - Fixed pulmonary hypertension
    - PVR > 5 Wood units
    - Transpulmonary gradient >15 mmHg
  - Cerebrovascular disease
  - Co-existent malignant or other life-limiting disease

End-stage heart failure is characterized by biventricular systolic and diastolic function with left ventricular ejection fraction (LVEF) 10–20%. Pulmonary hypertension (PHT), secondary to elevated LA pressure is common. Pulmonary vascular resistance (PVR) and transpulmonary gradient (TPG) are key determinants of outcome:

$$TPG = Mean\ PAP - PAWP$$
$$PVR = TPG/CO$$

A normal TPG is ~6mmHg, therefore a normal PVR is $6\,mmHg/5\,l\,min^{-1} = 1.2$ Wood units ($\sim96\,dyne \cdot s \cdot cm^{-5}$). Irreversible PVR >5 Wood units is associated with an increased incidence of post-transplantation RV failure. If PVR falls below 5 Wood units with medical treatment, the risk may be considered acceptable. A TPG >15 mmHg is associated with unacceptably high mortality and is an absolute contraindication to heart transplantation.

The effects of LV failure and increased PVR on LV and PA pressure waveforms are shown in Figure 40.1.

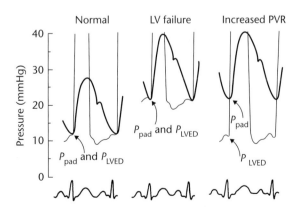

Figure 40.1 LV and PA pressure waveforms. In LV failure the PA diastolic (PAD) pressure and LVEDP are elevated, whereas increased PVR results in a large pressure gradient (i.e. PAD > LVEDP) (From Benumof JL. Anaesthesia for Thoracic Surgery, 2nd edition. Philadelphia: WB Saunders 1995.)

Anaesthetic management

Preoperative assessment

Thorough assessment in the transplant clinic should identify most potential anaesthetic problems. Despite the fact that recipients are often admitted to hospital only a few hours before surgery, cancellation of the procedure solely for anaesthetic reasons is extremely rare. Premedication is usually impractical as timings are generally provisional rather than fixed. Although many patients may have eaten within 6 h, it is unusual to encounter patients who have fasted <3 h. Liquid antacid and an H_2-blocker may be given to reduce the risk of aspiration. It is important that immuno-suppressive drugs and prophylactic antibiotics are administered in accordance with unit protocol.

Induction and maintenance

The overall approach is the same as that for a patient with severely impaired LV function. Use of an 8F central venous sheath allows rapid fluid administration and facilitates subsequent PAFC insertion. Given that the RIJ will be used for obtaining biopsies to monitor rejection, some centres prefer to use the LIJ vein for the operation. The maintenance of cerebral, renal and splanchnic perfusion is of greater importance than balancing myocardial oxygen demand and supply. Post-induction hypotension is common and should be treated aggressively with a combination of fluids, vasopressors and inotropes. Sensitivity to inotropes may be reduced. The use of aprotinin should be considered in patients undergoing repeat sternotomy.

Monitoring

Use of a PAFC before explantation is not routine as it rarely alters management. The catheter may be difficult to insert, may cause significant dysrhythmia, and must be withdrawn to <15 cm before heart explantation. TOE offers major advantages over the PAFC during surgery and provides valuable information about donor heart function. The PAFC may, however, be of use in the early post operative period.

Post-implantation

Following de-airing and reperfusion of the donor heart, isoproterenol ($5-10\,\mu g\,kg^{-1}min^{-1}$ for up to 5 days) is used to provide chronotropic support (target HR $\sim$ 100) and mild pulmonary vasodilatation. As the output of the donor heart is largely rate dependent, epicardial atrioventricular (A–V) sequential pacing should be initiated if isoproterenol is ineffective alone. Taking care not to disrupt surgical anastomoses, a

PAFC may be advanced at this stage with the help of the surgeon. Persistent hypotension in the presence of normal or elevated filling pressures should be treated with further inotropic support. Anaesthetic goals in the post CPB period are summarised below.

> Sinus rhythm (HR $\sim$ 100) – epicardial pacing as required.
> Avoidance of hypoxaemia, hypercarbia and metabolic acidosis.
> Maintenance of normal LV and RV filling pressures.
> Expectant management of ventricular dysfunction.
> Early consideration of ventricular assist in persistent ventricular failure.

Right ventricular failure

Patients with established PHT are at increased risk of donor heart dysfunction. TOE will reveal RV dilatation and a small, hyperkinetic LV. The therapeutic approach consists of inotropic support and vasodilatation. Hypoxia, hypercarbia and metabolic acidosis must be avoided. Owing to its effect on PVR, enoximone is a useful adjunct. Inhaled nitric oxide (NO) (up to 20 ppm) or epoprostenol (prostacyclin – PGI_2; $2-50\,ng\,kg^{-1}\,min^{-1}$) may be considered in refractory cases.

If ventricular failure persists despite maximal inotropic and vasodilator therapy, mechanical circulatory support with either an intra-aortic balloon or a ventricular device should be considered as a 'bridge to recovery'.

Coagulopathy

An increasing proportion of patients presenting for heart transplantation will have been taking anticoagulants before surgery. It is, therefore, important to have blood products (red cells, FFP and/or platelets) readily available after CPB.

The transplanted heart

The transplanted heart is initially denervated. In the absence of adrenergic and vagal efferents, the Frank–Starling mechanism and levels of circulating catecholamines and metabolites (e.g. lactate, H^+) dictate cardiac performance. Resting HR is usually higher than normal and rises to a lesser degree during exercise. Paradoxically, ischaemic injury to the SA or AV nodes may produce severe bradycardia. Up to 20% of transplanted patients will require a permanent pacemaker.

Immunosuppression

Cyclosporin, azothioprine, mycophenolate, antilymphocyte globulin and corticosteroids are the most widely used drugs. Regimens vary considerably from centre to centre. Chronic immunosuppression may lead to a variety of complications:

- *Infection* Predominantly bacterial and viral (~90%), and fungal and protozoal (~10%). Risk greatest in the 1st month. Incidence decreases rapidly after 6 months. Lungs and blood are most common sites of infection.
- *Neoplasia* Lymphoproliferative disorders.
- *Myelosuppression* Anaemia, thrombocytopenia, leucopaenia.
- *GI* Haemorrhage, cholelithiasis/cholecystitis, pancreatitis (azathioprine, mycophenolate).
- *Renal* Impaired tubular function, hypertension.
- *Metabolic* Diabetes, osteoporosis.
- *Other* Hirsutism (cyclosporin), gingival hyperplasia, obesity, cataract.

Rejection

Eighty-five per cent of patients undergo at least one episode of rejection during the first 3 months following transplantation. Typical presenting features include breathlessness, fatigue and reduced exercise tolerance. Low-grade fever, atrial flutter/AF and weight gain despite fluid restriction should also arouse diagnostic suspicion. After 6 months the risk dramatically decreases. Transvenous endomyocardial biopsy remains the diagnostic test with the greatest sensitivity and specificity.

Acute and chronic rejection can occur any time. An increase in LV wall thickness with impaired LV function may be apparent on echocardiography. Elevated troponin I, a lymphocytosis and the presence of circulating lymphoblasts suggest rejection. Treatment typically consists of high-dose immunosuppression.

Allograft vasculopathy

Initially thought to be a form of rejection, cardiac allograft vasculopathy (CAV) is the main cause of death after the first year of transplantation and ultimately limits long-term survival. Although immunological factors are thought to be involved, postulated aetiologies include donor ischaemia time, gender, age and recipient coronary artery disease, hyperlipidaemia and cytomegalovirus (CMV) infection. CAV is a vascular disease that involves all vessels of the transplanted heart including veins and leads to lumen obliteration. Angiographic evidence of CAV is seen in 10–20% patients at 1 year and 30–50% at 5 years. Retransplantation, the only definitive therapy, is limited by shortage of donor organs and poorer survival.

Key points

- RV failure is likely to occur if hearts are transplanted into patients with PVR >5 Wood units.
- A TPG >15 mmHg is associated with high postoperative mortality and is therefore a contraindication to heart transplantation.
- Maintaining perfusion pressure and oxygen delivery to the key organs is the primary goal in the pre-CPB period.
- Good quality organ donor management, which includes myocardial protection, is essential during the retrieval operation.
- The proportions of heart transplant recipients surviving 1, 5 and 10 years are approximately 90%, 70% and 50%, respectively.

Further reading

Benumof SL. Anaesthesia for Thoracic Surgery, 2nd edition. Philadelphia: WB Saunders, 1995

PAEDIATRIC CARDIAC ANAESTHESIA

GENERAL PRINCIPLES 41

I.A. Walker & J.H. Smith

Congenital heart disease occurs in approximately 8:1000 live births and may be associated with recognizable syndromes or chromosomal abnormalities in 25% of cases. Abnormalities are often complex affecting structure and function. Surgery may be corrective or palliative and can be staged. Over half of these operations occur in the first year of life. The timing of surgery is dictated by the severity of the lesion, the need to avoid the development of pulmonary vascular disease or the complications of cyanotic heart disease.

There are significant differences in infant and adult physiology that have a bearing on the conduct of anaesthesia for children with congenital heart disease. This chapter will address these differences in physiology and some general principles of anaesthesia for paediatric cardiac surgery.

Normal neonatal physiology

Newborn infants have a high metabolic rate and oxygen consumption. This is reflected in a high resting RR and CI (neonate: $300\,ml\,kg^{-1}min^{-1}$, adult $70–80\,ml\,kg^{-1}min^{-1}$). They have limited capacity to increase SV in response to increased filling and the resting HR is near maximal (Table 41.1). Neonates are exquisitely sensitive to negative inotropic or chronotropic agents.

The sarcoplasmic reticulum in neonatal myocytes is poorly developed. Calcium for cardiac contraction is derived from the extracellular fluid and infants do not tolerate ionized hypocalcaemia. There is a relative imbalance of sympathetic and parasympathetic nervous systems at birth and neonates are prone to vagal reflexes.

The infant lung is relatively non-compliant, the ribs horizontally placed and relatively compliant. The lower airways are small and easily obstructed by secretions. Infants are consequently prone to respiratory failure.

Other important factors to consider include immature renal function, temperature regulation, hepatic function and drug, particularly opiate, metabolism.

Transitional circulation

In utero blood bypasses the fetal lung via two shunts, the foramen ovale and the ductus arteriosus. With the first few breaths, there is a dramatic reduction in PVR and closure of fetal shunts. Pulmonary vasodilatation continues during the first few weeks of life, due to thinning of smooth muscle in the media of the pulmonary arterioles. PVR reaches adult levels by a few weeks of age (Figure 41.1). During this time the pulmonary vasculature remains reactive and stimuli such as hypoxia, hypercarbia and acidosis will cause pulmonary vasoconstriction and possibly reopen the ductus arteriosus (see below). Persistent pulmonary hypertension (PPHN) of the newborn may result; hypoxia may become critical and require treatment with inhaled nitric oxide or in extreme cases, extracorporeal membrane oxygenation (ECMO).

Closure of the ductus arteriosus occurs in two phases. Functional closure occurs within 2–4 days in nearly all healthy infants under the influence of increasing PaO_2, falling $PaCO_2$ and prostaglandins. Anatomical

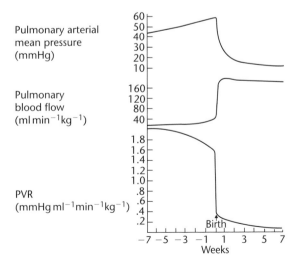

Figure 41.1 Perinatal changes in pulmonary haemodynamics. Reprinted with permission from Rudolph AM, 1996.

Table 41.1 Normal ranges for RR, HR and systolic BP according to patient age

Age	RR (bpm)	HR (bpm)	Systolic BP (mmHg)
Newborn	40–50	120–160	50–90
Infant (<1 year)	30–40	110–160	70–90
Pre-school (2–5 years)	20–30	95–140	80–100
Primary school (5–12 years)	15–20	80–120	90–110
Adolescent (>12 years)	12–16	60–100	100–120

closure of the ductus arteriosus due to fibrosis occurs within the first 3 weeks of life.

Continued ductal patency may occur due to prematurity (inadequate ductal smooth muscle) or in sick infants under the influence of excessive endogenous prostaglandin released in response to stimuli such as hypoxia (causing relaxation of ductal smooth muscle). A large duct may result in cardiac failure due to excessive pulmonary blood flow; diastolic BP will be low and may be associated with impaired renal or intestinal blood flow (possible renal impairment or necrotizing enterocolitis). Prostaglandin synthetase inhibitors such as indomethacin promote closure of the duct.

Duct-dependent circulation

In certain situations, continued ductal patency may be required for survival of the neonate (Table 41.2). In this situation prostaglandin E2 infusion will be required and should be continued until definitive surgery. High doses of prostaglandin infusion can result in apnoeas, fevers and systemic vasodilatation. Where prostaglandin infusion has been continued long term (for instance, a premature neonate awaiting surgery), it should be remembered that prostaglandins are effective pulmonary vasodilators and may have to be weaned gradually post surgery.

Infants with a *duct-dependent systemic circulation* typically present with cardiac failure or collapse during the 1st week of life as the duct closes and shunting from the pulmonary to systemic circulation is lost. Treatment requires resuscitation with inotropes and fluids and institution of prostaglandin infusion prior to definitive surgery.

Infants with *duct-dependent pulmonary circulation* become cyanosed after duct closure and the loss of left to right shunting across the duct. Cyanosis will be unresponsive to increased FiO_2 and pulmonary blood flow must be restored with prostaglandin infusion before a definitive surgical procedure for example, valvotomy or systemic to pulmonary shunt is performed.

Table 41.2 Conditions dependent on continuing patency of the ductus arteriosus

Duct-dependent	Conditions
Systemic circulation	Critical coarctation, critical AS, HLHS
Pulmonary circulation	Pulmonary atresia, critical pulmonary stenosis, tricuspid atresia
'Mixing'	Transposition of the great arteries

Infants with *duct-dependent 'mixing'* have two parallel closed loop circulations and are dependent on mixing between the right and left side. Prostaglandin infusion and balloon atrial septostomy will be required where there is inadequate intracardiac mixing.

Balancing systemic and pulmonary circulations in neonates

Appropriate balance between systemic blood flow and pulmonary blood flow can be crucial, particularly in the neonate when alteration in direction of shunt blood flow may cause dramatic changes in saturation or CO.

Oxygen is a potent pulmonary vasodilator in neonates, while hypercarbia and acidosis cause pulmonary vasoconstriction. High FiO_2 and hyperventilation may be beneficial in infants with reduced pulmonary blood flow. Conversely, they may have a detrimental effect in infants with high pulmonary blood flow, or with balanced systemic and pulmonary shunts.

Exposure of neonates with large left to right shunts (e.g. large VSD) to high FiO_2 will cause pulmonary hyperaemia and worsening cardiac failure. Infants in cardiac failure preoperatively should be given sufficient inspired oxygen to maintain SaO_2 in the low 90s only.

Similarly, neonates with a duct-dependent systemic circulation (see previous page) or with high volume, high pressure shunts (e.g. AV septal defect, truncus arteriosus, large Blalock-Taussig (B-T) shunt), may have balanced shunts between systemic and pulmonary circulation. Ventilation with 100% oxygen may cause a marked fall in PVR, excessive left to right shunting and a fall in systemic perfusion leading to hypotension and metabolic acidosis. Strategies should be adopted to improve CO (e.g. fluids, inotropes) and reduce pulmonary blood flow. Ventilation in theatre should be with air (or for cyanotic lesions, sufficient oxygen to maintain SaO_2 in the mid 80s), and with moderate hypercarbia. Conversely, a marked fall in SVR should be avoided as this may result in increased right to left shunting and critical cyanosis. Inotropic support may be required to increase SVR and CO, thus improving pulmonary blood flow. Similar principles should be followed postoperatively in the ICU, particularly after the first stage Norwood procedure for hypoplastic left heart syndrome (HLHS).

SVR should be maintained in infants with large right to left shunts, such as tetralogy of Fallot. Excessive vasodilatation on induction of anaesthesia may result in worsening cyanosis; vasoconstrictors may be required. Extreme right to left shunting is seen in the 'spelling Fallot' due to spasm of the RVOT infundibulum in the presence of excess catecholamines. Measures to overcome infundibular spasm and increase pulmonary blood flow are required. These include adequate sedation, hyperventilation with 100% oxygen, a fluid bolus, bicarbonate or phenylephrine – the latter to reverse the direction of the shunt across the VSD and improve forward flow to the lungs. Propranolol may also be considered to reduce infundibular spasm.

SVR must be maintained in infants with left (or right) ventricular outflow obstruction. A fall in SVR may lead to critical hypoperfusion of the hypertrophied ventricle. A reduction in PVR may be beneficial in infants with RV hypertrophy.

Cardiopulmonary interactions

Positive pressure ventilation is generally beneficial to infants in cardiac failure due to poor myocardial function or left to right shunts (reduced work of breathing and afterload, improved oxygenation and CO_2 clearance), with attention to the FiO_2, as above. However, hyperventilation at high pressures or volumes may increase PVR by over-distension of lung, disproportionately reducing the cross-sectional area of the pulmonary vasculature.

Breathing spontaneously with a negative intrapleural pressure will augment systemic venous return to the right heart and improve pulmonary blood flow. This fact is utilized in the postoperative management of patients with cavo-pulmonary connections.

Surgical strategy

The timing of surgical repair is dictated by the functional impact of the cardiac lesion. Urgent balloon septostomy may be indicated in neonates with transposition. Duct-dependent lesions require corrective or palliative surgery within days of birth. Similarly, infants with obstructed total anomalous pulmonary venous drainage (TAPVD) may present with extreme cyanosis and cardiac failure requiring urgent corrective surgery.

Systemic arterial to pulmonary shunts such as the B-T shunt (subclavian artery to main PA) are performed in infancy for conditions associated with low pulmonary blood flow such as severe tetralogy of Fallot or pulmonary atresia. Definitive corrective surgery is performed, usually in the first year, after further growth of the pulmonary arteries.

Conditions involving left to right shunts increase pulmonary blood flow and cause cardiac failure and pulmonary hypertension (PHT). Typically, high volume shunts cause heart failure as the PVR falls to adult levels at a few weeks of age (e.g. large VSD). Continued high pulmonary blood flow will result in irreversible changes in the pulmonary vasculature and will severely limit treatment options. Early surgery is therefore indicated. PA banding may be performed in infants with high pulmonary blood flow not suitable for early definitive surgery (e.g. multiple VSDs). Low volume shunts (e.g. ASD) may be closed when the child is older to avoid irreversible PHT in adult life.

Palliative surgery to create a univentricular circulation is performed in conditions where there is only a single functional ventricle or great vessel (univentricular AV connection – double inlet ventricle, HLHS, tricuspid atresia or severe pulmonary atresia with intact ventricular septum). Pulmonary blood flow may initially be provided with a B-T shunt in the neonatal period while the PVR remains high. Systemic venous shunts are performed after the PVR falls – initially a Glenn shunt (SVC to PA), followed by an IVC to PA anstomosis to complete the Fontan circulation (or total cavopulmonary venous connection (TCPC)) (see Chapter 43).

Closed cardiac surgery

Cardiac operations may be 'closed' or 'open'. Open operations are performed on CPB and are discussed in the next chapter. Closed operations are usually on the main vessels of the heart and do not require CPB. The four commonest indications for closed operation in neonates and infants are:

- Ligation of a patent ductus arteriosus (PDA) via left thoracotomy.
- Repair of coarctation via left thoracotomy.
- PA banding via sternotomy or thoracotomy. PA banding is a temporary measure to prevent PHT and is reversed at the time of definitive surgery.
- Systemic to pulmonary shunts for example, B–T shunt via sternotomy or thoracotomy.

Cyanosis

Children with cyanotic heart disease maximize tissue oxygen delivery by becoming polycythaemic and having a mild metabolic acidosis (causing right shift of the oxygen dissociation curve). Progression of cyanosis is reflected in an increase in haematocrit and venesection and haemodilution may be indicated. There is a risk of thromboembolism, including cerebral infarction, which is exacerbated by dehydration. Prolonged preoperative starvation must therefore be avoided. The prothrombotic tendency is partially compensated for by a mild coagulopathy – clotting factors should be available post bypass.

Key points

- Neonates have limited cardiopulmonary reserve and reactive pulmonary vasculature during the 1st weeks of life.
- Prostaglandin infusion may be required for duct-dependent circulation prior to surgery.
- Manipulations of PVR and SVR have an important effect on balanced circulation; ventilation strategies should be carefully considered.
- Cardiac operations in children may be open or closed, depending on the abnormality.
- Children with cyanotic heart disease require careful perioperative care.

Further reading

Côté, Todres, Goudsouzian, Ryan (Eds). *A Practice of Anaesthesia for Infants and Children*, 3rd edition. Pennsylvania: Saunders, 2001.

Rudolph AM, Rudolph CD, Hoffman JIE (Eds). *Rudolph's Pediatrics*. 21st edition. Norwalk, Connecticut: Appleton and Lange, 1996.

Sumner E. Anaesthesia for patients with cardiac disease. In: Sumner E, Hatch DJ (Eds). *Paediatric Anaesthesia*, 2nd edition. London: Arnold, 2000.

I.A. Walker & J.H. Smith

Paediatric cardiac anaesthetists work as part of specialized multidisciplinary teams. The anaesthetist requires a thorough understanding of congenital cardiac lesions, the planned surgery, the management of CPB and familiarity with anaesthetizing small infants for major surgery. It is not for the occasional practitioner.

The anaesthesia plan should be formulated in the light of all preoperative investigations and discussions. The predominant cardiac lesion should be considered on the basis of pathophysiology (Table 42.1), myocardial reserve, and an assessment of the nature of shunt or obstructive lesions and the impact of alteration of SVR or PVR.

Children with uncomplicated procedures such as closure of ASD or VSD may be suitable for a 'fast track' approach and this should be taken into account in planning anaesthesia. Children having a Fontan procedure (cavopulmonary connection) may benefit from early extubation as pulmonary blood flow is improved with spontaneous ventilation. Children who are in cardiorespiratory failure preoperatively, are unstable or who have large left to right shunts and are at risk for postoperative pulmonary hypertension, will require postoperative ventilation.

Preoperative assessment

The child must be evaluated carefully in the light of cardiological investigations. Symptoms of cardiac failure should be sought – poor feeding, sweating and grunting in young infants, recurrent chest infections, failure to thrive and poor exercise tolerance in older children. Signs of cardiac failure in young infants include tachycardia, tachypnoea and hepatomegaly (but

Table 42.1 Pathophysiology of congenital heart lesions

	Example	Comment
Acyanotic lesions		
Left to right shunt		May lead to congestive cardiac failure and
Restrictive	Small ASD, VSD, PDA	pulmonary hypertension, depending
Non-restrictive	Large ASD, VSD, PDA, AVSD	on the magnitude of the shunting
Obstructive	AS, coarctation, interrupted aortic arch, HLHS, PS, MS, TS	Severity of lesion determines age at presentation – neonates may be critically ill
Regurgitant	AR, MR, MV prolapse, TR, PR	
Cyanotic lesions		
Transposition of the great arteries	With ASD, PDA or VSD, ±LV outflow obstruction	May require BAS for survival if inadequate mixing. Presence of LV outflow obstruction determines surgical options
Right to left shunt	Tetralogy of Fallot, critical PS, pulmonary atresia (±VSD), tricuspid atresia	Severity of cyanosis depends on degree of obstruction through the right heart
Common mixing	TAPVD (+ASD, ±VSD, PDA, CoA), truncus arteriosus, double inlet ventricle (single ventricle), double outlet ventricle	Cyanosis may not be severe if lung blood flow unobstructed, but congestive heart failure will be present

AVSD, atrioventricular septal defect; HLHS, hypoplastic left heart syndrome; TAPVD, total anomalous pulmonary venous drainage; CoA, coarctation of the aorta (modified from Archer and Burch. *Paediatric Cardiology: An Introduction* 1998. Reprinted by permission of Hodder Arnold).

rarely peripheral oedema). In children with cyanotic heart disease baseline SaO_2 should be recorded and in children with tetralogy of Fallot, a history suggestive of hypercyanotic episodes. It is obviously important to exclude intercurrent infection as a cause of worsening symptoms.

Note should be made of associated disorders, particularly those affecting the airway. DiGeorge syndrome (22q11 deletion) causes 5% of cardiac anomalies, is associated particularly with truncus arteriosus and interrupted aortic arch and often results in thymic aplasia and neonatal hypocalcaemia. The immunological defect necessitates the use of irradiated blood products to prevent graft versus host disease (GVHD).

This is obviously a time of enormous stress for the family. There should be a detailed and sympathetic discussion with the parents (and child if appropriate), concerning invasive monitoring, the need for postoperative intensive care, blood transfusion, analgesia and sedation. It is our normal practice for parents to accompany the child to the anaesthetic room with a member of the nursing staff, if they wish – discussions should focus on their role and what to expect.

Premedication

Premedication of the young infant is not necessary, although chloral hydrate may be considered if the child has frequent hypercyanotic 'spells'. Older children may be premedicated with oral midazolam or temazepam, provided there are no contraindications such as upper airway obstruction or limited cardiac reserve. Topical local anaesthesia is a routine; amethocaine gel (Ametop®) is suitable for infants from 6 weeks of age. Preoperative fasting instructions are no food or milk for 6 h preoperatively, clear fluids up to 2 h preoperatively – this may avoid preoperative discomfort and intraoperative hypoglycaemia.

Induction

At the very minimum, a pulse oximeter should be applied before induction. Full monitoring should be instituted as soon as the child will tolerate it. Infants who are unstable should be anaesthetized in the operating theatre.

The choice of induction agent depends on the cardiac lesion. Children with less severe lesions (e.g. ASD, small VSD) will tolerate induction with judicious doses of propofol or thiopental. Inhalational induction with sevoflurane is routine for infants, although

extreme care should be taken in sick infants with severe cyanosis or cardiac failure, as they will not tolerate the myocardial depressant effects of the volatile agents. Anaesthesia may be maintained with isoflurane, and continued during CPB. Inhalational induction in the cyanosed child is only slightly prolonged compared to those with left to right shunt. Nitrous oxide may be used for induction, but then discontinued – it is a myocardial depressant and may increase PVR. Air should be available on the anaesthetic machine if required for infants with balanced shunts.

Ketamine is a safe alternative to inhalational agents, and is commonly used in sick patients. It causes an increase in CI, SVR and PVR, although a rise in PVR may be avoided with effective airway control. It has a direct myocardial depressant effect that is usually offset by inhibition of norepinephrine uptake. The myocardial depressant effect may be evident in children on long-term inotropic therapy with depleted catecholamine stores.

High dose fentanyl anaesthesia is also suitable for infants with limited myocardial reserve. It will limit the stress response to surgery, but doses above $50\,\mu g\,kg^{-1}$ probably confer no additional benefit and may result in hypotension. Doses higher than $1–2\,\mu g\,kg^{-1}$ should only be given incrementally with invasive monitoring.

Uncuffed ETTs are traditionally used to secure the airway. Cuffed tubes are available down to size 3.0 and may be useful if lung compliance poor or if a thoracotomy is to be performed (e.g. for coarctation repair or Blalock-Taussig (B-T) shunt).

Some advocate regional anaesthesia for paediatric cardiac surgery to reduce the stress response, improve postoperative recovery and reduce hospital costs. Others believe the risk of an epidural haematoma in a child who will be heparinized far outweighs the benefits. It is suggested that the risk of epidural haematoma is minimized by ensuring normal preoperative coagulation, abandoning difficult insertions or those where blood returns through the needle or epidural catheter. Heparin administration should be delayed until at least 60 min after needle placement and the catheter removed only in the presence of normal coagulation.

Vascular access and monitoring

The long saphenous vein is useful for peripheral vascular access. Sites for arterial access include the radial, femoral, axillary or brachial arteries. The arterial line and SaO_2 monitor should be in the right arm for coarctation repair, whereas vessels in the ipsilateral arm should not be cannulated prior to a B–T shunt. NIBP monitoring on the leg is useful after coarctation repair.

The internal jugular vein, cannulated using standard landmarks or with ultrasound guidance, is usually used for central venous access. Double or triple lumen catheters (4 F or 5 F) are available in various lengths. The internal jugular vein should not be used in infants with univentricular physiology who may have a Fontan procedure in the future as thrombosis of the neck veins will make this impossible. The femoral vein should be used as an alternative, with a small monitoring line in the internal jugular vein to reflect PA pressure for example, after a Glenn shunt. The left internal jugular vein should be avoided in children with a persistent left SVC as it commonly drains into the coronary sinus. Transthoracic lines may be placed to measure LA or PAP post CPB.

Core and peripheral temperatures are both measured. The nasopharyngeal temperature gives a measure of brain temperature – a peripheral probe should be placed on the foot. Overhead radiant heaters may be useful in the anaesthetic room, although overheating should be avoided and moderate hypothermia may be protective in infants undergoing coarctation repair.

Cardiopulmonary bypass

The difference in management of CPB in children compared to adults reflects differing physiology and complexity of intracardiac surgery. Cannulation will usually be bicaval. Pump flow rates are relatively high reflecting the increased metabolic rate of small infants. Perfusion pressures are maintained at 30–60 mmHg at normothermia and vasoconstrictors are rarely required. The volume of the pump is large relative to the circulating volume of infants – citrated blood is added to the pump prime to avoid excessive haemodilution (and calcium to avoid hypocalcaemia).

CPB may be conducted at normothermia, moderate hypothermia (25–32°C), deep hypothermia (15–20°C) or deep hypothermia with circulatory arrest. Deep hypothermic circulatory test (DHCA) is reserved for neonates and infants with complex lesions when the aortic and venous cannulae are removed to improve surgical access. Deep hypothermia also allows for periods of low pump flow to improve the surgical field.

There is significant risk of neurological morbidity in infants undergoing DHCA, possibly related to air or particulate emboli. Periods of circulatory arrest are best combined with periods of low flow. Circulatory arrest of up to 30–40 min may be tolerated during deep hypothermia. Uniform cooling is important and inadequate cooling time (<18 min) is associated with worse outcomes. Vasodilatation during cooling may be useful. Cerebral protection may be improved using pH control of acid–base balance (pH-stat) prior to circulatory arrest (associated with cerebral vasodilatation), and alpha-stat control at other times (cerebral autoregulation preserved). Icepacks are placed over the head during circulatory arrest to prevent rewarming. Hyperglycaemia should be avoided.

- *pH-stat* During cooling prior to circulatory arrest.
- *alpha-stat* At other times.

Weaning

Rewarming after AXC removal allows for spontaneous return of myocardial electrical activity. VF is uncommon in children and if persistent, may reflect poor myocardial preservation. De-airing should be meticulous to avoid coronary and cerebral air embolism – the lungs are ventilated to increase LA filling. Ventilation is recommenced as the heart starts to eject, with prior suctioning of the tracheal tube. Temporary pacing wires are inserted as a routine as intracardiac surgery may affect the conducting system.

Vasodilators (e.g. SNP, phentolamine or GTN) aid rewarming. Inotropic support is usual in infants and should be started at about 30°C after removal of the cross clamp. While dopamine is commonly used, dobutamine is preferable if the PVR is elevated. Phospho–diesterase-III (PDE-III) inhibitors (e.g. milrinone) are increasingly used in the setting of pulmonary hypertension (PHT) or RV dysfunction, with a loading dose being given during CPB. Combining a PDE inhibitor with either dopamine or epinephrine is useful in the presence of poor ventricular function or after ventriculotomy (Table 42.2). Volume overload in the small non-compliant ventricle must be avoided.

Post bypass management

Modified ultrafiltration

Modified ultrafiltration (MUF) is useful in children <20 kg weight. It is started prior to protamine administration. Blood is taken from the aorta, passed through an ultrafilter and returned to the RA. The process usually takes 15–20 min and is continued until the haematocrit is about 40% – as much as 500 ml of fluid may be removed. MUF increases haematocrit and colloid osmotic pressure, removes extracellular water (including myocardial oedema), reduces transfusion requirements and improves haemodynamic function. It also

Table 42.2 Common cardiac drug dosages in paediatric cardiac practice

Drug	Dilution	Dose
Dopamine	$3\,mg\,kg^{-1}$ in 50 ml 5% dextrose	$1\,ml\,h^{-1} = 1\,\mu g\,kg^{-1}\,min^{-1}$ Dose range $5–10\,\mu g\,kg^{-1}\,min^{-1}$
Dobutamine	$3\,mg\,kg^{-1}$ in 50 ml 5% dextrose	$1\,ml\,h^{-1} = 1\mu g\,kg^{-1}\,min^{-1}$ Dose range $5–10\,\mu g\,kg^{-1}\,min^{-1}$
Epinephrine	$0.03\,mg\,kg^{-1}$ in 50 ml 5% dextrose	$1\,ml\,h^{-1} = 0.01\,\mu g\,kg^{-1}\,min^{-1}$ Dose range $0.01–0.5\,\mu g\,kg^{-1}\,min^{-1}$
Norepinephrine	$0.03\,mg\,kg^{-1}$ in 50 ml 5% dextrose	$1\,ml\,h^{-1} = 0.01\,\mu g\,kg^{-1}\,min^{-1}$ Dose range $0.01–0.5\,\mu g\,kg^{-1}\,min^{-1}$
Milrinone	$0.3\,mg\,kg^{-1}$ in 50 ml 5% dextrose	$1\,ml\,h^{-1} = 0.1\,\mu g\,kg^{-1}\,min^{-1}$ Dose range $0.375–0.75\,\mu g\,kg^{-1}\,min^{-1}$ Loading dose $50–100\,\mu g\,kg^{-1}$ in 20 min
Isoprenaline	$0.03\,mg\,kg^{-1}$ in 50 ml 5% dextrose	$1\,ml\,h^{-1} = 0.01\,\mu g\,kg\,min^{-1}$ Dose range $0.01–0.5\,\mu g\,kg^{-1}\,min^{-1}$
SNP	$3\,mg\,kg^{-1}$ in 50 ml 5% dextrose	$1\,ml\,h^{-1} = 1\,\mu g\,kg^{-1}\,min^{-1}$ Dose range $0.5–5\,\mu g\,kg^{-1}\,min^{-1}$
GTN	$3\,mg\,kg^{-1}$ in 50 ml 5% dextrose Maximum concentration $1\,mg\,ml^{-1}$	$1\,ml\,h^{-1} = 1\,\mu g\,kg^{-1}\,min^{-1}$ Dose range $0.5–5\,\mu g\,kg^{-1}\,min^{-1}$
10% Calcium gluconate		Bolus dose $0.1\,ml\,kg^{-1}$
Phenylephrine		Bolus dose $1\,\mu g\,kg^{-1}$

reduces PVR, improves cerebral function and may reduce the levels of vasoactive cytokines.

Haemostasis

Diffuse coagulopathy is common in neonates after CPB. This is due to a combination of immature hepatic function, haemodilution by the pump prime (minimum prime volume 500 ml, blood volume of a neonate 240 ml) and activation of clotting by the large non-endothelialized surface of the CPB circuit. Operations tend to be long, pump flow rates are high, DHCA is often used, and relatively large volumes of blood are salvaged and returned to the CPB circuit. Thrombocytopenia and hypofibrinogenaemia are common and platelets and cryoprecipitate (or FFP) are ordered routinely. Mild coagulation defects are also common in children with cyanotic heart disease.

Aprotinin may reduce bleeding after reoperation but its use in patients undergoing DHCA or venous shunts (e.g. bi-directional Glenn shunt) remains controversial. It may have a useful anti-inflammatory effect but a test dose should be given because of the risk of anaphylaxis. Tranexamic acid and ε-aminocaproic acid may also be useful.

Transoesophageal echo

TOE is useful before CPB identify defects, and after CPB to assess contractility and the integrity of the surgical repair. Considerable expertise is required to interpret the image in complex lesions. Smaller infants can have epicardial echocardiography.

Delayed sternal closure

The chest may be left open after neonatal surgery if there is evidence of cardiac tamponade after primary chest closure. Delayed primary closure is usually possible on the ICU after 24–72 h.

Pulmonary hypertensive crisis

All newborns and those with high pulmonary blood flow (e.g. truncus arteriosus, atrioventricular septal defect (AVSD) and total anomalous pulmonary venous drainage (TAPVD)) are at risk of postoperative PHT. A monitoring line may be inserted into the main PA during surgery. During a pulmonary hypertensive crisis there may be a sustained rise in PA pressure (>65% systemic), or the PA pressure may be suprasystemic. It will usually respond to inhaled nitric oxide (NO) (20 ppm) but higher doses may be required. Standard management also includes moderate hypocapnia, avoidance of acidosis, ventilation in 100% oxygen and additional sedation and paralysis. The usual duration of therapy is 24–48 h.

Right heart failure

RV failure may be a consequence of surgical ventriculotomy, poor myocardial preservation (particularly with pre-existing RVH), transient PHT, raised transpulmonary gradient or anatomical problems subsequent to the surgery, such as an obstructed outflow tract. It is important to rule out the latter with an on-table echo or early postoperative catheter.

Treatment strategies include those for PHT, if indicated, careful volume loading (RA pressures 15–16 mmHg) and epinephrine combined with PDE inhibitors. Failure to respond to high dose inotropes may require the use of extracorporeal membrane oxygenation (ECMO) or a ventricular assist device (VAD).

Transfer to intensive care

Transfer of the child back to intensive care may be a hazardous process – lines may be displaced and haemodynamic instability may occur due to bleeding. The child should be fully monitored at all times. Finally, it is important that the anaesthetist transfers the wealth of information they have gleaned about the patient during the perioperative period over to the intensive care team in an effective manner.

Key points

- Anaesthetic and CPB strategies must take into account age of child, pathophysiology of cardiac lesion and planned surgical procedure.

- The volume of the pump is large compared to circulating volume of infant.
- DHCA may be required in neonates with complex lesions.
- MUF improves outcome post bypass in infants.
- Neonates with high pulmonary blood flow are at risk of pulmonary hypertensive crisis post bypass.

Further reading

Gaynor JW. Use of ultrafiltration during and after Cardiopulmonary bypass in children. *J Thorac Cardiovasc Surg* 2001; **122(2)**: 209–211.

Goldman AP, Delius RE, Deanfield JE, Macrae DJ. Nitric oxide is superior to prostacyclin for pulmonary hypertension after cardiac operations. *Ann Thorac Surg* 1995; **60(2)**: 300–306.

Laussen P. Optimal blood gas management during deep hypothermic paediatric cardiac surgery: alpha stat is easy, but pH stat may be preferable. *Paediatric Anaesthesia* 2002; **12(3)**: 199–204.

D.J. Barron & K.P. Morris

Patent ductus arteriosus

Incidence

Common: Persistence inversely proportional to gestational age. Incidence >80% in infants <1 kg birth weight.

Associations

Prematurity, diaphragmatic hernia, transposition of great arteries (TGA), Fallot's and pulmonary atresia.

Anatomy

Remnant of the distal portion of the sixth left aortic arch. Connects main PA to descending thoracic aorta (Figure 43.1).

Physiology

Carries ~90% of RV output *in utero*. Left to right (L–R) shunt increases as PVR falls following birth. Functional (reversible) closure within 15 h of birth. Permanent closure occurs within 3 weeks in term infants. Risk of endarteritis (often termed duct-related endocarditis). Haemodynamic impact of patent ductus arteriosus (PDA) dependent on size:

- Small PDA may go undetected.
- Large PDA may cause severe heart failure. Excessive pulmonary blood flow may exacerbate respiratory distress syndrome, precipitate pulmonary haemorrhage and compromise weaning from the ventilator. 'Run-off' from the aorta results in a low diastolic pressure and 'steal' from the systemic circulation. Reduced mesenteric blood flow may result in necrotizing enterocolitis.

Diagnosis

Continuous machinery murmur. Echocardiography confirms duct and direction of shunting; LA: aortic diameter ratio reflects degree of L–R shunting.

Management

According to duct dependence (see Chapter 41).

- *Medical*: treatment with indomethacin or another NSAID may result in duct closure. Often combined with fluid restriction and diuretics.
- *Trans-catheter closure*: may be undertaken in the catheter laboratory (Cath lab) in large infants or child.
- *Surgical*: Necessary if medical treatment fails or is contraindicated (renal impairment, GI or other haemorrhage). Duct is ligated or closed with a clip via left thoracotomy without CPB.
  - *Complications*: inadvertent ligation of left PA or descending aorta, damage to recurrent laryngeal nerve or thoracic duct, reduced pulmonary compliance. Inotropes rarely required for ventricular dysfunction and poor perfusion.

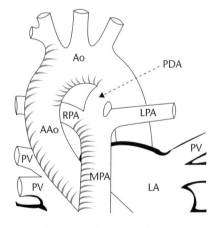

Figure 43.1 The patent ductus arteriosus.

Coarctation of the aorta

Incidence

6% of all congenital heart disease.

Associations

Turner's syndrome, bicuspid AV (up to 40%), VSD.

Anatomy

Narrowing of aorta in the region of the ductal insertion (i.e. distal to the left subclavian artery). Can occasionally occur proximal to the left subclavian.

Physiology

Presentation depends on severity of narrowing:

- Severe coarctation of the aorta (CoA) presents in a neonate as the duct closes. Aorta virtually occluded causing circulatory collapse, acute LV failure and loss of lower limb pulses.
- Moderate CoA presents more subtly with degree of LV failure in childhood (rare).
- Less severe CoA presents with chance finding of murmur or upper limb hypertension.

Management of the neonate

Prostaglandin E (PGE) infusion. This reopens the duct and re-establishes flow to the lower body. Ductal tissue is often involved in CoA, so the severity of CoA

may also be reduced with PGE. Neonates usually have considerable heart failure. May require full resuscitation with ventilation/inotropic support. Condition can usually be stabilized with these measures. Rarely the duct will not reopen and surgery is required as an emergency.

Surgery

Via left thoracotomy; ~1% perioperative mortality for isolated CoA. Repaired either with resection and end-to-end anastamosis or with subclavian flap angioplasty (Figure 43.2). Both have excellent results, the former is regarded by most as the gold standard. Sacrificing the subclavian artery in the neonate does not cause limb ischaemia and at worse may result in reduced limb growth. Repair of hypoplastic aortic arch may require bypass via sternotomy.

Postoperative management

Monitor femoral pulses. Echo to assess LV function and confirm adequate arch repair. May have postoperative hypertension, requiring treatment (β blocker). 0.5% risk of paraplegia due to spinal cord ischaemia. Record lower limb function when muscle relaxants are stopped.

Aortic interruption is an extreme form of CoA. Usually associated with a VSD and commonly associated with 22q11 deletion. Requires repair on bypass via sternotomy. Much higher-risk condition.

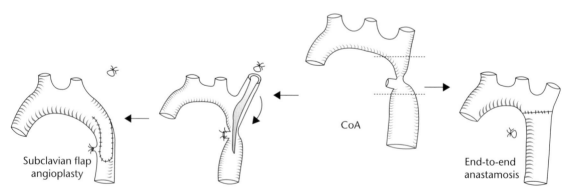

Figure 43.2 Surgery of coarctation of the aorta.

Atrial septal defect

Incidence

8% of all congenital heart disease.

Associations

Holt-Oram, maternal rubella and Down's (primum defect) syndromes.

Anatomy

Defects occur at different sites (Figure 43.3). Secundum ASDs are the most common – the majority of *secundum* defects can be closed with a device in cath lab. All other types of defects require surgical closure. Primum ASDs are a type of atrioventricular septal defect (AVSD) page 235 (Figure 43.5).

Physiology

L–R shunt causing volume load on pulmonary circulation. Most children are symptomless but plethoric lungs may predispose to chest infections and failure to thrive. Very large shunts may result in effort intolerance. Pulmonary hypertension is *not* associated with isolated ASDs in children.

Surgery

Suture closure of small defects, autologous pericardium or prosthetic patch closure of larger defects.

Postoperative care

Surgery is generally of low risk and children can be weaned and extubated shortly after surgery. Sinus venosus ASD repair involves the root of the SVC and there is a risk of causing SVC obstruction. If face looks plethoric or SVC pressure is high, arrange echo/contrast evaluation. Nodal rhythms may occur with high atrial incisions (e.g. sinus venosus ASD).

Some units 'fast track' ASD repairs to the ward on the day of surgery. Appropriate monitoring must be continued on the ward.

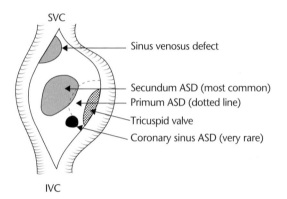

Figure 43.3 View inside right atrium.

Ventricular septal defect

Incidence

30% of all congenital heart disease.

Associations

VACTERL syndrome and *coarctation*. Remember that many other complex forms of congenital heart disease include a VSD (e.g. truncus, pulmonary atresia and Fallot).

Anatomy

Schematic of the ventricular septum viewed from the right side is given in Figure 43.4.

Physiology

The majority of VSDs do not require intervention and either close spontaneously or are so small as to not warrant closure. Perimembranous VSDs are unlikely to close spontaneously and the most likely to need surgical closure. Large VSDs cause heart failure and failure to thrive in neonates/infants and are the most common indication for repair.

'Unrestrictive' VSD means there is no Doppler gradient across the VSD on echo. This means that the VSD must be large and the pressure within the RV is at systemic level, leading to pulmonary hypertension. Pulmonary hypertension should completely reverse as long as the defect is closed before 6 months of age.

Less common indications for closure are:

- moderate VSDs in older children that have failed to close and continue to produce a significant shunt ($Q_P : Q_S > 1.5 : 1$);
- small VSDs that have been associated with an episode of endocarditis;
- small perimembranous VSDs that have resulted in aortic valve prolapse into the defect, with aortic regurgitation.

Surgery

1–2% mortality for isolated VSD. Most VSDs are closed via the RA using a prosthetic patch.

Postoperative management

Patients are usually neonates/young infants with considerable heart failure preoperatively. Regular diuretics and vasodilators help offload the LV. *Check rhythm*: atrioventricular node is adjacent to perimembranous VSDs and variable degrees of heart block can be seen. All patients should have atrial and ventricular pacing wires available. Block is usually transient (a few hours) but can be permanent (1–2%). Any patient who is pacemaker dependent should have thresholds checked daily. Rising threshold alerts to need for urgent wire replacement. Echo should be performed postoperatively to assess LV function, to exclude any residual VSD and to estimate the RV pressure. Pulmonary hypertensive crises are a potential risk but uncommon in simple VSD repair. Older children (>6 months) with large VSDs are at a greater risk.

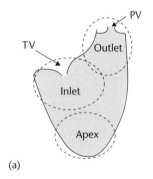
(a)

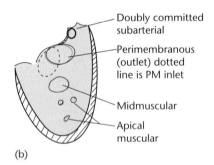
(b)

Figure 43.4 Schematic of ventricular septum viewed from right side. a) ventricular septum can be divided into inlet, apex and outlet portions, b) sites in which VSDs are found.

Atrioventricular septal defect

Atrioventricular septal defect (AVSD) is also called atrioventricular canal defect or endocardial cushion defect. AVSDs may be complete (cAVSD) or partial (pAVSD).

Incidence

4% of all congenital heart disease.

Associations

Both cAVSDs and pAVSDs are strongly associated with Down's syndrome. Within the UK ~75% of patients with cAVSD and ~30% of patients with pAVSD have Down's syndrome.

Anatomy

There is a defect in the centre of the heart with a single valve (the common AV valve) straddling both ventricles and a hole above and below it. In pAVSD, the VSD component has closed leaving only an ASD (Figure 43.5).

Physiology

- *cAVSD*: Behaves like a large VSD (i.e. L–R shunt leading to high pulmonary blood flow and heart failure in neonates). In addition, the common AV valve can be regurgitant, adding to the heart failure. All require surgical closure before 6 months of age. Later repair is associated with significant risk of irreversible pulmonary hypertension.

- *pAVSD*: Also called Primum ASD. The ventricular component has closed, there is less of an L–R shunt and generally children are not in heart failure. Repair generally before 5 years of age.

Surgery

cAVSD ~5% perioperative mortality; pAVSD ~1% perioperative mortality. The VSD is closed with one patch, the ASD with another, sandwiching the valve between them. Surgery recreates two separate atrioventricular (A-V) valves. However, anatomically the valve between the LA and LV is not a true mitral valve (referred to as the 'left A-V valve') (Figure 43.6). Repair of cAVSD in babies without Down's syndrome is typically more complicated (poor A-V valve function) compared to babies with Down's syndrome.

Postoperative management

LA line is useful and PA line is inserted where concern exists about postoperative pulmonary hypertension. Echo to exclude residual VSD, look at LV function and atrioventricular valve function. Confirm rhythm, risk of heart block. Babies usually in marked heart failure preoperatively with pulmonary congestion, may take time to wean from ventilator. Risk of pulmonary hypertension. Management of pulmonary hypertension is described in chapter 44. pAVSDs are generally uncomplicated but most have had a left atrioventricular valve repair and should have an echo to document the result.

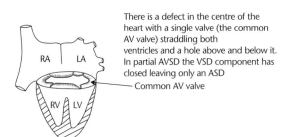

There is a defect in the centre of the heart with a single valve (the common AV valve) straddling both ventricles and a hole above and below it. In partial AVSD the VSD component has closed leaving only an ASD — Common AV valve

Figure 43.5 Anatomy of atrioventricular septal defect.

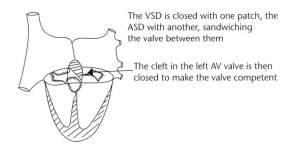

The VSD is closed with one patch, the ASD with another, sandwiching the valve between them

The cleft in the left AV valve is then closed to make the valve competent

Figure 43.6 Surgery of atrioventricular septal defect.

Fallot's tetralogy

It is also called Tetralogy of Fallot, TOF and Fallot.

Incidence and Associations

6% of all congenital heart disease. 22q11 deletion.

Anatomy

The key anatomical features of perimembranous VSD with aortic over-ride and multilevel RV outflow obstruction are highlighted in Figure 43.7. Coronary artery anatomy is important: 2–4% have anomalous LAD crossing in front of the PA. Repair requires a conduit to jump over the anomalous coronary. Absent pulmonary valve (PV) syndrome is a rare type of Fallot with similar intracardiac anatomy but no true PV, just a membrane. The PAs beyond the valve have marked post-stenotic dilatation and may cause compression of the airways and bronchomalacia. Treatment is similar but involves plication of the aneurysmal central PAs and respiratory assessment.

Physiology

The degree of cyanosis depends on severity of RVOT obstruction and tends to gradually worsen with age. Cyanotic neonates are usualy palliated with a Blalock-Taussig (B-T) shunt (see page 243). Stable *infants* are usually repaired around 1 year of age. β blockers may help relieve infundibular muscle spasm and reduce degree of cyanosis.

Surgery

4–5% early mortality. Muscle bundles in the RVOT are resected and the VSD is closed, usually via0 the right atrium. If transannular incision is required then the PV is sacrificed leaving a degree of pulmonary regurgitation (60–80% of cases) (Figure 43.8).

Postoperative management

Rhythm disturbances and low cardiac output can occur.

Junctional tachycardias are common and may be nodal or His bundle in origin. An atrial wire study (Figures 44.1 and 44.2) may identify dissociated p waves suggesting His bundle tachycardia. Management of junctional ectopic tachycardia is discussed in Chapter 44.

Restrictive physiology may lead to a low cardiac output state and RV failure.

- Due to a non-compliant, small RV chamber leading to predominantly diastolic dysfunction.
- A pathognomonic echo finding is forward flow in the pulmonary artery during ventricular diastole; atrial systole results in opening of the pulmonary valve as a consequence of pressure transmission through the stiff, non-compliant RV.
- Residual structural RVOT obstruction must be excluded on echo.
- Treatment is by increasing preload to RAP ~ 10–15 mmHg.
- Inodilators such as milrinone are preferred to epinephrine which may worsen RV diastolic function.
- PA forward flow and pulmonary regurgitation are adversely affected by positive-pressure ventilation; shorten inspiratory time relative to expiratory time, possible role for negative-pressure ventilation.
- Marked capillary leak often with high ascitic losses. Peritoneal dialysis (PD) may be needed.
- Consider return to theatre for residual RVOT obstruction, placement of competent valve into RVOT or creation of an ASD to allow R-L shunt.

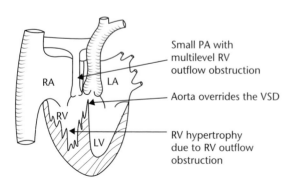

Figure 43.7 Anatomy of Tetralogy of Fallot.

Small PA with multilevel RV outflow obstruction

Aorta overrides the VSD

RV hypertrophy due to RV outflow obstruction

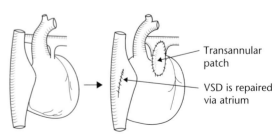

Figure 43.8 Surgery of Tetralogy of Fallot.

Transannular patch

VSD is repaired via atrium

Pulmonary atresia

Complex group of conditions and may have areas of lung supplied by major aorto-pulmonary collateral arteries (MAPCAs). Can be divided into three groups:

1 with intact ventricular septum
2 with VSD, without MAPCAs
3 with VSD and MAPCAs.

Incidence

1.5% of all congenital heart disease.

Associations

22q11 deletion.

With intact ventricular septum

A 'dead-end' ventricle which can vary from normal size to hypoplastic. Management depends on size of RV.

- *Normal size*: Perforation and balloon dilatation of PV (cath lab) with or without surgical opening of RVOT.
- *Small*: Modified B-T shunt with or without opening of RVOT to encourage forward flow through RV.
- *Very small (hypoplastic)*: Modified B-T shunt.

Coronary fistulae or sinusoids – the 'dead-end' ventricle leads to enormous intra-cavity pressures that may squeeze blood backwards into the coronaries and create fistulae. Fortunately rare but if present cannot risk relieving the RVOT without causing coronary ischaemia (RV-dependent coronary circulation).

With VSD, without MAPCAs

It is effectively an extreme form of Tetralogy of Fallot. Duct dependent at birth requiring PGE infusion and modified B-T shunt. Postoperative management of a B-T shunt is detailed on page 243. Complete repair is managed as per Tetralogy of Fallot, using RV–PA conduit.

Postoperative management

Majority follow single ventricle route, initially with modified B-T shunt. If RVOT has been opened beware of restrictive RV physiology (see TOF on page 236).

With VSD and MAPCAs

- Pulmonary blood supply is from large collateral vessels arising from the aorta.
- Surgery aims to join the MAPCAs together (unifocalization), reconnect them to the native PAs (if present), insert an RV–PA conduit and close the VSD (Figure 43.9). This usually requires a combined thoracotomy and sternotomy approach.
- May require several staged procedures. VSD often left open until confident that PVR will be low enough for RV to cope.

Postoperative management

Will remain cyanotic postoperatively if VSD left open. Operated side may have considerable collapse/contusion to the lung. Previously poorly perfused areas may suffer reperfusion injury with localized oedema, congestion and haemorrhage: management includes positive end-expiratory pressure (PEEP) and diuretics. Any increase in PAP/PVR usually a consequence of small PAs and is seldom reactive; unlikely to respond to inhaled NO. RV will be non-compliant, may show restrictive physiology.

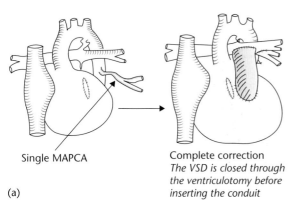

Single MAPCA

Complete correction
The VSD is closed through the ventriculotomy before inserting the conduit

(a)

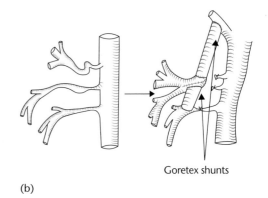

Goretex shunts

(b)

Figure 43.9 (a) Repair or PA/VSD with a single MAPCA. (b) Example of unifocalization of three major MAPCAs to the right lung.

Transposition of the great arteries

It is also called 'transposition' or TGA. D-TGA is the most common variety and the type requiring neonatal correction. L-TGA is very complex, often called congenitally corrected TGA (ccTGA) and not relevant to most practices.

Incidence

5% of all congenital heart disease.

Anatomy

It has many variants, but 'simple' transposition implies the ventricular septum is intact (as opposed to TGA/VSD) (Figure 43.10). Circulations are in parallel rather than in series. Coronary arteries arise from the anterior positioned aorta. Risk factors:

- Abnormal coronary artery patterns, especially intramural.
- Side-by-side great vessels (rather than anterior–posterior).
- Presence of additional lesions – CoA or VSD.
- Age >10 days slight risk, >42 days major risk.

Physiology

Cyanotic. Reliant on patent foramen ovale (PFO) and PDA to allow mixing. Presence of a VSD may improve mixing. In TGA with intact ventricular septum the LV muscle mass will begin to regress once PVR falls. Presence of VSD prevents this as ventricular pressures are both at systemic level. Rare combinations such as TGA/VSD/PS may be well-balanced cyanotic circulations and not require any early intervention.

Initial management

PGE infusion to maintain patency of PDA. May require ventilation. Cardiologists perform balloon atrial septostomy to enlarge PFO and improve mixing. Sometimes done on ICU under echo guidance. In cases with an intact ventricular septum aim to perform surgery within first 10 days of life before LV muscle mass regresses. Late presentations (>4/52) may consider PA banding to 'train the LV' prior to switch (increase muscle mass).

Surgery

The arterial switch procedure. It is complex and has 5% early mortality. The great arteries are divided and switched. The coronaries are transferred separately onto the neo-aorta. Note from Figure 43.11 that the PA ends up in front of the aorta (Lecompte manouvre).

Postoperative care

LV tends to be non-compliant and small changes in preload cause marked changes to LA pressure. Kinking or malposition of coronaries can result in coronary ischaemia. If there are ST changes or rhythm problems perform 12-lead ECG. Echo on return to ITU should look for:

- LV function and regional contractility.
- LVOT and RVOT, residual VSD.
- Neo-aortic regurgitation.

Vasodilators help non-compliant LV to relax. Infants with large duct may have high pulmonary blood flow preoperatively and need regular diuretics. Older switches (>4/52) may require prolonged inotropic support to 'retrain' LV. Branch PA stenosis may develop as late complication.

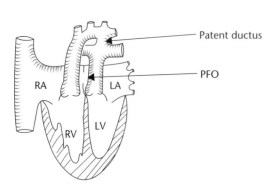

Figure 43.10 Anatomy of transposition of the great arteries.

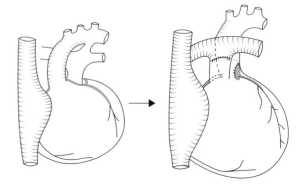

Figure 43.11 The arterial switch procedure.

Truncus arteriosus

It is also called common arterial trunk and 'truncus'.

Incidence

1.5% of all congenital heart disease.

Associations

22q11 deletion (DiGeorge syndrome)

Anatomy

Single ventricular outflow tract (arterial trunk) with a multi-leaflet truncal valve and VSD. Pulmonary arteries arise from the arterial trunk via a main pulmonary artery (type 1) or via separate origins for right and left PAs (types 2 & 3) Figure 43.12.

Complex variants:

- Truncus with interrupted arch.
- Disconnection of the left PA (supplied by a ductus).

Risk factors:

- Regurgitant truncal valve.
- Presentation in severe heart failure.
- Complex variants.

Physiology

Unrestricted pulmonary blood flow – present in neonate with heart failure. Mild cyanosis due to mixing of bloodstreams – mild due to high pulmonary blood flow.

Surgery

High-risk surgery with 10–15% early mortality. VSD closure, disconnection of PAs from trunk, RV–PA conduit (Figure 43.13).

Postoperative management

High-risk procedure, chest may be left open. LAP and PA pressure (PAP) monitoring lines essential. Risk of pulmonary hypertension – aim for mean PAP <1/2 mean systemic pressure. Management of pulmonary hypertension includes control of $PaCO_2$, inhaled NO and phenoxybenzamine (which may have been given perioperatively). Echo should record – LV and RV function, truncal (i.e. aortic) regurgitation, exclude residual VSD, RVOT flow and flow into branch PAs. Use irradiated blood unless 22q11 deletion has been excluded.

In the absence of a PA line, PAP can be estimated from the velocity of regurgitant TR jet and CVP (see Bernoulli Equation Chapter 24).

$$PAP = CVP + 4 \times Velocity_{TR}^{2}$$

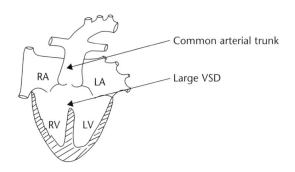

Figure 43.12 Anatomy of truncus arteriosus.

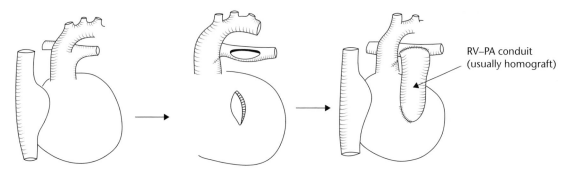

Figure 43.13 Surgery of truncus arteriosus.

Total anomalous pulmonary venous drainage

It is also called 'TAPVD', 'TAPVC'.

Incidence

1.5% of all congenital heart disease.

Anatomy

Pulmonary veins do not drain back to the LA, but to a separate collecting chamber that drains into the systemic venous circulation (Figure 43.14).

Physiology

Cyanotic. Kept alive due to a PFO allowing R–L flow. Key to the condition is whether or not the drainage is *obstructive*. When the pathway is unobstructed the infant will be cyanosed but well. Obstructed pathways lead to pulmonary hypertension, pulmonary congestion, tachypnoea and profound cyanosis. CXR appearance of diffuse pulmonary oedema.

Cor triatriatum is a condition in which there is a membrane within the LA between the pulmonary veins and the mitral valve. If the opening in this membrane is (small or absent), presentation in neonates will be similar to 'TAPVD'. Treatment is surgical resection of the membrane.

Management

Obstructed cases present in the neonatal and will often need ventilation. Urgent surgical decompression is needed. All types can be surgically repaired by restoring the pulmonary veins to the LA and dividing a superior or inferior draining vein. 5–10% early mortality risk depending on degree of obstruction. There is a risk of recurrent pulmonary vein stenosis which is associated with poor outcome.

Postoperative care

Pulmonary hypertension is high risk in any obstructed case. Monitor PAP. Surgeon may leave a small PFO if concerned about pulmonary hypertension. This will allow R–L shunt if high PAP and lead to desaturation. LV tends to be non-compliant because it has not been used to normal preload. Thus may run high LA and be very sensitive to volume. Obstruction at level of anastamosis will lead to pulmonary venous congestion. Consider re-operation if Doppler pulmonary vein flow looks obstructive.

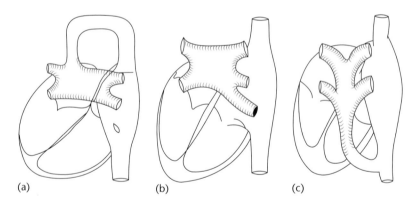

(a)   (b)   (c)

Figure 43.14 Three anatomical variants of TAPVD as seen from *behind* the heart. (a) Supracardiac: the most common. (b) Cardiac: drain to coronary sinus; least likely to be obstructive. (c) Intracardiac: less common, but most are obstructive.

Hypoplastic left heart syndrome

This is also called 'HLHS'.

Incidence

1.5% of all congenital heart disease, *but* accounts for 40% of all neonatal cardiac deaths.

Associations

None, though potential gene loci recently identified.

Anatomy

Variety of subtypes with varying degrees of hypoplasia of the LV and LVOT, classically occurs with mitral and aortic atresia.

Physiology

HLHS is characterised by an inability of the LV to support the systemic circulation. Thus the RV supports the systemic circulation via the PDA. Condition is fatal without surgery. Problems balancing parallel circulations are discussed later in this chapter and on Chapter 58.

Preoperative management

Often present with profound circulatory collapse requiring preoperative ventilation, inotropes and vasodilators to improve systemic circulation/limit pulmonary blood flow. PGE infusion to keep duct open. Aim for a *balanced* circulation (i.e. $Qp:Qs$ of ~1, aim for SaO_2 ~ 75–80% if no forward flow through LVOT.

Surgery

The Norwood procedure (Figure 43.15): High risk – 25–35% perioperative mortality.

- RV supports both the systemic and pulmonary circulations. Surgery secures a controlled source of pulmonary blood supply via Goretex shunt and repairs any systemic outflow tract stenosis.
- Recent modification uses RV–PA conduit to supply pulmonary blood flow instead of modified B-T shunt (Sano modification).

Postoperative management

Fragile postoperatively. Chest usually left open. CVP line gives common atrial pressure. Avoid hyperventilation and high F_iO_2 – these lead to pulmonary vasodilatation, increased $Qp:Qs$ and compromised systemic circulation. Aim for SaO_2 75–80%. Monitor blood lactate and central venous saturation (SvO_2) to assess systemic perfusion. Aim for SvO_2 45–60%, requires $Qp:Qs$ ~1 (see Figure 43.16). Use vasodilators and inotropes to improve systemic perfusion. Echo to assess RV function, degree of TR and arch repair. *Do not* hand ventilate with 100% oxygen. Always use air/oxygen mix to match F_iO_2 on ventilator. Chest closure can decrease RV compliance and cause deterioration over next few hours. Re-echo and maintain high vigilance following closure.

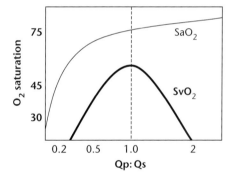

Figure 43.16 Balancing systemic and pulmonary flow in a Norwood circulation.

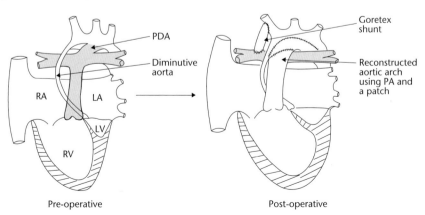

Pre-operative   Post-operative

Figure 43.15 The Norwood procedure.

Surgical procedures

Staged palliation of a functionally univentricular heart

A number of lesions are not suitable for a two ventricle repair and are managed with a series of 2 or 3 palliative procedures. Examples include mitral atresia, tricuspid atresia, some forms of pulmonary atresia, double inlet left ventricle and hypoplastic left heart syndrome.

In the neonatal period surgery may be required to optimise pulmonary blood flow.

- If there is inadequate pulmonary blood flow or a duct dependent pulmonary blood flow, a pulmonary shunt may be inserted.

- If pulmonary blood flow is high, a band is placed around the pulmonary artery and tightened to increase resistance and reduce flow to the lungs.

Pulmonary vascular resistance is high in the newborn period and falls over the first few months of life.

If a cavopulmonary ('venous') shunt was created in the newborn period the high pulmonary vascular resistance would result in excessively highly SVC pressure and low pulmonary blood flow – hence an arterial (modified BT) shunt is initially needed that provides a higher driving pressure and guarantees adequate pulmonary blood flow.

Pathways of palliative operations for a univentricular heart are summarised below.

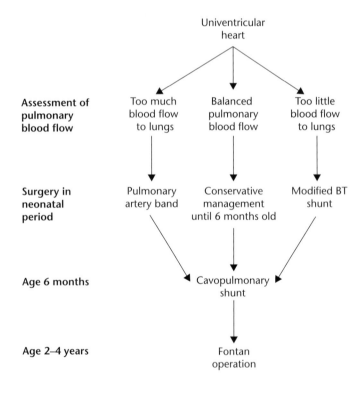

Arterial shunt

It is also called shunt, modified Blalock–Taussig (BT) shunt, systemic–PA shunt and central shunt.

Physiology

Used to *augment pulmonary blood flow* in a variety of conditions with inadequate pulmonary blood flow. Some conditions have bi-ventricular anatomy. (e.g. Fallot's, pulmonary atresia/VSD, TGA/ VSD/PS). Others have functionally single ventricle anatomy (e.g. tricuspid atresia/TGA/PS, pulmonary atresia/ intact ventricular septum). Behaviour following the shunt is influenced by the underlying anatomy; patients with bi-ventricular anatomy are usually more stable and tolerate the volume load of the shunt better.

Many neonates are duct dependent preoperatively and receiving PGE infusion (see Chapter 41). The duct will remain open for some time postoperatively even after the PG infusion is stopped – this may have the effect of 'flooding' the lungs until the duct closes. Blood flow through the shunt will be influenced by the shunt radius and length:

$$\text{Flow} \propto \text{radius}^4/\text{length}.$$

Typical sizes 3.5 mm–4.0 mm though these may need to be modified in the light of PA size and PVR.

Surgery

Variety of approaches and techniques (Figure 43.17). Most common and most widely used is the *modified B-T shunt* performed via a thoracotomy. Can be left or right sided. Generally performed on the side of the innominate artery (usually right). Performed without CPB unless child is very unstable or part of a more complex repair. Original description of B-T shunt divided subclavian artery and anastamosed it directly to PA. Modification uses a synthetic graft between subclavian/innominate artery and PA. Central shunt implies a shunt between the *aorta* and the PAs. Can be performed via a thoracotomy (classical Waterstone/ Potts) or via sternotomy, performed on or off bypass. Most common type of central shunt now is a modified type using a Gortex shunt between the aorta and the central PAs.

Postoperative management

Establish the underlying anatomy.

- Single or bi-ventricular anatomy?
- Any other source of pulmonary blood supply other than the shunt? Duct still open?

Shunts that require CPB imply unstable haemodynamics and need careful monitoring. Shunts with underlying bi-ventricular anatomy tend to run stable course. Need to balance Qp:Qs in functionally single ventricle. If shunt is the only source of pulmonary blood flow aim for 75–80% saturation (Qp:Qs ~ 1) (see Figure 43.16). Too small shunt or obstructed shunt results in hypoxaemia; trial of inhaled nitric oxide may be helpful in differentiating structural shunt problem versus high PVR (latter is reactive and responds to inhaled nitric oxide). Too high shunt flow leads to low diastolic pressure, pulmonary congestion and volume overload of ventricle. Attempts to reduce pulmonary blood flow by increasing PVR seldom effective, lowering SVR with vasodilators more effective at balancing Qp:Qs. Surgical revision of shunt may be necessary. Start heparin infusion on return to ICU when stabilised and no bleeding ($10\,\text{IU}\,\text{kg}^{-1}\text{h}^{-1}$).

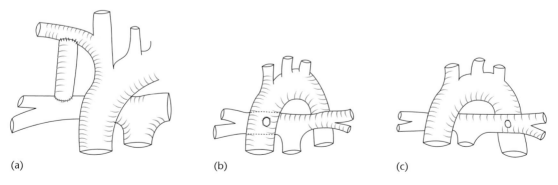

(a)   (b)   (c)

Figure 43.17 (a) Modified B-T shunt. (b) Waterstone shunt. (c) Potts shunt.

Pulmonary artery banding

PA banding is performed in a variety of different conditions.

Major indication is to *limit pulmonary blood flow*. The band protects the lungs from high pressure and flow in the following situations:

1 Bi-ventricular heart with multiple VSDs not suitable for surgical closure or for large VSD/AVSD in a neonate if felt to be high risk to repair.
2 CoA + VSD where the CoA is the critical lesion and is repaired via a thoracotomy. The band can also be placed via the thoracotomy.
3 Functional single ventricle anatomy with excessive (unobstructed) pulmonary blood flow (e.g. tricuspid atresia with TGA/VSD). See 'Staged palliation of a functionally single ventricle' on page 242.

Rarely a PA band is performed to 'train' the sub-pulmonary ventricle in infants with TGA in preparation for arterial switch. This may be required in late presentations in which the LV muscle mass has regressed. The band places an afterload on the ventricle and stimulates hypertrophy (Figure 43.18).

Physiology

Depends on the underlying anatomy. In groups 1 and 2, the band reduces the degree of heart failure by reducing the L–R shunt across the VSD. Any shunting remains predominantly L–R and so SaO_2 will remain 95–100%. In group 3, the band reduces pulmonary blood flow and so increases systemic flow at the expense of reducing SaO_2.

Surgery

Does not require CPB. Can be placed either via midline sternotomy or via left thoracotomy.

Postoperative management

Depends on *underlying anatomy*. In groups 1 and 2 aim for $SaO_2 \sim 95$–100. Generally well tolerated. Group 3 will be cyanotic and may be haemodynamically unstable. Aim for SaO_2: 75–80%. Echo to look at: gradient across band, ventricular function (can cause rapid ventricular failure if band too tight) and atrioventricular valve function (band can increase atrioventricular valve regurgitation in AVSD). Bands placed for VSDs are tighter (Doppler velocity 3–4 m s^{-1}) than bands in the single ventricle setting (velocity 2.5–3 m s^{-1}). Babies with high PVR may show a deceptively small gradient because distal PAP is high rather than the PA band loose.

PA banding performed to 'train' the LV in a baby with TGA may be complicated by hypoxaemia due to a failure of mixing of systemic and pulmonary circulations. May need addition of a modified B–T shunt. The stressed sub-pulmonary ventricle (LV) may fail postoperatively as a result of excessive afterload. Echo to assess degree of ventricular dilatation and monitor for a rise in LAP or signs of falling CO.

PA banding patients can be very unstable. Since the procedure is relatively minor, there is a tendency to regard the patients as low risk when the converse can be true.

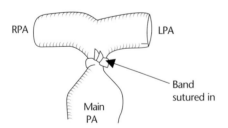

Figure 43.18 Pulmonary artery banding.

Bi-directional cavopulmonary shunt and the Fontan procedure (total cavopulmonary connection)

Staged palliative procedures for children with functionally single ventricle circulation, 5% of all congenital heart disease (e.g. tricuspid atresia, double inlet LV, HLHS, unbalanced AVSD, PA/IVS).

Physiology

These procedures involve connecting the systemic veins directly into the pulmonary circulation, thus bypassing the right side of the heart completely. They rely on *venous pressure* to drive pulmonary blood flow and are only possible if PVR is low. A failing ventricle or a high PVR may preclude these procedures.

Bi-directional cavopulmonary shunt

Also called cavopulmonary (CP) shunt, modified Glenn, Hemifontan. A bidirectional cavopulmonary shunt is carried out around 6 months of age. The SVC is anastamosed to the PA, IVC return remains to the RA (Figure 43.19). If the patient previously had an arterial shunt this is usually taken down. In other patient groups a decision is taken whether to ligate the main pulmonary artery or to leave some antegrade pulmonary blood flow. Original Glenn operation involved direct anastamosis of SVC to isolated right PA.

Postoperative management

Arterial saturation typically 80–85%. SVC line and IVC (or common atrial) line. SVC pressure equates to PAP (typically 12–16 mmHg). The difference between PAP and atrial/IVC pressure gives the trans-pulmonary gradient (TPG). TPG <8–10 mmHg generally implies low PVR and a favourable outcome.

If high TPG (>15 mmHg) must exclude a mechanical holdup, that is, anastamotic or PA narrowing, or clot at the anastamosis. If no obstruction then consider inhaled NO to reduce PVR. SVC pressure/PAP may be high (>20 mmHg) with a normal TPG as a consequence of a high atrial pressure, secondary to ventricular dysfunction. Management aimed at lowering atrial pressure (vasodilator, inotrope) will lead to a lowering of SVC pressure/PAP. Haemodynamics are generally good since the volume loading of the ventricle is substantially reduced by this procedure. Hypertension is common and may require treatment. *Aim to wean positive-pressure ventilation and extubate as soon as possible* as this will reduce intrathoracic pressure and improve pulmonary blood flow. Aim to get SVC line out as soon as possible to reduce risk of clot. High SVC pressure may result in pleural effusions (sometimes chylothorax), head and neck venous congestion and headache.

Total cavopulmonary connection

Also called TCPC or 'Fontan'. Children have almost always had a previous bi-directional cavopulmonary shunt (BCPS). Very rarely performed as a single procedure. 5–7% early mortality.

The completion of the Fontan procedure, usually before school age, connects the IVC blood flow to the pulmonary artery. Surgery has evolved over time to reduce postoperative complications, particularly atrial dysrhythmias:

1 RA directly anastamosed to PA (original Fontan procedure; no longer performed)
2 Lateral tunnel formed within RA to direct IVC flow to PA.
3 External conduit used to direct IVC return to PA. Fenestration preserves adequate ventricular output at the expense of a degree of hypoxaemia and has improved outcome (Figure 43.20).

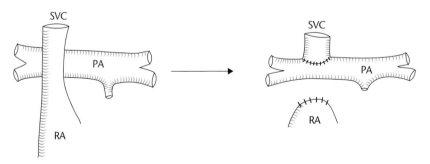

Figure 43.19 The bi-directional cavopulmonary shunt.

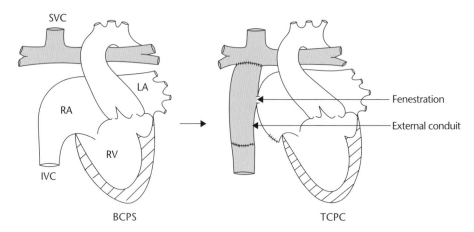

Figure 43.20 Completion of a total cavopulmonary connection in a patient with HLHS.

Postoperative management

Similar principles to management of BCPS. SVC and IVC pressures are now equal and both need to be relatively high to drive blood through the pulmonary circulation. A low PVR is essential. SVC/IVC pressure is no longer a marker of ventricular preload. These patients often require a lot of volume which should be titrated to atrial pressure. A separate line will give common atrial pressure. PAP typically 12–16 mmHg, TPG ideally <10 mmHg.

Fenestration causes some obligate R-L shunt, degree of shunting proportional to TPG and size of fenestration.

Low PVR/favourable haemodynamics generally associated with SaO_2 >90%. *Ideally aim for early weaning and extubation* – associated with increased pulmonary blood flow but *do not* wean/extubate a patient with unstable haemodynamics. Anticoagulate early due to sluggish venous circulation.

Echo assessment should assess ventricular function, the degree of R-L shunting across the fenestration and assess any ventricular outflow tract obstruction (reduced ventricular volume load may unmask outflow tract obstruction).

F.E. Reynolds & K.P. Morris

This chapter highlights the similarities and differences between paediatric and adult cardiac critical care.

Routine postoperative care

Direct measurement of cardiac output (CO) is rarely undertaken in paediatric critical care. If specific problems have been anticipated, direct LA and PA pressure monitoring may have been instituted during surgery. Indirect measures of CO and oxygen delivery (DO_2) (i.e. blood lactate and SVC/IVC SO_2) are more commonly utilized. Interpretation of blood lactate values (normal $<2\,\mathrm{mmol\,l^{-1}}$) should take into account the complexity of surgery – elevated levels should normalize after surgery. Blood lactate $>5\,\mathrm{mmol\,l^{-1}}$ implies inadequate DO_2 and is predictive of adverse outcome. Decline in mixed venous (or SVC or IVC) SO_2 should raise suspicion of a low CO state.

Blood transfusion may be required to ensure an optimal Hb level. Aim for a Hb $>10\,\mathrm{g\,dl^{-1}}$ in children with non-cyanotic defects, $12\text{–}14\,\mathrm{g\,dl^{-1}}$ in those with cyanotic heart defects. Chest drain blood loss should be $<4\,\mathrm{ml\,kg^{-1}}$ in the first hour, $<2\,\mathrm{ml\,kg^{-1}}$ in the second hour and $<1\,\mathrm{ml\,kg^{-1}\,h^{-1}}$ thereafter. Re-exploration of the chest for excessive bleeding is infrequent in paediatric practice. Whenever possible, coagulopathy should be corrected prior to re-exploration.

Early postoperative transthoracic echocardiography is routinely performed in many paediatric units. The criteria for weaning from ventilatory support are broadly similar to those for adults. Tracheal extubation is considered once bleeding is minimal and the patients is warm and haemodynamically stable. IV opioids are typically used to provide postoperative analgesia.

Common problems

Low cardiac output state

Low cardiac output state (LCOS) may be the consequence of inadequate preload, impaired LV or RV function, high afterload or an abnormal heart rhythm. LCOS may manifest as haemodynamic instability, poor perfusion, oliguria, hyperlactataemia and metabolic acidosis. The presence of a residual cardiac defect must be excluded.

Preload: Higher RA pressures may be required to maintain adequate CO following right-heart procedures (e.g. Fallot's tetralogy) because of reduced RV compliance. Similarly, a higher LA pressure (LAP) is required following left-heart procedures (e.g. total anomalous pulmonary venous drainage (TAPVD)). It is important to realize that the administration of small fluid volumes may result in large LAP changes.

Contractility: Myocardial dysfunction may result from incomplete myocardial protection and the systemic inflammatory response to CPB. Metabolic derangements (acidosis, hypocalcaemia), injury of the conducting tissue, ventricular wall (e.g. ventriculotomy) or coronary artery disruption (e.g. Fallot's and arterial switch operations) may also impair cardiac function.

In adult myocardium, excitation–contraction coupling is mediated by the release of cytosolic (e.g. intracellular) Ca^{2+}, whereas in neonates cytosolic Ca^{2+} levels are lower and contraction is dependent on extracellular Ca^{2+}. For this reason neonates are particularly susceptible to hypocalcaemia.

The choice of inotrope is dictated by the tone of the pulmonary and systemic circulations. Traditionally, dobutamine, dopamine or epinephrine have been the first-line choice, although the phosphodiesterase (PDE) inhibitors are becoming increasingly popular.

Afterload: Excessive vasoconstriction increases LV work and may reduce CO. Vasodilatation may be achieved using GTN or SNP, although phenoxybenzamine (a non-competitive α-blocker with a long half-life) is still widely used in paediatric cardiac surgery.

If, despite maximal therapy, LCOS persists, further investigation to exclude a residual defect (i.e. echocardiography, cardiac catheterization) is mandatory. The following may be considered:

- chest reopening to reduce constriction of the heart and allow time for myocardial oedema to resolve;
- cooling the patient to 34°C to reduce oxygen demand;

- ventricular assist device (VAD) or extracorporeal membrane oxygenation (ECMO);
- intra aortic balloon counter pulsation.

Dysrhythmia

Bradycardia: Surgery near conducting tissue (e.g. atrioventricular septal defect (AVSD) repair) may result in bradycardia. Persistent complete heart block mandates permanent pacemaker insertion, whereas conduction defects secondary to oedema usually only require temporary pacing.

Tachycardia: It may be the result of increased automaticity or re-entry phenomena. The risk is increased by metabolic abnormalities (K^+, Mg^{2+}, Ca^{2+} and PO_4^-), pyrexia and sympathomimetic drugs.

Ventricular dysrhythmias: They are rare in paediatric practice and often reflect myocardial ischaemia or ventricular dysfunction. Haemodynamically unstable VT or VF requires immediate direct current (DC) cardioversion.

SVT is more common. Accurate diagnosis is the key to determining appropriate therapy. A 12-lead ECG, supplemented with an atrial ECG from temporary pacing wires may yield the diagnosis. An atrial ECG amplifies atrial activity, allowing easier differentiation between atrial and ventricular excitation (Figures 44.1 and 44.2).

Adenosine, which slows or blocks AV conduction, aids diagnosis and may terminate re-entrant tachycardias. Synchronized DC cardioversion or overdrive pacing may also be used.

Junctional ectopic tachycardia: Results from increased automaticity with variable haemodynamic consequences. The diagnosis is confirmed by atrial ECG and lack of response to adenosine and overdrive pacing. Amiodarone may be required when haemodynamic compromise is significant, whereas a stable patient can be observed. Induced hypothermia may slow the rate and allow AV sequential pacing at a greater rate.

Haemorrhage and tamponade

Causes and features of haemorrhage and tamponade are similar to adults (see Chapter 52). As in adults, echocardiography may fail to reveal tamponade and delay re-operation.

Neurological injury

The mechanism of neurological injury after cardiac surgery is multifactorial. It may present as seizure activity, encephalopathy or focal neurological deficit. Seizures and chorea are more common in the paediatric population.

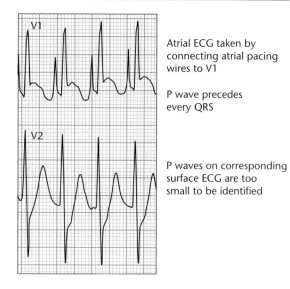

Atrial ECG taken by connecting atrial pacing wires to V1

P wave precedes every QRS

P waves on corresponding surface ECG are too small to be identified

Figure 44.1 Atrial (V1) and surface (V2) ECGs in normal sinus rhythm – P waves are amplified by atrial ECG.

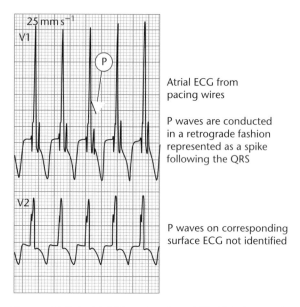

Atrial ECG from pacing wires

P waves are conducted in a retrograde fashion represented as a spike following the QRS

P waves on corresponding surface ECG not identified

Figure 44.2 Atrial (V1) and surface (V2) ECGs in nodal tachycardia. The retrograde P waves amplified by atrial ECG are seen after the QRS complex.

Renal dysfunction

Oliguria and renal impairment – leading to hyperkalaemia, acidosis and fluid overload – are common after surgery. In contrast to the adult population, haemofiltration or haemodialysis are rarely required. Hyperkalaemia and fluid overload usually responds to diuretic therapy. The combination of IV frusemide ($0.2–1.0\,mg\,kg^{-1}h^{-1}$) and oral metolazone (a thiazide), is useful. The criteria for institution of renal replacement therapy are the same as those for adults, however peritoneal dialysis is more commonly used. A peritoneal catheter may be inserted at the time of surgery in high risk infants. Mortality rate is increased in infants who require dialysis postoperatively.

Hypothermia

A high surface area to volume ratio makes children more vulnerable than adults to heat loss. Moderate and profound degrees of hypothermia are more commonly used in paediatric surgical practice, and immediate postoperative hypothermia is almost inevitable. Meticulous attention to the adequacy of rewarming and prevention of heat loss following CPB and during transport is necessary.

Controlled hypothermia may be used therapeutically to slow dysrhythmias, to limit oxygen demand in LCOS, or to ameliorate hypoxic ischaemic brain injury following cardiac arrest.

Hyperthermia should be avoided. Deleterious effects include: tachycardia, increased metabolic rate and exacerbation of neurological injury.

Pulmonary hypertension

Pulmonary hypertension (PHT) may complicate the postoperative course of some operations. It is particularly likely when a period of high pulmonary blood flow has caused muscular hypertrophy of the PAs. The condition is characterized by an increase in PVR and increased PA and RV pressures resulting in RV dysfunction and worsening of any right to left shunt.

> **Features of pulmonary hypertensive crisis:**
> - rising PA pressure – exceeding systemic arterial pressure;
> - rising CVP;
> - falling LAP;
> - falling systemic BP;
> - ventricular septal wall encroaching on LV cavity.

Therapy is directed at reducing PVR and supporting RV function. Adequate sedation and muscle relaxation should be ensured. Ventilation should be optimized to avoid hypoxaemia and hypercarbia. Inhaled nitric oxide (NO) (5–20 ppm) may be beneficial. Although adverse effects at low NO concentrations are rare, methaemoglobin and NO_2 concentrations must be monitored. Other drug treatments include: prostacyclin, sildenafil, phenoxybenzamine and dipyridamole.

Ventilation

General principles of mechanical ventilation are similar to adult practice with attention to limiting FiO_2 and avoiding lung injury. In the absence of significant lung disease positive end-expiratory pressure (PEEP) is usually set at 4–6 cmH$_2$O and tidal volume at 8–10 ml kg^{-1}. Ventilator rates are greater than those used routinely in adults and are age dependent: neonates 25–35 bpm, infants 15–25 bpm, older child 12–20 bpm. Ventilation is adjusted to maintain normocapnia. Oxygenation may be problematic in the presence of a residual right to left shunt.

Control of $PaCO_2$ is particularly important in cases of PHT in which an increase in $PaCO_2$ will increase PVR and may precipitate a pulmonary hypertensive crisis. In patients with pulmonary blood flow supplied by an arterial shunt (parallel circulation, e.g. Blalock–Taussig shunt) hyperventilation and a fall in $PaCO_2$ will lower PVR and increase pulmonary blood flow, potentially at the expense of systemic blood flow. In contrast, hypoventilation will increase PVR, lower pulmonary blood flow and result in increasing hypoxaemia. In these groups of patients, a volume control mode of ventilation will result in a more stable $PaCO_2$, as minute ventilation will vary over time with changes in lung compliance if a pressure control mode is used.

Following a bi-directional cavopulmonary shunt or Fontan procedure pulmonary blood flow is dependent on a gradient between systemic venous pressure and common atrial pressure, and is very dependent on intrathoracic pressure. During mechanical ventilation antegrade pulmonary blood flow may cease during inspiration. The optimum ventilation strategy includes a short inspiratory time (long I:E ratio), low/normal PEEP and the lowest achievable peak inspiratory pressure. As soon as the patient is stable they should be weaned and extubated. Negative pressure ventilation has been used in difficult situations.

Malnutrition

In contrast to the average adult cardiac surgical patient, preoperative malnutrition or 'failure to thrive' – secondary to heart failure and prolonged hospitalization – is common in paediatric patients. Postoperative fluid restriction, feed intolerance or necrotizing enterocolitis may further exacerbate the situation. Enteral feeding should be introduced as soon as practicable.

As in adults, total body water is increased following CPB. Modified ultrafiltration following CPB may be used in smaller children (see Chapter 42).

Infection

Gross sternal wound infection and mediastinitis are uncommon in the paediatric cardiac surgical patients. A prolonged delay before chest closure, with either opposed skin edges or a Gortex® membrane covering the heart, increases the potential for infection.

Patients with a congenital defect of cellular or humoral immunity (e.g. Di George syndrome) are also at greater risk of infection.

Systemic inflammation

SIRS is associated with capillary leak, oedema and impaired pulmonary and renal function. Therapy is supportive and the patient may require ventilation and renal replacement therapy until they resolve.

Outcome

Overall operative mortality for the correction of congenital heart disease is about 5% in the UK. The perioperative mortality for surgical ASD closure is <1%, whereas mortality for first stage palliation of hypoplastic left-heart syndrome is >25%. Co-existing congenital and acquired conditions are important co-determinants of outcome.

Key points

- Paediatric and adult cardiac surgical critical care have many facets in common. The variety of conditions encountered is much greater in paediatric practice.

- A detailed knowledge of anatomy and pathophysiology is needed, as management of individual complex lesions is very different.
- Management should be co-ordinated by the ICU team in close collaboration with cardiologists and surgeons.
- Low CO or deviation from expected clinical course should prompt exclusion of a residual lesion.

Further reading

Chang AC, Hanley FL, Wernovski G, Wessel DL. *Pediatric Cardiac Intensive Care*. Baltimore: Williams & Wilkins, 1998.

Appendix

Resuscitation drug doses
- Epinephrine 0.1 ml kg^{-1} 1 in 10,000 (1st dose)
- Epinephrine 0.1 ml kg^{-1} 1 in 1,000 (2nd dose for circulatory collapse)
- Atropine 20 μg kg^{-1}
- Sodium bicarbonate 1 mmol kg^{-1} (2 ml kg^{-1} of 4.2% solution)
- 10% calcium gluconate 0.3 ml kg^{-1}
- Amiodarone 5 mg kg^{-1}
- 10% dextrose 5 ml kg^{-1}

45

D. Gifford & S.J. Gray

History

1813	Le Gallois describes the concept of extracorporeal circulation (ECC)
1885	Von Frey and Gruber build the first extracorporeal oxygenator
1930s	Gibbon begins experiments with ECC/ oxygenation in cats
1953	First successful clinical use of CPB by Gibbon to close an ASD
1954	Lillehei employs cross circulation to facilitate correction of congenital cardiac lesions; extracorporeal oxygenation was achieved by cannulating the femoral vessels of a parent
1956	DeWall develops the first disposable bubble oxygenator for clinical use
1978	BioMedicus introduces the first centrifugal pump

Modern CPB systems consist of numerous disposable components connected together with polycarbonate connectors and silicone, latex or polyvinyl chloride (PVC) tubing. The basic components of the system are illustrated in Figure 45.1. CPB systems for clinical use are considerably more complex (Figure 45.2).

Blood pumps

Two types of pumps are available, namely roller and centrifugal.

Roller pumps

Rollers remain in contact with the tubing in the pump head 'raceway' for 180–210° of travel. As the pump head rotates, the tubing is squeezed against a back-plate propelling fluid forward. When stopped, these rollers act as a valve, preventing back-flow (Figure 45.3). Pump stroke volume is determined by (1) tubing internal diameter (ID) and (2) pump head diameter. Pump flow ($l\,min^{-1}$) is the product of SV and pump speed in revolutions per minute (RPM). Most pumps are calibrated to display pump flow rather than RPM. The degree of tube compression is critical – excessive occlusion induces haemolysis and increased tubing wear, whereas under-occlusion reduces the effective pump flow.

In addition to driving blood through the oxygenator, roller pumps are also used to provide variable cardiotomy suction (returning shed blood from the operative site to the venous reservoir) and deliver cardioplegic solutions.

Centrifugal pumps

Two types of centrifugal pump are available, namely nested cones constrained vortex and vertical vane impellor (Figure 45.4). The more commonly used vertical impellor is more energy efficient and requires a lower priming volume than the nested cone type.

Rapidly spinning components impart kinetic energy to the blood, propelling it forward by vortex displacement. Although the transmission of gases is impeded – because they receive much less kinetic energy than denser blood – potentially lethal gaseous embolism may still occur. As they are completely non-occlusive, fluid can flow in either direction; therefore, the arter-ial line must be clamped whenever the pump is not running.

Centrifugal pumps are both pre- and afterload dependent, their output being dependent on filling and outflow impedance (Figure 45.5). This in part explains why there is no direct relationship between pump speed and output, and the need for an independent measure of flow, such as an electro-magnetic probe.

In contrast to roller pumps, centrifugal pumps cause less trauma to erythrocytes and platelets, and reduce the risk of embolization of damaged tubing fragments. These favourable characteristics have led to their use

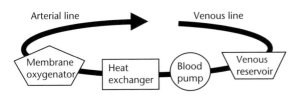

Figure 45.1 The basic components of a CPB system.

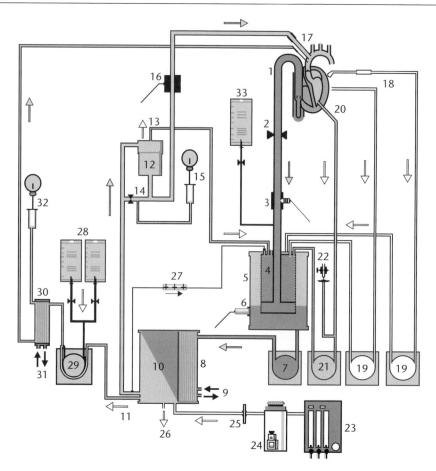

Figure 45.2 Schematic diagram of a typical CPB system: (1) venous line, (2) venous line clamp, (3) venous oxygen saturation meter, (4) cardiotomy filter, (5) venous reservoir, (6) reservoir-level detector, (7) main blood pump, (8) oxygenator heat exchanger, (9) water inlet and outlet for heat exchanger, (10) membrane oxygenator, (11) oxygenated blood outlets, (12) arterial line filter, (13) arterial filter vent, (14) arterial filter bypass, (15) arterial line pressure, (16) arterial bubble detector, (17) arterial line cannula, (18) sucker ends, (19) suction pumps, (20) vent, (21) vent pump, (22) vent suction controller, (23) gas supply and blender, (24) anaesthetic vaporizer, (25) gas filter, (26) oxygenator gas outlet, (27) blood sample/injection ports, (28) cardioplegia solution (CP), (29) CP pump, (30) CP heat exchanger, (31) CP water inlet and outlet, (32) CP pressure monitor and (33) fluid transfusion.

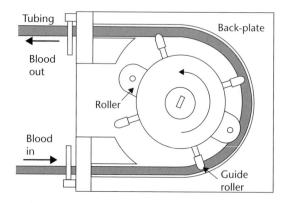

Figure 45.3 Twin roller pump head.

for short-term ventricular assist and mechanical (kinetic) assist for venous drainage in some specialized cardiac procedures.

Oxygenators

In addition to oxygenating venous blood, oxygenators remove carbon dioxide (CO_2) and permit the administration of volatile anaesthetic agents during CPB. The introduction of disposable bubble oxygenators in the 1950s rapidly led to the worldwide development of cardiac surgery. In the modern era, bubble oxygenators have largely been superseded by membrane oxygenators.

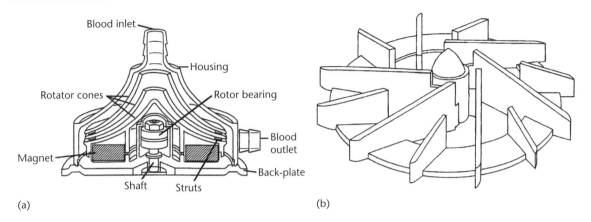

(a)
(b)

Figure 45.4 (a) Cross section of centrifugal (BioMedicus) pump heed and (b) detail of vertical blade impellor pump rotor.

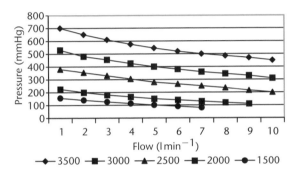

Figure 45.5 BioMedicus centrifugal pump pressure–flow characteristics at various speeds (in rpm).

Bubble oxygenators

Gas exchange is achieved across the large blood–gas interface produced by 'bubbling' oxygen directly through venous blood. Bubble size has an impact on the efficiency of both oxygenation and CO_2 removal. Oxygenation is improved with smaller bubbles (greater surface area to volume ratio), whereas CO_2 transfer is more efficient with larger bubbles (CO_2 tension rises faster in smaller bubbles). Bubble size selection is therefore a compromise. To avoid aero-embolism, the oxygenated blood 'froth' is passed through a silicone anti-foam-coated filter to remove bubbles before entering the arterial reservoir and being pumped back to the patient (Figure 45.6). The ever present risk of air embolism, embolism of anti-foam particles, and a tendency to greater haemolysis and complement activation have made this type of oxygenator obsolete.

Membrane oxygenators

Unlike the bubble oxygenator, the blood and gas phases in a membrane oxygenator are separated by a semi-permeable membrane – much like they are in the

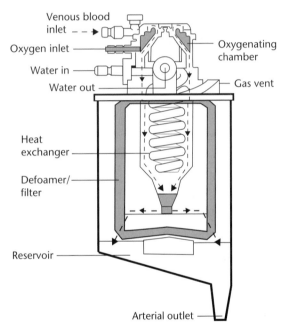

Figure 45.6 Cross section of a typical bubble oxygenator.

lung. Gas transfer is either by transmembrane diffusion or via micro-pores ($<0.1\mu m$ diameter) produced by stretching polypropylene. The membrane can take the form of flat sheets ($100–150\,\mu m$ thick) or hollow fibres ($100–200\,\mu m$ ID).

In modern hollow fibre oxygenators, the blood flows over the fibres (Figure 45.7) and gases pass through them. Eddies induced in the blood continually bring more red cells to the gas exchange surface. Nitrogen is relatively insoluble and is therefore largely confined in the gas phase. The oxygen/air mixture is used to regulate the PaO_2, and fresh gas flow determines $PaCO_2$. As the membrane oxygenator design imposes

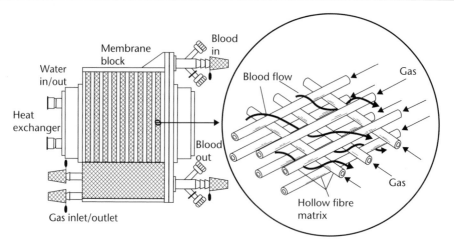

Figure 45.7 Cross section of typical membrane oxygenator block.

a much greater resistance to blood flow than bubble oxygenators, they must be placed after the blood pump (Figure 45.8).

During operation micro-porous membranes quickly develop a proteinaceous coating when blood first comes into contact with it, preventing a direct blood–gas interface. With prolonged use however, 'plasma breakthrough' into the gas pathway reduces gas exchange efficiency, limiting device life to hours rather than days. In contrast, diffusion membranes may operate efficiently for several days or weeks.

Although the maximum oxygen transfer capacity of a membrane oxygenator is only 20–25% that of the lungs, it should be borne in mind that this is achieved with an exchange surface area ~6% that of the lungs.

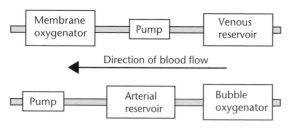

Figure 45.8 The contrasting arrangements of oxygenator, blood pump and reservoir in CPB systems employing membrane versus bubble oxygenator.

Heat exchangers

Heat exchangers are typically incorporated into oxygenators and cardioplegia delivery systems. In most systems, non-sterile water is circulated from a large heated/cooled reservoir through the heat exchanger in a counter-current fashion. The blood and water pathways are usually separated by coated stainless steel or aluminium that has been 'finned' or folded to maximize the surface area for heat transfer. Heat exchangers in oxygenators are normally placed proximal to the membrane to minimize the risk of micro-bubble generation during rapid rewarming.

Venous and arterial reservoirs

A large capacity (3000–4000 ml) reservoir is always positioned proximal to the main blood pump in any CPB circuit to buffer fluctuations in venous return. Reservoirs are described as being either 'open' or 'closed' to the atmosphere.

Hard shell (open) reservoirs are more commonly used as they allow for the inclusion of a large capacity filter to manage cardiotomy suction, and filter venous blood. Although collapsible bag (closed) reservoirs eliminate the blood–air interface present in open systems, a separate cardiotomy filter/reservoir is required, which increases blood contact surface area and complexity of the circuit. Closed systems offer the advantage of protection against gross air entrainment but do not prevent air being pulled out of solution. Once gross air entrainment has occurred, it can be difficult to remove from the reservoir safely.

Cannulae

The range of cannulae available to the cardiac surgeon is huge. Owing to their size, venous cannulae are usually reinforced or armoured with an integral wire spiral to prevent kinking (Figure 45.9).

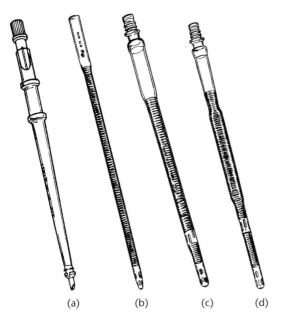

Figure 45.9 Examples of cannulae used in adult cardiac surgery: (a) straight aortic cannula, (b) single venous cannula suitable for caval cannulation, (c) round two-stage venous cannula and (d) oval two-stage venous cannula. Courtesy of Medtronic Inc.

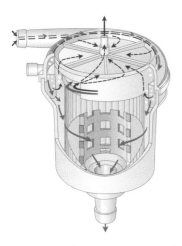

Figure 45.10 A typical auto-venting arterial line filter. Courtesy of Pall Biomedical, UK.

Tubing

The diameter of CPB tubing is a trade-off between resistance to flow and priming volume. The principle determinates of tubing size are the patient size, site of cannulation and pressure drop. Venous tubes are invariably of larger diameter than arterial tubes to optimize passive venous drainage.

Arterial line filters and bubble traps

Screen filters of 20–40 μm pore size provide a final stage of protection against systemic gas and particulate embolization. Although they provide excellent protection against gross air embolism, protection against micro-bubble embolism is dependent on continuous venting of accumulated gas. The bubble trapping properties of these devices are greatly aided by their architecture (Figure 45.10): the blood inlet is normally offset so that the blood flow creates a centrifugal effect, trapping the less dense air bubbles in the centre long enough for them to rise to the top of the filter to be removed. The gas-free blood then exits from the bottom of the device.

The incorporation of leucocyte-depleting filters has been shown to reduce the inflammatory response to CPB and the incidence of postoperative wound infection. Leucocyte depletion of blood cardioplegia solutions may also limit free-radical-induced myocardial injury.

Safety features

Modern CPB systems incorporate a number of features designed to protect both the patient and the circuit, and aid patient management during use. Several systems incorporate computerized record-keeping and can interface with haemodynamic monitors.

Additional ports permit:

- administration of crystalloids, colloids, blood products and drugs;
- arterial and venous blood sampling for blood-gas/biochemical analysis;
- venting of blood to a secondary reservoir, if the primary reservoir overfills;
- incorporation of a haemoconcentrating device (e.g. haemofilter, see below);
- re-circulation of arterialized blood through the oxygenator (i.e. shunting) in certain clinical situations.

Monitors, which provide early warning of impending problems and may automatically alter pump controls, include:

- The venous oxygenator saturation monitor – providing a global estimate of CPB adequacy.
- The venous reservoir-level detector/alarm – alerting the perfusionist to a fall in venous return and the risk of venous air entrainment.
- The arterial line pressure monitor/alarm – alerting the perfusionist to the risk of circuit/patient

barotraumas. It may indicate clot formation or arterial cannula malposition. The monitor can also be used to measure proximal aortic pressure when the pump is not running.

- The arterial line bubble detector/alarm – alerting the perfusionist to the presence of air-embolism. It may indicate gross venous air entrainment, arterial line filter failure or loss of membrane integrity.
- An oxygen analyser in the oxygenator gas supply line.
- Venous and arterial line temperature monitors.
- In-line arterial blood-gas monitoring.

In the event of main power supply failure a battery backup or manual hand-crank can be used to maintain the output of the primary pump.

Heparin bonded circuits

The highly acidic nature of heparin lends itself to ionic or covalent bonding to plastics. Coating the internal surfaces of an extracorporeal circuit with heparin theoretically improves biocompatibility, reduces the need for systemic anticoagulation, and reduces postoperative bleeding.

Although heparin-coated circuits are widely used in liver transplantation and extracorporeal life support, controversy surrounding adequate systemic heparinization has limited its application in cardiac surgery.

Haemofilters

The design of modern CPB systems allow the optional inclusion of ultra-filtration devices to passively remove excess fluid and electrolytes. Hollow fibre semi-permeable membranes have high efficiencies, removing up to $180\,\mathrm{ml\,min}^{-1}$ and filtering molecules up to 20,000 Daltons (e.g. low molecular weight heparin). Metabolite removal can be enhanced by diafiltration.

Key points

- CPB circuits should be constructed to achieve minimum prime volumes without inducing blood trauma.
- Apart from systemic blood flow, roller and centrifugal pumps have specialized ancillary rolls in CPB that are not interchangeable.
- Additional functions of the CPB circuit include blood and air scavenging from the operative field, cardioplegia delivery and blood filtration.
- Only diffusion membrane oxygenators have operational lives extending into days.
- Heat exchangers are integral to other CPB components.
- Heparin-coated CPB circuits provide theoretical patient management advantages that have yet to be conclusively demonstrated in practice.
- Haemofilters on CPB circuits can remove large volumes of fluid including some heparin.

S. Colah & S.J. Gray

Failure to wean a patient from CPB at the first attempt is a relatively common occurrence. Fortunately, in most cases it is temporary and merely delays a successful clinical outcome. In the vast majority of cases, weaning difficulty can be attributed to myocardial ischaemia secondary to prolonged aortic cross-clamp time, inadequate myocardial protection, coronary embolism or MI. Less common causes include extremes of vascular resistance, prosthetic valve malfunction, anastomotic strictures (e.g. in transplantation) and retained surgical swabs (e.g. atrial compression).

Regardless of aetiology, the key to successful termination of CPB in this situation is the recognition that there is a problem, the identification of its causes and the timely institution of remedial therapy. In order to prevent ventricular distension and inadequate coronary perfusion, reinstitution of CPB should be considered. Generally speaking, conditions impeding successful weaning can be considered as either correctable or non-correctable by the anaesthetist (Table 46.1).

Table 46.1 Causes of failure to wean from CPB

Correctable
Impaired myocardial contractility
Air embolism
Dysrhythmia
Hypothermia
Metabolic/acid–base
Preload
Respiratory
Extremes of SVR and PVR
Profound haemorrhage
Gross anaemia
Monitoring artefact

Non-correctable
Acute myocardial infarction
Inadequate surgical correction
New anatomical defect
Prosthetic valve malfunction

Coronary perfusion ↑

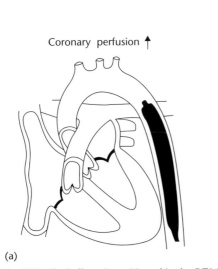

Cardiac work ↓
Myocardial O₂ consumption ↓
Cardiac output ↑

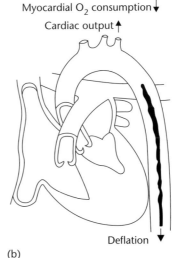

Deflation ↓

(a)   (b)

Figure 46.1 The IABP. The balloon is positioned in the DTA just distal to the origin of the left subclavian artery. During diastole, the balloon is rapidly filled with helium and impedes blood flow to the distal aorta. The rise in proximal aortic pressure augments coronary perfusion pressure. The balloon is deflated at the end of diastole (before the onset of isovolumic LV contraction) resulting in reduced LVEDP. Courtesy of Datascope Corp, NJ, USA. (a) Inflation, diastole and (b) deflation, systole.

Correctable causes

Impaired ventricular performance

Dysfunction may be systolic or diastolic; effect LV or RV; and be regional or global. TOE is invaluable in assessing the extent and severity of ventricular dysfunction and response to intervention. Myocardial stunning secondary to prolonged myocardial ischaemia, or inadequate myocardial protection or revascularization, usually responds to a further period of CPB and inotropes. A minimum period of 10–15 min coronary reperfusion following AXC removal should precede any attempt to wean from CPB. Spasm of native coronary arteries or arterial bypass conduits, which may cause significant ventricular dysfunction, usually responds to nitrates.

Air embolus

The incidence of air embolism is increased following procedures in which the left-heart is opened (e.g. aortic, mitral valve, aortic valve and LV aneurysm surgery). The right coronary artery (RCA) is more commonly affected as its anterior aortic ostium lies superiorly in the supine patient. RV distension and conduction abnormalities may be the first clinical indications of air embolism. TOE may reveal a regional wall motion abnormality (RWMA) and myocardial 'air contrast' (increased echo reflectivity) in the RCA territory. In practice, vasopressors are used to treat mild myocardial dysfunction, whereas allowing the heart to eject while on partial CPB may be necessary if myocardial dysfunction is severe.

Dysrhythmia

It is futile attempting to terminate CPB in the presence of untreated asystole, bradycardia, VT or VF. Atropine and epicardial pacing are the first-line treatments for bradydysrhythmias. Persistent ventricular dysrhythmias require cardioversion in the first instance. An underlying physical or metabolic cause should be actively sought before resorting to an anti-dysrhythmic drug (e.g. lidocaine, amiodarone). New-onset AF or other SVT may respond to synchronized, transatrial cardioversion, whereas unstable nodal rhythms may be converted to sinus rhythm by isoproterenol.

Hypothermia

Ventricular irritability, dysrhythmia and contractile dysfunction are more common at temperatures <34°C.

Metabolic

Increased or decreased K^+, decreased Mg^{2+} and increased H^+ may induce dysrhythmia, impair myocardial contractility and increased PVR.

Preload

Inadequate ventricular preload leads to reduced CO. Over enthusiastic elevation of atrial pressures risks ventricular distension, MR, TR and cardiac failure. TOE assessment of LV end-diastolic area (LVEDA) is a better guide to preload optimization than CVP monitoring.

Respiratory

Inadvertent failure to restart mechanical ventilation may occur, particularly after repeated attempts to wean from CPB. Severe bronchospasm apparent at the termination of CPB is a rare but potentially lethal complication. The management of this complication requires continuation of CPB, avoidance of lung distension (which may damage a mammary artery graft), bronchoscopy (to exclude airway obstruction), aggressive treatment with several bronchodilators (e.g. isoflurane, epinephrine, β_2-agonists, aminophylline, ketamine, $MgSO_4$) and steroids.

Extremes of SVR or PVR

CPB provides a ready opportunity to accurately calculate SVR. To calculate SVR in 'traditional' Wood units, the following formula is used:

$$SVR = (MAP - CVP)/Pump\ flow$$

The figure obtained can be converted to $dyne \cdot s \cdot cm^{-5}$ by multiplying by 80. For example; when MAP = 65 mmHg, CVP = 5 mmHg and pump flow is $5 l min^{-1}$, the SVR = 12 Wood units or 960 $dyne \cdot s \cdot cm^{-5}$.

Assuming that SVR does not markedly change during weaning from CPB, an estimate of CO can be made using MAP, CVP and calculated SVR. A target SVR of 10–14 Wood units (800–1120 $dyne \cdot s \cdot cm^{-5}$) with a CVP of 5 mmHg will generate an MAP in the range 55–75 mmHg with a CO of $5 l min^{-1}$. Reduced tissue perfusion and increased myocardial work secondary to excessive afterload (i.e. SVR > 20) may lead to acidosis and myocardial ischaemia. In addition, increased vascular sheer stress may cause aortic dissection during decannulation and worsen bleeding from suture lines. An excessively low afterload (i.e. SVR < 6) may result in inadequate coronary perfusion and depressed CO.

Profound haemorrhage

Bleeding from posterior structures or suture lines can be difficult to deal with. Elevating or rotating the heart around its base may impede venous return and dramatically reduce CO. Assessment and surgical repair may be more safely carried out on CPB.

Gross anaemia

A haematocrit <20% is undesireable as low oxygen-carrying capacity coupled with low CO may lead to tissue hypoxia and acidosis. The haematocrit may be elevated by reducing crystalloid administration, red cell transfusion, diuretic administration or haemofiltration.

Monitoring artefact

Unexplained hypotension may be due to problems with invasive monitoring. Zero-drift, damping, line occlusion, transducer misplacement and other causes of inaccuracy must be excluded before the administration of vaso-active drugs. A large discrepancy between peripheral arterial pressure and CPB arterial line pressure (monitored by the perfusionist) should prompt the use of direct aortic pressure monitoring using a 21G needle and a separate manometer line and transducer.

Causes uncorrectable by anaesthetist

Acute myocardial infarction

A difficult diagnosis to make intraoperatively. Diagnosis suggested by persistent, new, severe RWMA (i.e. akinesia or dyskinesia) in a coronary artery territory. Causes include distal coronary embolization, graft occlusion and incomplete revascularization. The surgeon may consider further revascularization on CPB.

Inadequate surgical procedure

More common in surgery for congenital heart disease. Incomplete myocardial revascularization may cause problems, particularly in redo surgery.

New anatomical defect

Iatrogenic mitral stenosis, new ASD or LVOT obstruction may arise following MV surgery. Similarly, a basal VSD is a recognized complication of surgery for hypertrophic obstructive cardiomyopathy.

Prosthetic valve malfunction

Large paravalvular leaks, impeded leaflet opening due to prolapse of subvalvular tissue and inadvertent use of a mitral prosthesis in the aortic position (and vice versa).

Pharmacological support

Having excluded and treated reversible causes of failed weaning from CPB, administration of inotropic agents should be considered. Both systemic and pulmonary vascular resistance, as well as institutional preference largely dictate drug selection. Inotropes are discussed in Chapter 10.

Mechanical support

Intra-aortic balloon counter-pulsation is a common intervention undertaken in all cardiac surgical centres. In contrast, the use of mechanical univentricular or biventricular assist is restricted to designated specialist centres.

Intra-aortic balloon pump

The IABP may be used to augment pharmacological therapy or when drugs alone have resulted in failure to wean from CPB. The device is normally inserted via the femoral artery and the tip sited in the descending thoracic aorta, just distal to the left subclavian artery (Figure 46.1). Correct positioning may be confirmed by TOE or CXR. The device improves LV performance by augmenting coronary perfusion and reducing LVEDP (Figure 46.2).

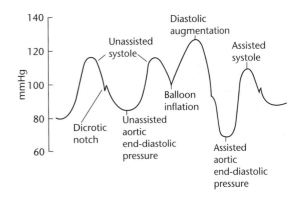

Figure 46.2 Proximal aortic pressure waveforms without and with IABP augmentation. Balloon inflation takes place at the dicrotic notch (AV closure). Balloon deflation takes place before AV opening so as not to impede LV ejection. Courtesy of Datascope Corp, NJ, USA.

Incorrect IABP positioning may result in left arm ischaemia (balloon too high/proximal) or renal ischaemia (balloon to low/distal). The most common complications are vascular injury and infection at the insertion site and lower limb ischaemia.

As the IABP does not interfere with cardiac surgery, insertion may be undertaken before induction of anaesthesia in high-risk patients and in patients with angina despite maximal medical therapy. Direct LA pressure monitoring and TOE facilitate weaning from CPB.

Ventricular assist devices

Unlike the IABP, which augments ventricular function, ventricular assist devices (VADs) may be used to take over ventricular systolic function. VADs may be used to replace the right (RVAD), left (LVAD) or both (BiVAD) ventricles in patients with severe cardiac failure as a 'bridge' to recovery or transplantation. In the setting of cardiac surgery, the indication for VAD insertion is persistent inability to wean from CPB despite maximal inotropic support, optimal ventricular fill-ing and full IABP augmentation. Occasionally, VAD insertion may be required in patients with resistant, haemodynamically unstable dysrhythmias.

Implantable	Thoratec II
	Baxter Novacor®
	Jarvik 2000
	Impella™
Paracorporeal	Thoratec I
Extracorporeal	Abiomed BVS 5000

Commercially available VADs can be classified as implantable, paracorporeal or extracorporeal. Blood flow is generated by either intermittent ejection of a 'stroke volume' or continuous 'axial' flow. All currently available systems suffer from the requirement for some degree of anticoagulation and an external power supply and the ever-present risks of infection and thromboembolism. It is essential that there is no ASD or PFO. The presence of significant AR following LVAD implantation results in recirculation and overestimation of true 'cardiac output'. A similar situation can arise following RVAD implantation in the presence of significant PR. Rather than repair of replace a regurgitant semilunar valve, most surgeons will opt for simple suture closure. Although valve opening is not required during full VAD support, this approach prevents spontaneous ventricular ejection.

Abiomed BVS 5000

Dual-chamber pump; pneumatic; LVAD, RVAD and BiVAD; flows up to $6 \, l \, min^{-1}$ (Figure 46.3):

- *Inflow* From atrium or ventricular apex by gravity into polyurethane 'atrial' and 'ventricular' bladders inside clear plastic housing.
- *Outflow* To aorta or PA. Compressed air causes the ventricular bladder to collapse and expel its contents. Two polyurethane valves maintain unidirectional flow.
- *Advantages* Relatively cheap. Easy to operate.
- *Disadvantages* Requirement for anticoagulation, haemorrhage, air entrainment, temporary solution (i.e. <14 days).

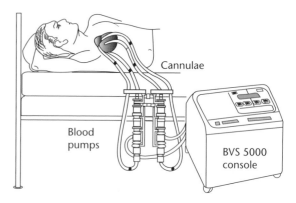

Figure 46.3 Abiomed BVS 5000.

Thoratec I

Single-chamber pump; pneumatic; LVAD, RVAD and BiVAD; flows up to $7.2 \, l \, min^{-1}$ (Figure 46.4):

- *Inflow* From atrium or ventricular apex by passive or active (negative pressure) filling of a flexible chamber within a translucent plastic housing.
- *Outflow* To aorta or PA. Compressed air causes the flexible chamber to collapse and expel its contents. Two prosthetic valves maintain unidirectional flow.
- *Advantages* A paediatric and adult biventricular solution. Biocompatible chamber lining. Approved for short- and long-term (bridge to transplant) use.
- *Disadvantages* Inconvenience and discomfort of paracorporeal location in long-term use.

Jarvik 2000

Axial flow rotary pump (8000–12,000 rpm); electrically powered; flows up to $5.0 \, l \, min^{-1}$ (Figure 46.5):

- *Advantages* Very small size (25 × 50 mm, weight <100 g). Implantable solution. Can be inserted

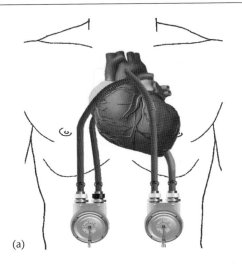

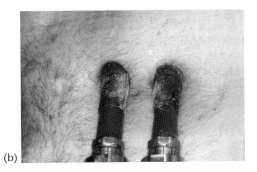

(a)   (b)

Figure 46.4 (a) Thoratec I and (b) xiphisternal cannula exit sites.

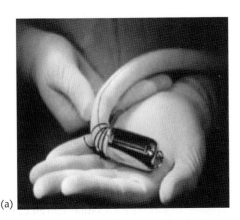

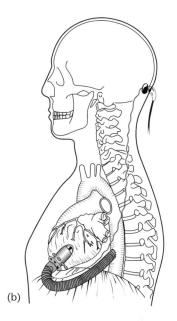

(a)   (b)

Figure 46.5 (a) The Jarvik 2000 blood pump (reprinted from Frazier OH. *J Congest Heart Failure Circ Suppl* 2000; **1**: 107–111, with permission of Isis Medical Media, Oxford). (b) Diagram of insertion site and route of subcutaneous power cable used by the Oxford team (reprinted from Westaby *et al. J Thorac Cardiovasc Surg* 1997; **114**: 467–474, with permission).

via a left thoracotomy. Lower infection risk. No valve, therefore reduced requirement for anticoagulation.

- *Disadvantages* Limited clinical experience.

Extracorporeal membrane oxygenation

In severe, life-threatening respiratory failure, extra-corporeal oxygenation of the blood allows the lungs to be rested. In contrast to paediatrics, where outcomes are good, the use of extracorporeal membrane oxy-genation (ECMO) in adults is invariably disappointing. A long-term extracorporeal blood circuit is used con-sisting of a roller or centrifugal pump, oxygenator and heat exchanger. Either veno-venous or veno-arterial support can be accomplished. Possible cannulation sites include the femoral vessels, central veins, right atrium and aorta.

Key points

- Myocardial stunning and inadequate myocardial protection or revascularization are common causes of failure to wean from CPB.
- Many of the causes of failure to wean from CPB are amenable to intervention by the anaesthetist.
- Intraoperative MI is difficult to diagnose in the operating theatre.
- The IABP is contraindicated in the presence of significant aortic regurgitation.
- The major risks associated with VAD implantation are haemorrhage, infection and thromboembolism.

Further reading

Baskett RJ, Ghali WA, Maitland A, Hirsch GM. The intraaortic balloon pump in cardiac surgery. *Ann Thorac Surg* 2002; **74(4)**: 1276–1287.

Richenbacher WE, Naka Y, Raines EP, Frazier OH, Couper GS, Pagani FD *et al.* Surgical management of patients in the REMATCH trial. *Ann Thorac Surg* 2003; **75(6 Suppl)**: S86–S92.

COAGULOPATHY DURING CARDIOPULMONARY BYPASS 47

J.H. Mackay & J.E. Arrowsmith

Coagulation pathways

Coagulation is a complex dynamic process involving enzymatic and cellular mechanisms, vascular and inflammatory processes and humoral responses. Traditionally this system has been divided into intrinsic and extrinsic pathways ending in a final common pathway, which leads to the formation of fibrin clot. In practice, there is much interaction between the intrinsic and extrinsic pathways, as well as with platelet activation, and fibrinolytic and inflammatory mechanisms.

Extrinsic system

The binding of factor VII to tissue factor (a transmembrane glycoprotein (GP) derived from macrophages and subendothelial cells) yields factor VIIa, which catalyses the production of factors IXa and Xa. This highlights the interaction between extrinsic and intrinsic

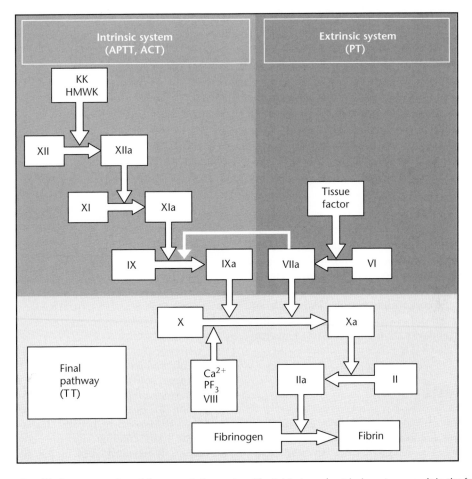

Figure 47.1 Simplified representation of the coagulation system. The intrinsic and extrinsic systems result in the formation of thrombin (factor IIa) and fibrin. KK, kallikrein; PF_3, platelet factor 3.

pathways. Warfarin and other coumarins inhibit the hepatic synthesis of vitamin K-dependent factors (i.e. II, VII, IX and X).

Intrinsic (contact) system

Activation occurs when factors XII and XI, high-molecular-weight kininogen (HMWK) and prekallikrein come together on a negatively charged surface, to produce factors XIIa and XIa. Factor XIIa formation is amplified by a positive feedback loop. Unfractionated heparin acts as an anticoagulant by inducing a conformational change in antithrombin (antithrombin III), a non-specific protein serease inhibitor. The heparin–antithrombin complex inhibits factors XIa, Xa, IXa and IIa, as well as trypsin, plasmin and kallikrein. Adequate anticoagulation ensures the presence of overwhelming numbers of heparin–antithrombin complexes, which immediately scavenge any thrombin before it can interact with fibrinogen, platelets, endothelium or leucocytes. Heparin induces a 1000-fold increase in the affinity of antithrombin for thrombin, but has little direct anticoagulant effect itself.

Common pathway

The first step involves the formation of factor Xa, which catalyses the conversion of prothrombin (factor II) to thrombin, which in turn leads to the conversion of fibrinogen to fibrin (Figure 47.1).

Role of platelets

In the presence of vascular injury interruption of the normally antithrombogenic endothelial surface leads to platelet adhesion, activation and aggregation. von Willebrand factor (vWF) binds to collagen in the disrupted endothelial basement membrane and acts as an adhesive site for platelets. Activated platelets have a procoagulant surface, which accelerates many of the key steps in the coagulation cascade. Degranulation results in further adhesion and activation as well as the attraction and activation of leucocytes. The characteristics of platelets are shown in Table 47.1.

Fibrinolysis

The proteolytic degradation of fibrin by plasmin controls the extent and location of clot formation within the circulation. The delicate balance between coagulation and fibrinolysis is determined by the rate at which plasminogen is converted to plasmin under the influence of plasminogen activators (Figure 47.2).

Table 47.1 The characteristics of platelets

General	2–3 μm diameter
	Non-adhesive surface (if undamaged)
	No nucleus – contain RNA but no DNA
	Half-life 9–10 days
Surface receptors	
GP	GP Ib: binds vWF
	GP Ia/IIa: binds collagen
	GP IIb/IIIa: binds fibrinogen and fibronectin
Other	Thrombin, thromboxane, serotonin, α_2-adrenergic
Contents	
α-granules	Procoagulants: PF_4, βTG, factor V
	Anticoagulants: plasminogen
	Adhesive proteins: vWF, fibrinogen
	Growth factors: PDGF
β-granules	ATP, ADP, serotonin

PF_4, platelet factor 4; βTG, beta thromboglobulin; PDGF, platelet-derived growth factor; ATP, adenosine triphosphate; ADP, adenosine diphosphate; GP, glycoprotein.

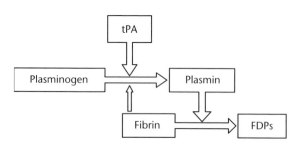

Figure 47.2 Fibrinolysis. The conversion of plasminogen to plasmin is catalysed by activators, such as tissue and urokinase plasminogen activators (tPA and uPA, respectively). The rate of conversion is increased 500-fold in the presence of fibrin. FDPs, fibrin degradation (split) products.

Tissue plasminogen activator (tPA) is the principle plasminogen activator in humans. It is constantly secreted from endothelium and removed from the circulation by binding with plasminogen activator inhibitors (PAIs) and by hepatic clearance. By occupying the lysine-binding sites on plasminogen and fibrinogen, lysine analogues inhibit fibrinolysis by inhibiting the action of tPA on plasminogen. One of the many actions of aprotinin is the inhibition of plasminogen activators.

Coagulopathy in cardiac surgery

Any form of surgery or trauma that results in tissue injury will result in the activation of procoagulant and anticoagulant systems. Cardiac surgery adds the additional stresses of blood contact with foreign surfaces; dilution, sequestration and consumption of clotting factors; platelet activation and destruction; hypothermia and deliberate anticoagulation. At the onset of CPB, circulating levels of most clotting factors are reduced by ~40%, although factor V (proaccelerin) levels may fall by 80%. Although some postoperative bleeding is to be expected, excessive bleeding may have a surgical or haematological aetiology (Table 47.2).

Heparin administration prior to CPB causes significant platelet dysfunction by inhibiting thrombin and stimulating fibrinolysis. The institution of CPB, when tPA and plasmin levels rise and PAI levels fall, accentuates this fibrinolytic effect. After surgery, normalization of tPA levels and elevation of PAI levels yields a hypofibrinolytic state. Although heparin competitively inhibits factors IXa, Xa and XIIa, it does not limit activation of the coagulation cascade and does not entirely abolish thrombin generation. The end result is the consumption of coagulation factors in the absence of clot formation. Loss of platelet α-granules during CPB prevents platelet adhesion with vWF. Similarly, a reduction in GP IIb/IIIa receptor expression reduces platelet aggregation.

Prophylaxis

Owing to the significant morbidity and mortality associated with excessive bleeding, prophylactic measures are frequently employed. The level of evidence supporting the use of these measures is highly variable. Although the withdrawal of aspirin and clopidogrel

Table 47.2 Causes of coagulopathy after cardiac surgery. The risk of coagulopathic bleeding is increased by endocarditis and prolonged CPB

Quantitative platelet problem	Destruction, haemodilution, sequestration, activation, consumption
Qualitative platelet problem	Damage, aspirin, clopidogrel, GP-IIb/IIIa inhibitors, NSAIDs, uraemia
Coagulation factor deficiency	Haemodilution, consumption, liver disease, congenital
Altered enzyme kinetics	Hypothermia
Anaemia	Haemorrhage, haemodilution
Anticoagulants	Residual heparin, excessive protamine
Altered factor clearance	Hepatic and renal hypoperfusion, hypothermia

Table 47.3 Strategies to reduce perioperative blood loss and transfusion requirements during cardiac surgery

Strategy	Comments	Efficacy
Antiplatelet drugs	Avoid for 10–14 days prior to surgery	+/−
Anticoagulation	Convert warfarin to heparin Consider vitamin K, FFP, cryoprecipitate if pathological	+
Anaemia	Correct preoperatively Consider iron salts, vitamin B_{12}, folate, erythropoietin, transfusion	+
Lysine analogues	Reduce perioperative blood loss Reduction in blood product usage less clear	+
Aprotinin	Reduces perioperative blood loss and blood product usage Widely used in high-risk cases	++
DDAVP	von Willebrand's disease, uraemia, cirrhosis	+
ANH	Removal of autologous whole blood (10 ml kg^{-1}) prior to heparinization and retransfusion following administration of protamine	+/−
Cell salvage	Cardiotomy blood filtered, washed and returned to the circulation Pericardial and pleural blood contains increased tPA, fibrinogen and FDPs	+/−
Transfusion policy	Institutional protocols for investigation of bleeding and use of all blood products	+
Blood products	Routine use of FFP and platelets in patients at increased risk of coagulopathy or with clinical evidence of coagulopathy	+/−

FDPs, fibrin-degradation products; DDAVP, desmopressin (1-desamino-8-D-arginine vasopressin); ANH, acute normovolaemic heamodilution.

before surgery is widely practised, there are reports that these drugs do not increase transfusion requirements. Furthermore, aspirin withdrawal may increase the risk of an adverse cardiac event. When used, it is recommended that lysine analogues be administered before CPB but after heparinization. The evidence supporting the routine use of acute normovolaemic haemodilution (ANH) is conflicting. Reasons why ANH is not more widely practised include: acute haemodynamic instability, the deleterious effects of acute anaemia, and a lack of efficacy (a venesection volume of $10\,ml\,kg^{-1}$ may be too small). The combination of ANH and perioperative cell salvage may reduce

transfusion requirements but their impact on bleeding complications is unclear (Table 47.3).

Diagnosis

The diagnosis of coagulopathy is usually made on the basis of clinical suspicion and the results of near-patient tests. Laboratory tests may be a useful guide to management but their value is often limited by the time interval between sending a sample and receiving a report (Table 47.4).

Activated clotting time

Heparin prolongs the ACT in a dose-dependent fashion, and ACT measurement is the most widely used monitor of anticoagulation during cardiac surgery. Typically celite (dicromatous earth) or kaolin (clay) is used to accelerate whole blood coagulation and the formation of fibrin detected by automated point-of-care equipment. ACT measurement is simple, quick and inexpensive, and yields reproducible results. Any process that influences the conversion of fibrinogen to fibrin (e.g. hypothermia or haemodilution) may prolong the ACT.

Heparin greatly prolongs the celite-ACT in the presence of aprotinin and an ACT of 400 s may not represent anticoagulation adequate for CPB. It is recommended that the ACT be maintained at >750 s when celite-ACT monitoring is used. In contrast, the kaolin-ACT

Table 47.4 Routine perioperative coagulation tests

Tests	Normal values
Platelets	
Platelet count	$150\text{--}400 \times 10^9\,l^{-1}$
Coagulation	
ACT	90–140 s
PT	12–15 s (INR 1.0–1.3)
APTT	35–45 s
Thrombin time (TT)	<14 s
Fibrinogen	$>2\,g\,l^{-1}$
Fibrinolysis	
Fibrin(ogen) split products	$<10\,mg\,l^{-1}$
D-dimers	

INR, International normalized ratio.

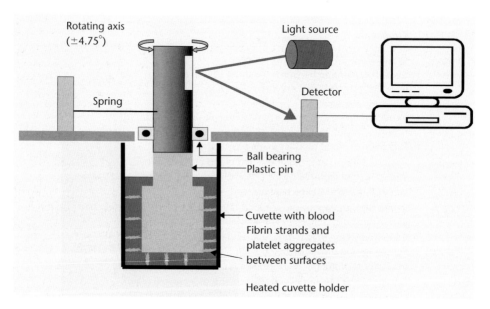

Figure 47.3 Principles of TEG. In this system, the central pin rotates while the cuvette remains stationary. The force required to rotate the pin in the blood sample increases as the blood clots. Reproduced with permission of Sysmex UK Ltd.

is largely unaffected by clinical doses of aprotinin. It is essential that the anaesthetist knows which type of ACT activator/accelerator is present.

Thromboelastography

In contrast to conventional laboratory tests, thromboelastography (TEG) measures the speed, quality and stability of clot formation, giving a global overview of clotting and fibrinolysis. TEG can be performed at the point of care and the results used to target the treatment of coagulopathy (Figure 47.3).

Whole blood is placed in a cup (cuvette) then a pin is lowered into the blood. Alternating rotational force is applied to one component of the system (either the cup or the pin, depending on the manufacturer) and the torque transmitted from the rotating to the

stationary component via the sample is measured. Initially, the blood is liquid and no torque is transferred through the system. When fibrin strands form, torque is transferred between components and as more fibrin strands form and the clot becomes more established, the transfer of torque increases until it reaches a maximum level. Eventually fibrinolysis

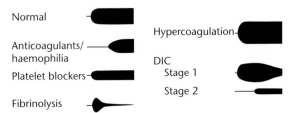

Figure 47.5 Normal and abnormal TEGs.

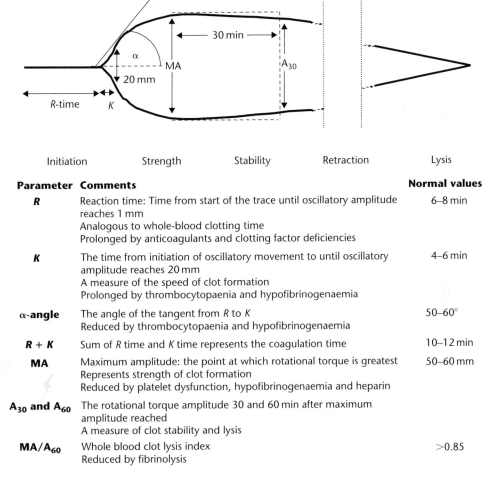

Parameter	Comments	Normal values
R	Reaction time: Time from start of the trace until oscillatory amplitude reaches 1 mm Analogous to whole-blood clotting time Prolonged by anticoagulants and clotting factor deficiencies	6–8 min
K	The time from initiation of oscillatory movement to until oscillatory amplitude reaches 20 mm A measure of the speed of clot formation Prolonged by thrombocytopaenia and hypofibrinogenaemia	4–6 min
α-angle	The angle of the tangent from R to K Reduced by thrombocytopaenia and hypofibrinogenaemia	50–60°
R + K	Sum of R time and K time represents the coagulation time	10–12 min
MA	Maximum amplitude: the point at which rotational torque is greatest Represents strength of clot formation Reduced by platelet dysfunction, hypofibrinogenaemia and heparin	50–60 mm
A$_{30}$ and A$_{60}$	The rotational torque amplitude 30 and 60 min after maximum amplitude reached A measure of clot stability and lysis	
MA/A$_{60}$	Whole blood clot lysis index Reduced by fibrinolysis	>0.85

Figure 47.4 The TEG and derived parameters.

Table 47.5 Suggested therapy for excessive bleeding after cardiac surgery based on the results of tests of coagulation

Test	Usual therapy	Comments
ACT $> 140\,s$	Protamine	? Residual heparin
		Consider TEG $\pm$ heparinase
Increased APTT	Protamine $\pm$ FFP	
Increased PT, fibrinogen normal	FFP	
Increased PT, decreased fibrinogen	Cryoprecipitate	
Platelets $< 100 \times 10^9\,l^{-1}$	Platelet concentrate	
APTT and PT normal	Consider TEG, surgical	Coagulopathy unlikely
Fibrinogen normal	re-exploration or platelets	
TEG: $MA/A_{60} < 0.7$	Lysine analogue	Fibrinolysis

Anaemia (e.g. Hb $< 8.5\,g\,dl^{-1}$) should be treated with packed red cells.

occurs and torque transmission decreases as clot is broken down. From the resulting TEG a number of parameters may be derived (Figure 47.4).

The addition of reagents, such as heparinase, to the reaction cuvette allows detection of coagulation abnormalities that may be masked by heparin. Many commercially available systems allow two or more samples (i.e. with and without heparinase) to be analysed simultaneously. This allows coagulation to be assessed during CPB. Following protamine administration, the presence of residual heparin produces a difference in the TEG R-time that is usually obvious with 10–12 min. Normal and abnormal TEGs are shown in Figure 47.5.

Treatment

Whenever possible the treatment of coagulopathic bleeding after cardiac surgery should be based on objective evidence and locally derived guidelines (Table 47.5). Despite the relatively poor sensitivity and specificity of routine laboratory tests of coagulation, an APTT, prothrombin time (PT) and fibrinogen assay should be requested along with a blood count. Where available, TEG should be performed in parallel.

Key points

- Excessive bleeding after cardiac surgery may be due to loss of vascular integrity, coagulopathy or both.
- Despite the traditional separation of the coagulation pathways, there is considerable interaction between the intrinsic and extrinsic systems.
- Increased tPA mediates increased fibrinolytic activity during CPB.
- TEG provides a rapid assessment of coagulation and permits early therapeutic intervention.

Further reading

Jeske W, Pifarré R, Wolf H, Fareed J. An overview of blood coagulation. In: Pifarré R (Ed.). *New Anticoagulants for the Cardiovascular Patient*. Philadelphia: Hanley & Belfus, Inc., 1997; pp. 9–37; ISBN 1-56053-220-3.

McGill N, O'Shaughnessy D, Pickering R, Herbertson M, Gill R. Mechanical methods of reducing blood transfusion in cardiac surgery: randomised controlled trial. *Br Med J* 2002; **324(7349)**: 1299–1305.

Shore-Lesserson L, Manspeizer HE, DePerio M, Francis S, Vela-Cantos F, Ergin MA. Thromboelastography-guided transfusion algorithm reduces transfusions in complex cardiac surgery. *Anesth Analg* 1999; **88(2)**: 312–319.

Speiss BD (Ed.). *The Relationship between Coagulation, Inflammation and Endothelium – A Pyramid Towards Outcome*. SCA Monograph. Baltimore: Lippincott, Williams & Wilkins, 2000; ISBN 0-781-72758-8.

R.J. De Silva & A. Vuylsteke

Up to 2% of patients may suffer morbidity and mortality as a direct consequence of CPB. The whole-body systemic inflammatory response to sepsis (SIRS) is characterized by pathological hypotension, fever of non-infectious origin, DIC, diffuse tissue oedema and injury, and in extreme cases, multi-organ failure. Surgical trauma, endotoxaemia, the CPB system and ischaemia–reperfusion injury (IRI) all contribute to the development of SIRS (Figure 48.1).

Ischaemia–reperfusion injury and the neutrophil

Myocardial and lung ischaemia during CPB can be partially offset by the use of systemic hypothermia and cardioplegia. IRI describes tissue injury that paradoxically occurs after resumption of normal tissue perfusion following a period of ischaemia. Neutrophils cause damage during IRI by the production of toxic substances during the metabolism of oxygen and the secretion of proteolytic enzymes from their granules. In order to cause this damage, activated neutrophils must sequentially undergo a process of contact and adhesion with endothelium, extravasation from the vasculature and migration through the affected tissue. Intercellular adhesion molecules (ICAMs), selectins and cytokines, such as interleukin (IL)-8, all play an important part in this process. The observation that IRI-induced tissue injury is markedly reduced in neutrophil-depleted animals suggests a pivotal role for the neutrophil.

Reactive oxygen metabolites

Depletion of high-energy phosphates (i.e. adenosine triphosphate (ATP)) in ischaemic tissue leads to a build-up of reactive oxygen metabolites, such as hydrogen peroxide, hypochlorus acid and the superoxide anion. Under normal conditions, hypoxanthine is oxidized to xanthine by xanthine dehydrogenase using nicotinamide adenine dinucleotide (NAD). In ischaemic tissue however, xanthine dehydrogenase is converted to xanthine oxidase and levels of hypoxanthine rise (Figure 48.2). Upon reperfusion, xanthine oxidase utilizes the now available oxygen to convert hypoxanthine to xanthine with the generation of large amounts of oxygen free radicals, which overwhelm endogenous scavenging systems and cause damage to cellular components. The resulting tissue injury leads to increased vascular permeability and chemotaxis.

Arachidonic acid metabolites

Arachidonic acid metabolites are generated as a consequence of free radical release and phospholipase A_2 activation (Figure 48.3). Leukotrienes and thromboxane A_2 result in further neutrophil attraction and activation, and produce local vasoconstriction.

Is the neutrophil essential for ischaemia– reperfusion injury?

Despite evidence supporting the pivotal role of the neutrophil in IRI, animal studies have shown that IRI is not totally abolished by neutrophil depletion. Neutrophil depletion appears to have a much greater impact on late IRI (i.e. >4 h after reperfusion) than early IRI (<30 min after reperfusion). This observation suggests a bimodal pattern of neutrophil involvement

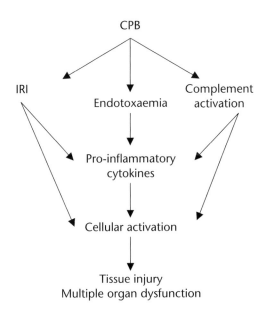

Figure 48.1 An overview of the inflammatory response to CPB.

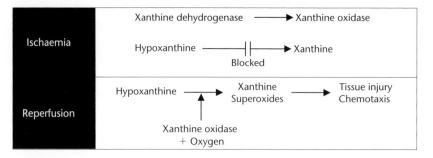

Figure 48.2 Hypoxanthine and xanthine oxidase accumulation during ischaemia results in excessive superoxide anion production during reperfusion.

in this model, with early IRI occurring via a neutrophil-independent mechanism. Other cell types such as mast cells, may in part mediate early IRI.

Endotoxaemia

Plasma levels of endotoxins – lipopolysaccharides (LPSs) derived from the cell membranes of Gram-negative bacteria – are known to rise during CPB. Splanchnic vasoconstriction leading to gut mucosal ischaemia and bacterial translocation, make the gut the most likely source of endotoxaemia during CPB. The magnitude of endotoxin release is highly variable and may be related to CPB duration. Pulsatile CPB may be associated with lower levels of endotoxaemia than non-pulsatile CPB.

Once in the circulation, LPS is bound to LPS-binding protein (LBP), levels of which dramatically increase during endotoxaemia. LPS–LBP complexes are a 1000 times more potent at activating macrophages than LPS alone. Activated macrophages liberate tumour necrosis factor (TNF) and protein kinase, thus propagating the inflammatory process (Figure 48.4). The physiological effects of TNF include hypotension, fever, increased production of acute phase proteins and reduced serum albumin levels.

Contact activation

Blood–gas interfaces and exposure of blood to the components of the CPB system result in the activation of three interconnected plasma protease pathways, namely the kinin–kallikrein pathway, the fibrinolytic-coagulation pathway and the complement system.

The kinin–kallikrein pathway

When bound to anionic surfaces, inert Hageman factor (factor XII) becomes factor XIIa and factor XIIf.

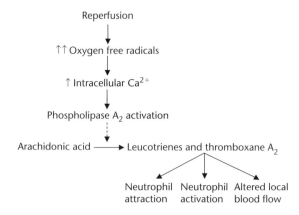

Figure 48.3 The role of products of arachidonic acid metabolism in neutrophil-mediated IRI.

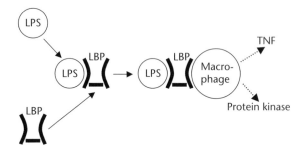

Figure 48.4 The role of endotoxaemia in the inflammatory response to CPB. Circulating LPS is bound to LBP. This complex activates macrophages resulting in TNF and protein kinase release.

In the presence of high-molecular-weight kininogen (HMWK), factor XIIa converts prekallikrein to kallikrein (KK), and generates more of factor XIIa via a positive-feedback mechanism. KK cleaves surface-bound HMWK to yield bradykinin, a potent vasodilator that promotes smooth muscle contraction and capillary permeability. This potentiates neutrophil-mediated endothelial permeability causing tissue

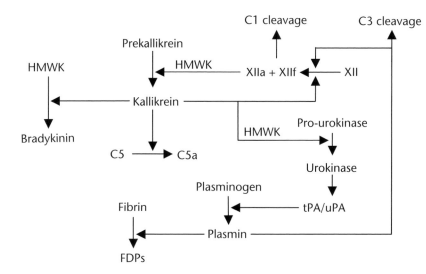

Figure 48.5 The interaction of plasma proteases during contact activation.

oedema. KK and factor XIIa cause neutrophil activation, resulting in reactive oxygen metabolite formation and neutrophil aggregation (Figure 48.5). Heparin retards the inactivation of factor XIIa and KK, thereby propagating the inflammatory response.

The fibrinolytic pathway

Under normal conditions, fibrin clots formed at the site of surgical incision are eventually dispersed by plasmin. Bradykinin production during CPB promotes endothelial secretion of tissue plasminogen activator (tPA), which converts plasminogen to plasmin. In the presence of HMWK, KK cleaves pro-urokinase to yield urokinase. Urokinase activates urokinase plasminogen activator (uPA), resulting in increased plasmin formation. In the presence of plasmin, fibrin is proteolytically digested into pro-inflammatory fibrin split (degradation) products (FDPs). These inhibit further fibrin production and are implicated in platelet and endothelial dysfunction. Plasmin activation of factor XII forms a positive-feedback loop.

The complement system

The complement system consists of over 20 plasma proteins. The host-defence functions include: chemotaxis, inflammation, opsonization, neutralization, lymphocyte activation, degranulation (mast cells, basophils and eosinophils) and lytic complex formation. Complement activation, leading to C3 cleavage, may occur by either 'classical' or 'alternative' pathways (Figure 48.6).

Cleavage of C3 leads to the production of C3a and C3b which stimulate the release of histamine and other inflammatory mediators from mast cells, basophils and eosinophils, leading to increased vascular permeability and smooth muscle contraction. In addition, C3a is

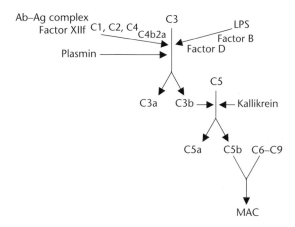

Figure 48.6 Activation of the complement pathway. Factor XIIf (via C1 activation), plasmin and kallikrein can activate complement. C3a and C5a are the so-called anaphylatoxins. Ab-Ag, antibody-antigen.

thought to cause tachycardia, coronary vasoconstriction and reduced cardiac contractility. C5a acts as a powerful chemo-attractant for neutrophils, as well as stimulating neutrophil aggregation, adhesion and activation. Due to their potent actions, C3a and C5a are also known as anaphylatoxins. C3b interacts with membrane-bound C5b and components C6–C9 to form the membrane attack complex, which has the ability to activate platelets and 'punch' holes in bacterial cell walls.

Although CPB results in complement activation by the alternative pathway, protamine–heparin complexes may also activate complement by the classical pathway. Plasma levels of the products of complement activation rise within 2 min of the onset of CPB, and show a second peak after removal of the cross clamp and during rewarming. Levels return to normal 18–48 h after uncomplicated surgery. A strong correlation has been shown between peak C3a levels after CPB and MOF.

Therapeutic intervention

Pharmacological strategies

The impact of corticosteroids on the inflammatory response to CPB has been the subject of considerable research for over 30 years. Corticosteroids greatly enhance the release of the anti-inflammatory cytokines (e.g. IL-10) and reduce pro-inflammatory cytokine mRNA translation and release, endothelial selectin expression, and neutrophil integrin expression. Although these effects are greatest with administration just before the onset of CPB, there are no large-scale studies conclusively demonstrating any improvement in clinical outcome.

In addition to their haemostatic properties, protease inhibitors (e.g. aprotinin, ulinastatin, nafamstat) have been shown to reduce the levels of pro-inflammatory cytokines and reduce the upregulation of integrins in a dose-dependent fashion.

Antioxidants (e.g. tocopherols, desferrioxamine, allopurinol) have long been considered as a means of reducing the tissue injury and inflammation caused by reactive oxygen metabolites. The presence of free-radical scavenging mechanisms within erythrocytes suggests that blood cardioplegia should, at least in theory, be superior to crystalloid cardioplegia.

The goal of selective decontamination of the digestive tract is the reduction of bacterial translocation during surgery. Despite the potential benefits of this technique, logistical difficulties have ensured that the practice remains unpopular.

Other strategies

Heparin-coated CPB systems may reduce the inflammatory response by reducing the exposure of blood to foreign antigens. This is achieved by inhibiting granulocyte activation and reducing complement activation, platelet adhesion and pro-inflammatory cytokine release. Despite reducing the biochemical markers of inflammation, heparin-coated circuits have not conclusively been shown to improve clinical outcome.

Haemofiltration during CPB, particularly in the paediatric population, has been shown to improve outcome. Haemoconcentration and the selective removal of pro-inflammatory cytokines may explain this phenomenon. The use of leucocyte filters during CPB has been shown to improve pulmonary function, reduce cerebral embolism and reduce postoperative infective complications.

The future

Emerging evidence suggests that certain individuals are more vulnerable to the effects of systemic inflammation than others. In patients undergoing major cardiac and non-cardiac surgery, elevated preoperative levels of antibodies to endotoxin core antibody appear to confer a degree of protection from infective complications. Similarly, gender differences and cytokine (e.g. TNF, LBP, IL-1) gene polymorphisms appear to influence the magnitude of pro-inflammatory cytokine release following trauma, surgery and CPB. It is conceivable that preoperative genotyping may allow the identification of patients who might be better managed without CPB. Alternatively, pre-treatment with an anticytokine agent (e.g. antibodies to TNF and IL-1-receptor antagonist) might become possible. Given the complexities of the inflammatory response and past experience with monoclonal antibodies in sepsis, it is unlikely that any single therapy will be effective alone.

Key points

- Upto 2% of patients may suffer morbidity and mortality as a consequence of CPB.
- Surgical trauma, endotoxaemia, IRI and contact activation can induce a systemic inflammatory response.
- The neutrophil plays an important role in IRI.
- The clinical application of advances in molecular biology and genetics are as yet of unproven benefit.

Further reading

Hall RI, Smith MS, Rocker G. The systemic inflammatory response to cardiopulmonary bypass: pathophysiological, therapeutic, and pharmacological considerations. *Anesth Analg* 1997; **85(4)**: 766–782.

Mojcik CF, Levy JH. Aprotinin and the systemic inflammatory response after cardiopulmonary bypass. *Ann Thorac Surg* 2001; **71(2)**: 745–754.

Schroeder S, Borger N, Wrigge H *et al*. A tumor necrosis factor gene polymorphism influences the inflammatory response after cardiac operation. *Ann Thorac Surg* 2003; **75(2)**: 534–537.

Westaby S, Bosher C. Evolution of cardiopulmonary bypass and myocardial protection. In: Westaby S, Bosher C (Eds), *Landmarks in Cardiac Surgery*. London: Martin Dunitz, 1998.

CONTROVERSIES OF CARDIOPULMONARY BYPASS 49

A.C. Knowles & S.L. Misso

It is more than 50 years since the introduction of CPB into clinical practice. Despite considerable research the characteristics of 'optimal' CPB remain imprecisely defined. This chapter discusses the main areas of controversy (Table 49.1).

Table 49.1 Controversies in CPB management

CPB perfusion characteristics	Pressure versus flow
	Pulsatile versus non-pulsatile
Temperature	Normothermia versus hypothermia
Acid–base management	pH-stat versus alpha-stat
Priming fluids	Glucose versus no glucose

Pressure versus flow

Prolonged periods of hypotension and hypoperfusion are deleterious. Despite the fact that routine CPB perfusion pressures of 40–60 mmHg represent deliberate hypotension, the vast majority of patients appear to survive intact. When pressure falls below this range an increase in either pump flow or SVR is the usual response. The question of whether the perfusion pressure or the perfusion flow rate is more important for organ preservation remains unanswered.

At normocapnia, autoregulation maintains vital organ perfusion over a wide range of pressures (50–150 mmHg). During hypothermic CPB the lower limit of cerebral autoregulation falls to 20–30 mmHg. Children appear to tolerate pressures even lower than this. It follows, therefore, that cerebral hypoperfusion would be unlikely with MAP ≥40 mmHg. For most cases this remains the target pressure. It must be remembered that this cannot always be applied to an individual and in a significant proportion of the population the lower limit of autoregulation may well be 70–85 mmHg (Table 49.2).

In 1995, a randomized study of higher (80–100 mmHg) versus lower (50–60 mmHg) CPB pressure in 248 CABG patients showed that *combined* neurological and cardiac outcomes 6 months after surgery were significantly better in the higher pressure group. The study was criticized for analysing combined outcomes, using multiple comparisons, the high stroke rate (7.2%) in the lower pressure (control) group and being insufficiently powered to detect a 50% reduction in stroke rate. The following year, TOE findings in 75% of these patients were published and it became apparent that the incidence of high-grade aortic atheroma was greater in the lower pressure group (~30% versus 40%). From this intriguing and provocative study, it can be tentatively concluded that higher perfusion pressures may reduce the risk of stroke in patients with severe aortic atheroma (Table 49.3).

Studies examining the influence of CPB flow on cerebral blood flow (CBF) and metabolism have produced conflicting results. The only conclusion that can be drawn is that, within the bounds of usual clinical practice, modest changes in flow rate have little impact on CBF at normocapnia.

Table 49.2 Proposed advantages and disadvantages of low and high CPB perfusion pressure

Perfusion pressure	Advantages	Disadvantages
Lower (<60 mmHg)	↓ Incidence of emboli ↓ Haematological trauma ↓ Collateral warming of the heart Less blood in operative field	Cerebral and renal hypoperfusion
Higher (>80 mmHg)	Vital organ perfusion maintained In event of cerebral injury secondary to emboli, collateral flow is said to be pressure dependent	↑ Haematological trauma ↑ Risk of emboli ↑ Bleeding complications

Table 49.3 Patient groups which may benefit from a higher CPB perfusion pressure

Advanced atherosclerosis
Severe (grade IV and V) atheromatous disease of the DTA (visible on TOE) is a good marker of atheromatous disease near the aortic cannulation site (not well visualized with TOE).

Chronic hypertension
In patients with chronic, poorly controlled hypertension the pressure–flow autoregulation curve is shifted to the right, therefore a mean perfusion pressure much greater than 50 mmHg is required to maintain flow.

Cerebrovascular disease
Patients with cerebrovascular disease and those with a history of stroke are at greater risk of neurological injury.

Age >70
Increasing age does not affect cerebral autoregulation. However, there may be slower vasodilatation of cerebral resistance vessels during rewarming leading to transient episodes of metabolism–flow mismatch with resultant ischaemia. Unless there is co-existing atherosclerotic or hypertensive disease there is as yet no evidence that age *per se* is a reason for using high perfusion pressures.

Diabetes mellitus
These patients appear to have an impaired metabolism–flow coupling during CPB with possibly some loss of pressure–flow regulation. It has therefore been postulated but not proven that a higher pressure would be required during rewarming or during normothermic bypass.

DTA, Descending thoracic aorta.

Normothermic versus hypothermic

Studies suggesting that normothermic cardioplegia and CPB may improve myocardial protection during cardiac surgery have led to the use of so-called 'warm-heart' or normothermic techniques.

In 1994, the Toronto Warm Heart Investigators reported no increase in adverse neurological outcomes in patients maintained at normothermia during CPB, whereas the Atlanta group reported a marked increase in neurological injury. Based on patient numbers, however, evidence accumulated in subsequent studies suggests that the avoidance of hypothermia during CPB does not increase the risk of adverse neurological outcomes (Table 49.4).

Pulsatile versus non-pulsatile

It has long been thought that pulsatile CPB is beneficial by virtue of the fact that it is more physiological. The additional energy present in pulsatile flow increases capillary perfusion and enhances lymphatic drainage. A pulsatile flow profile can be generated with either a programmable roller pump or with an IABP during non-pulsatile CPB (Table 49.5). The contradictory conclusions of clinical studies may in part be explained by differences in the pressure–flow characteristics of pulsatile CPB employed.

Table 49.4 Reasons for failure to demonstrate hypothermic neuroprotection

- Normothermic CPB in many cases meant a temperature of ~35.5°C, which may have conferred a degree of neuroprotection.
- Inadvertent cerebral hyperthermia during rewarming during hypothermic CPB.
- Patients in both hypothermic and normothermic CPB groups were relatively normothermic at times of greatest cerebral vulnerability – aortic cannulation/ decannulation and onset/offset of CPB.

Table 49.5 Proposed benefits of pulsatile CPB

↑ Myocardial (subendocardial) perfusion, oxygenation and contractility
↑ Renal (cortical) blood flow and urine output
↑ Cerebral perfusion
↓ Catecholamine, renin, angiotensin, aldosterone and lactate levels
Preserved baroreceptors function
Maintenance of pancreatic β-cell function

In patients with *pre-existing* renal insufficiency, pulsatile CPB appears to be associated with improved postoperative renal function. The application of an AXC denies the ischaemic heart any potential benefit from pulsatile CPB. Any improvement in myocardial outcome may be

Table 49.6 The differences between the clinical applications of alpha-stat and pH-stat blood-gas management strategies

α-stat	pH-stat
So-called because the ionization state of enzymatic α-histidine–imidazole groups is maintained constant.	So-called because pH is maintained at ~7.4 regardless of blood temperature.
Blood-gas analysis results *not* corrected for temperature.	Blood-gas analysis results corrected for temperature.
Target = 'normal' blood gases at 37°C.	Target = 'normal' blood gases at *blood temperature*.
Temperature corrected hypocapnia and alkalosis tolerated.	Temperature uncorrected hypercapnia and acidosis tolerated.
No additional CO_2 administered to patient.	Additional CO_2 administered to patient.

Table 49.7 Advantages and disadvantages of alpha-stat and pH-stat blood-gas management strategies

	Advantages	Disadvantages
α-stat	Cerebral autoregulation preserved ↓ Cerebral micro-embolization ? ↓ Cerebral injury post-DHCA Improved myocardial function	? Risk of cerebral hypoperfusion
pH-stat	More uniform cerebral cooling ↑ H^+ reduces organ metabolism HbO_2 dissociation curve right shifted	Pressure passive CBF ↑ Cerebral micro-embolization ↑ Free radical-induced tissue damage

solely due to higher perfusion pressures during pulsatile CPB. In a Canadian study of 316 CABG patients, pulsatile CPB was associated with lower mortality and cardiovascular morbidity but no improvement in neurological and neuropsychological outcomes.

α-stat versus pH-stat

The solubility of a gas in a liquid is inversely proportional to temperature. As temperature falls, the total gas content remains unchanged but the proportion of dissolved gas in equilibrium with the gas phase (i.e. the partial pressure) falls. Automated blood-gas analysis undertaken at 37°C masks this fall in carbon dioxide (CO_2) partial pressure. When temperature corrected blood-gas measurements are used, hypothermic patients appear hypocapnic and alkalotic.

In nature, two blood-gas management strategies have emerged to maintain normal physiology during hypothermia. Poikilotherms (e.g. fish and reptiles) exhibit 'alpha-stat' blood-gas changes when exposed to different environmental temperatures. In contrast, mammals (e.g. bears) exhibit 'pH-stat' blood gases during hypothermic hibernation (Table 49.6).

During hypothermic CPB, blood vessels maintains their responsiveness to CO_2 and modulate organ blood flow accordingly. The impact of blood-gas management strategy on neurological, cardiac and renal outcomes following hypothermic CPB has generated considerable debate (Table 49.7).

Based on the results of laboratory and clinical studies, alpha-stat is recommended for adults undergoing uninterrupted hypothermic CPB, while pH-stat should probably be used during hypothermic CPB prior to deep hypothermic circulatory arrest (DHCA). The risk of neurological injury during DHCA appears, at least in part, to be due to incomplete brain cooling and insufficient metabolic rate reduction in during the early part of cooling. As cerebral autoregulation is lost as temperature falls, blood-gas management has progressively less influence on CBF.

The reduction in organ metabolism (O_2 consumption) associated with ↑H^+ (pH-stat) is attributed to acidosis-induced intracellular enzyme dysfunction and impaired O_2 utilization.

Glucose management

There is now consensus that hyperglycaemia prior to DHCA is deleterious and should be avoided. Debate continues regarding the continued use of CPB priming solutions containing glucose for patients undergoing CPB without circulatory arrest.

Supporters of glucose containing priming solutions argue that hyperglycaemia is unlikely to worsen *permanent* focal ischaemia caused by embolization of atheromatous debris. Adding glucose to priming solutions results in smaller crystalloid additions, reduced perioperative fluid retention and enhanced diuresis – all of which may improve lung function after surgery. Opponents argue that most CNS injuries involve some degree of reperfusion and that hyperglycaemia worsens ischaemic intracellular acidosis, neuronal regulation and mitochondrial adenosine triphosphate (ATP) generation thus exacerbating neurological injury.

Recent evidence that tight glucose control improves outcomes in critically ill patients poses a simple question: is the problem adding glucose, or failing to manage hyperglycaemia? If the latter is true, patients may enjoy the benefits of glucose, insulin and potassium therapy without additional cerebral risk.

Finally, the normothermic brain is likely to be more sensitive to the deleterious effects of hyperglycaemia than the hypothermic brain. It has been suggested that the hyperglycaemia and cerebral hyperthermia contributed to the higher incidence of adverse neurological outcomes in the Atlanta study (Martin, 1994).

Key points

- Higher perfusion pressures may reduce the risk of stroke in patients with diabetes mellitus, chronic hypertension or severe aortic atheroma.
- Patients are relatively normothermic at times of greatest cerebral vulnerability during cardiac surgery with hypothermic CPB.
- Alpha-stat is recommended for adults undergoing uninterrupted hypothermic CPB.
- Avoidance of hyperglycaemia may be more important in normothermic than hypothermic CPB.

Further reading

Gold JP, Charlson ME, Williams-Russo P, Szatrowski TP, Peterson JC, Pirraglia PA *et al*. Improvement of outcomes after coronary artery bypass: a randomized trial comparing intraoperative high versus low mean arterial pressure. *J Thorac Cardiovasc Surg* 1995; **110(5)**: 1302–1314.

Grigore AM, Mathew J, Grocott HP *et al*. Prospective randomized trial of normothermic versus hypothermic cardiopulmonary bypass on cognitive function after coronary artery bypass graft surgery. *Anesthesiology* 2001; **95(5)**: 1110–1119.

Henze T, Stephan H, Sonntag H. Cerebral dysfunction following extracorporeal circulation for aortocoronary bypass surgery: no differences in neuropsychological outcome after pulsatile versus nonpulsatile flow. *Thorac Cardiovasc Surg* 1990; **38(2)**: 65–68.

Hindman B. Con: Glucose priming solutions should not be used for cardiopulmonary bypass. *J Cardiothorac Vasc Anesth* 1995; **9(5)**: 605–607.

Kurth CD, O'Rourke MM, O'Hara IB. Comparison of pH-stat and alpha-stat cardiopulmonary bypass on cerebral oxygenation and blood flow in relation to hypothermic circulatory arrest in piglets. *Anesthesiology* 1998; **89(1)**: 110–118.

Martin TD, Craver JM, Gott JP *et al*. Prospective randomised trial of retrograde warm cardioplegia: myocardial benefit and neurological threat. *Ann Thorac Surg* 1994; **57(2)**: 298–304.

Metz S. Pro: Glucose priming solutions should be used for cardiopulmonary bypass. *J Cardiothorac Vasc Anesth* 1995; **9(5)**: 603–604.

Murkin JM, Martzke JS, Buchan AM *et al*. A randomized study of the influence of perfusion technique and pH management strategy in 316 patients undergoing coronary artery bypass surgery. II. neurologic and cognitive outcomes. *J Thorac Cardiovasc Surg* 1995; **110(2)**: 349–362.

O'Dwyer C, Prough DS, Johnston WE. Determinants of cerebral perfusion during cardiopulmonary bypass. *J Cardiothorac Vasc Anesth* 1996; **10(1)**: 54–64.

Patel RL, Turtle MR, Chambers DJ, James DN, Newman S, Venn GE. Alpha-stat acid–base regulation during cardiopulmonary bypass improves neuropsychologic outcome in patients undergoing coronary artery bypass grafting. *J Thorac Cardiovasc Surg* 1996; **111(6)**: 1267–1279.

Reves JG, White WD, Amory DW. Improvement of outcomes after coronary artery bypass. *J Thorac Cardiovasc Surg* 1997; **113(6)**: 1118–1120.

The Warm Heart Investigators: Randomised trial of normothermic versus hypothermic coronary bypass surgery. *Lancet* 1994; **343(8897)**: 559–563.

S.L. Misso & A.C. Knowles

Deep hypothermic circulatory arrest (DHCA) involves the use of systemic hypothermia ($\leq 18°C$) and the intentional cessation of the circulation for periods up to 60 min. The technique is used when the nature of the surgical procedure makes conventional CPB impractical or impossible (Table 50.1). DHCA produces a motionless, bloodless and cannula-free surgical field, allowing unobstructed surgical access.

Table 50.1 Cardiac and non-cardiac indications for DHCA

Cardiac
Repair of complex congenital cardiac anomalies
Aortic aneurysm, rupture or dissection
Aortic arch reconstruction

Non-cardiac
Hepatic and renal cell carcinoma
Repair of giant cerebral aneurysms
Resection of cerebral AV malformations
Pulmonary thromboendarterectomy

By reducing cellular metabolism, hypothermia preserves high-energy phosphate stores and protects organs from short periods of ischaemia. In the CNS, neuronal electrical activity and excitatory neurotransmitter release are both reduced. The putative benefits of hypothermia have to be balanced against a significant number of potential problems and complications (Table 50.2).

Safe period of circulatory arrest

While all organs are at risk of injury during DHCA, the brain is the most sensitive. The safe duration of DHCA at any given temperature is defined as the maximum period of continuous circulatory arrest that is not complicated by significant and permanent neurological injury. In general, neonates and infants tolerate longer periods of DHCA than adults. Most patients tolerate 30 min DHCA at 18°C, whereas only three-quarters of patients tolerate 45 min DHCA at this temperature.

The spectrum of neurological injury following surgery with CPB and DHCA is similar to that following cardiac surgery (see Chapter 57). Seizures and choreoathetosis may occur in up to 20% of paediatric patients.

Cerebral protection

Temperature

Hypothermia remains the single most important mechanism of cerebral protection. DHCA at 15–20°C provides the longest safe period of circulatory arrest. The application of external ice packs to the head delays brain rewarming during DHCA.

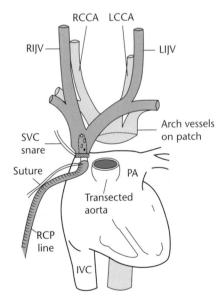

Figure 50.1 Retrograde cerebral perfusion (RCP) via a cannula in the SVC. A purse string suture is used to hold the cannula in place and a circumferential snare is used to prevent reflux of blood into the RA. Other cannulae have been omitted for clarity. RIJV, LIJV: right and left internal jugular veins, respectively; RCCA, LCCA: right and left common carotid arteries, respectively.

Table 50.2 Problems associated with profound hypothermia

General
Prolonged CPB

Circulation
↑ Plasma viscosity, ↓ erythrocyte plasticity
Vasoconstriction, impaired microcirculatory flow
Leftward shift of Hb O_2 saturation curve
Cold agglutinins may worsen regional perfusion and cause haemolysis

Cardiac
Cardiomyocyte K^+ loss and Na^+ gain ↑ Predisposition to dysrhythmias

Cerebral
Vasoconstriction
Risk of cerebral hyperthermia during rewarming

Gastrointestinal
Gastric dilatation and ileus; submucosal erosion and haemorrhage
Impaired hepatic thermogenesis; acute pancreatitis

Renal
↓ GFR; ↓ Na^+, water and glucose reabsorption; ↓ H^+ excretion

Metabolic
Impaired glucose metabolism and tendency to hyperglycaemia
Tendency to metabolic acidosis
Altered pharmacokinetics and pharmacodynamics

Coagulation
Impairs coagulation
↓ Platelet count
May cause DIC

GFR, glomerular filtration rate.

Haemodilution

Hypothermia-induced vasoconstriction and an increase in blood viscosity leads to impaired micro-circulatory flow and organ ischaemia. The rationale for haemodilution during hypothermic CPB is, therefore, improvement of the microcirculation. The optimal degree of haemodilution remains unclear. A haematocrit of <10% results in inadequate tissue oxygenation during cooling and risks tissue hypoxia during rewarming.

Acid–base management

Cerebral vasodilatation associated with pH-stat blood-gas management improves brain cooling and ensures more homogenous cooling of deeper brain structures. pH-stat may however, induce a cerebral metabolic acidosis and increase micro-embolization secondary

to increased cerebral blood flow (CBF). On theoretical grounds, switching from pH-stat to alpha-stat blood-gas management after cooling and prior to the onset of DHCA (the so-called 'crossover' management) has some appeal.

Glucose management

Accumulating evidence supports the notion that tight glycaemic control during DHCA is associated with improved clinical outcome (see Chapter 49).

Pharmacological

Pharmacological protection from cerebral ischaemia remains elusive and at present no drug is licensed for neuroprotection in cardiac surgery. Although various anaesthetic agents (e.g. thiopental, propofol and isoflurane) can induce EEG burst suppression and profoundly decrease cerebral metabolic rate (for oxygen) $CMRO_2$, their neuroprotective properties remain unproven (Table 50.3).

Surgical strategies

Selective antegrade cerebral perfusion

This technique involves selective cannulation of the brachiocephalic, axillary or carotid arteries. Oxygenated blood is pumped via a separate arterial line at $5–10\,ml\,kg^{-1}\,min^{-1}$ as long as perfusions pressure remains <150 mmHg. In addition to increasing complexity and crowding, the surgical field with cannulae, selective antegrade cerebral perfusion (SACP) is accompanied by the risk of cerebral embolization. An intact circle of Willis is required when unilateral SACP is employed. A misplaced cannula may result in inadequate cerebral perfusion while giving a false sense of security.

Intermittent cerebral perfusion

Intermittent systemic perfusion punctuated by ~20 min periods of DHCA has been used as an alternative strategy to prolong the total duration of DHCA. It is suggested that intermittent reperfusion preserves neurological tissue by replenishing cerebral high-energy phosphates and removing accumulated waste products.

Retrograde cerebral perfusion

Retrograde cerebral perfusion (RCP) technique, which relies on the fact that cerebral veins have no valves, involves the continuous administration of cold (10–15°C) oxygenated blood via a SVC cannula (Figure 50.1). Blood flow to the brain is most likely to

Table 50.3 Examples of drugs used for cerebral protection, despite considerable research, any neuroprotective properties remain unproven

Barbiturates (Thiopental)
Majority of non-DHCA studies suggest ↓ mortality but not ↓ stroke
Widely used pre-DHCA despite inconclusive evidence of efficacy
↓ $CMRO_2$, CBF and cerebral blood volume; may ↓ cerebral micro-embolization
At best produce little additional neuroprotection during DHCA

Propofol
Transient EEG burst suppression with ↓ CBF and ↓ $CMRO_2$ following $2–3\,mg\,kg^{-1}$
No evidence of improved clinical outcomes

Ca^{2+}-channel blockers
Improve CBF rather than ↓ abnormal influx of Ca^{2+} into cells
Improve outcome from subarachnoid haemorrhage but not head injury
Outcomes after CPB *worsed* by nimodipine in phase III study
No clinical information about use in DHCA

Glucocorticoids
↓ Liberation of inflammatory cytokine durings CPB
No impact on outcome following normothermic cardiac arrest

Other
Amino acid receptor antagonists (Mg^{2+}, remacemide)
Glutamate-release inhibitors (lignocaine, fosphenytoin)
Anti-proteases (aprotinin, nafamostat)
Free radical scavengers (mannitol, desferrioxamine)
Chlormethiazole and nicorandil

occur via the azygos veins because the internal jugular veins possess valves. The azygos vein has connections to the vertebral venous system and the venous plexus of the foramen magnum and intracranial sinuses. Massive shunting via the superficial and deep venous systems, including the internal and external jugular veins, may result in only a small fraction of the blood entering the SVC actually reaching the cerebral arteries. For this reason the exact levels of CBF and metabolic substrate delivery provided by RCP, have yet to be defined (Table 50.4). Suggested blood flow rates for RCP are $200–300\,ml\,min^{-1}$ with SVC pressure $<25\,mmHg$. Higher pressures associated with retrograde flow may increase the potential for cerebral oedema.

Theoretical advantages of RCP include: more homogenous brain cooling; washout of air bubbles, embolic debris and metabolic waste products; prevention of cerebral blood cell microaggregates; and delivery of O_2 and metabolic substrates to the brain. The prolongation of safe DHCA that can be achieved with RCP is less than that with SACP. RCP for $>60\,min$ is a significant predictor of permanent neurological dysfunction.

Conduct of anaesthesia

Most procedures requiring DHCA are complex and prolonged. Close coordination and cooperation

Table 50.4 Potential problems associated with antegrade and retrograde cerebral perfusion during DHCA

SACP
Embolization of air or plaque
Cannula malposition and inadequate CBF
Unilateral flow requiring flow through circle of
 Willis to contralateral side
↑ Complexity of surgery and crowding of the
 surgical field

RCP
↑ Intracranial pressure (ICP)
Cerebral oedema
Low level of substrate supply

between the anaesthetist, the perfusionist and the surgeon is essential. The risks of coagulopathy and significant haemorrhage should prompt early discussion of likely blood product requirements with the local transfusion service.

Prior to the onset of DHCA the emphasis should be on cardiovascular stability and maintenance of tissue O_2 delivery. Following the onset of CPB, systemic cooling proceeds in the presence of a beating heart. The onset of hypothermia-induced VF signals the need for AXC and administration of cardioplegia. The head is surrounded by ice packs during cooling.

Cooling continues until a stable core temperature of 15–20°C has been achieved for at least 20 min.

The optimal site for temperature monitoring is controversial, as gradients exist between all regions of the body. Temperature monitoring at several sites is advised to ensure uniform cooling. Nasopharyngeal temperature, which follows brain temperature relatively closely, is the preferred site for monitoring brain temperature. Bladder or rectal probes are often used to monitor core temperature.

At the onset of DHCA the pump is switched off and blood is allowed to drain from the patient via the venous line and cardiotomy line to provide a bloodless field. The time of onset of DHCA should be noted. As the IV administration of drugs during DHCA is at best pointless and at worst potentially dangerous, all infusions should be discontinued and any drugs for neuroprotection administered well *before* the pump is switched off.

Removal of the AXC and opening the aorta to the atmosphere exposes both the coronary and cerebral arteries to the risk of air embolism. At the end of DHCA therefore, adequate de-airing and precautions such as head-down tilt and flooding of the surgical field with crystalloid at 4°C should be undertaken. The time of termination of DHCA should be recorded.

Following a variable period of hypothermic reperfusion, slow rewarming commences with vasodilators, such as SNP, being used to promote homogeneous rewarming. Rewarming may take 45–90 min or more and should not be rushed. Hyperthermia, which exacerbates neurological injury following reperfusion, must be avoided at all costs. Infusions of anaesthetic agents are restarted to avoid the risk of awareness during rewarming. The metabolic acidosis that is invariably present following DHCA normally resolves with time if CPB is adequate.

Haemoconcentration by haemofiltration is usually undertaken during rewarming to remove excess body water and reduce the risks of cerebral ischaemia secondary to anaemia.

Key points

- Hypothermia is the single most important mechanism of cerebral protection during DHCA.
- Drugs with putative neuroprotective properties are widely used prior to DHCA despite an absence of convincing evidence of efficacy.
- Haemodilution is used to improve microcirculation.
- The use of continuous or intermittent cerebral perfusion techniques during DHCA may prolong the safe duration of circulatory arrest.

Further reading

Bonser RS, Wong CH, Harrington D, Pagano D, Wilkes M, Clutton-Brock T *et al.* Failure of retrograde cerebral perfusion to attenuate metabolic changes associated with hypothermic circulatory arrest. *J Thorac Cardiovasc Surg* 2002; **123**(5): 943–950.

Deeb GM, Jenkins E, Bolling SF, Brunsting LA, Williams DM, Quint LE *et al.* Retrograde cerebral perfusion during hypothermic circulatory arrest reduces neurologic morbidity. *J Thorac Cardiovasc Surg* 1995; **109**(2): 259–268.

Laussen PC. Optimal blood gas management during deep hypothermic paediatric cardiac surgery: alpha-stat is easy, but pH-stat may be preferable. *Paediatr Anaesth* 2002; **12**(3): 199–204.

Murkin JM. Retrograde cerebral perfusion: Is the brain really being perfused? *J Cardiothorac Vasc Anesth* 1998; **12**(3): 249–251.

D.J. Daly

Failure of tissue oxygenation represents an emergency during CPB. The principle causes are gaseous embolism, inadequate oxygenation and inadequate CPB flow.

Air (gas) embolism

> There are two types of perfusionist ... those that have pumped air, and those that will pump air.
>
> Old perfusionists' proverb

Massive aero-embolism (AE) is defined as the witnessed or likely entry of air into the circulation. The quoted incidence is $1:1000$ cases, which probably represents under-reporting. In 25% of recorded cases, massive AE leads to permanent injury or death.

Air can enter the circulation from the surgical field, from the CPB circuit and via indwelling venous and arterial cannulae. A degree of venous AE probably occurs in all patients undergoing CPB and appears to have few obvious sequelae.

Surgical field entrainment

This is by far the most common source of significant AE. Air enters the circulation when the heart is opened or when a loose atrial suture allows air to be entrained via the venous cannula. The inadvertent delivery of air with cardioplegia solutions may lead to coronary embolism. An aortic root or pulmonary vein vent, at high negative pressure, can draw air into the ventricle via a coronary arteriotomy. Valveless centrifugal pumps may allow retrograde siphoning of arterial blood and air entrainment via the arterial cannula.

Cardiopulmonary bypass air

The maintenance of an adequate volume in the CPB reservoir is a fundamental principle of perfusion. In the early days of CPB, without automatic reservoir level alarms, arterial line AE secondary to reservoir emptying was a relatively common. Advances in CPB circuit design, monitoring and alarm systems have dramatically reduced the likelihood of this event. Nowadays, CPB equipment includes venous and arterial line bubble detectors, and a system that automatically shuts off the pump when the reservoir volume falls below a critical level.

The transition from bubble to membrane oxygenators has significantly reduced the amount of gas deliberately added to the circulation during oxygenation. Punctured or misconnected lines and loss of membrane integrity may however lead to significant gas embolism.

Anaesthetic

Unprimed IV infusion lines and the use of pressurized infusion devices may result in the delivery of significant quantities of air. The practice of re-connecting partially used infusion bags greatly increases the risk of AE and should be avoided. AE of this type tends to occur before and after CPB, at times when the patient may already be haemodynamically unstable.

Physical principles

An understanding of the gas laws and the properties of air bubbles within the circulation are the keys to successful management (Table 51.1).

Nitrogen and oxygen are the main constituents of air. As oxygen is readily absorbed, the challenge is the enhancement nitrogen elimination. Hypothermia tends to reduce bubble size (Charles' law) and increase blood nitrogen solubility (Henry's law). Barometric and hydrostatic pressure (Boyle's law) prevent dissolved nitrogen leaving solution, while the partial pressure

---

Table 51.1 The gas laws

Charles' law states that at a constant pressure the volume of a given mass of gas varies directly with the absolute temperature.

Boyle's law states that at a constant temperature the volume of a given mass of gas varies inversely with the absolute pressure.

Henry's law states that at a particular temperature the amount of a given gas dissolved in a given liquid is directly proportional to the partial pressure of the gas in equilibrium with the liquid.

dictates any tendency to bubble formation (Henry's law). Self contained underwater breathing apparatus (SCUBA) divers know that too rapid an ascent can lead to the formation of nitrogen bubbles causing decompression illness (the bends).

The institution of hyperoxia ($PaO_2 \gg 13\,kPa$) gradually leads to nitrogen displacement (denitrogenation). The arteriovenous oxygen difference (i.e. $PaO_2 - PvO_2$) reflects the gradient favouring nitrogen absorption. A nitrogen bubble, 4 mm in diameter (i.e. 0.025 ml), takes $\sim$10 h to disappear while breathing air, but <1 h while breathing 100% oxygen. As with anaesthetic gas elimination, the rate of denitrogenation is cardiac output dependent.

Management

As massive AE is rare, it is essential that anaesthetists are aware of the possibility and the goals of management *before* they encounter the problem for the first time. For this reason many centres have developed their own management protocols with action plans for the anaesthetist, surgeon and perfusionist. The clinical scenario also lends itself well to simulation (Tables 51.2 and 51.3).

The fundamental principles of good management are early diagnosis, good communication and rapid institution of measures of proven or likely benefit.

Most management plans include retrograde cerebral perfusion (RCP) on the grounds that cerebral AE will have occurred. After the CPB pump is stopped and the line clamped, the surgeon will usually clamp the aortic cannula, cut the arterial line close to the cannula and assist the perfusionist to refill the line. This practice reduces the risk of aortic injury caused by decannulation and subsequent recannulation. The primed arterial line is then connected to the RA or SVC, retrograde perfusion commenced at $1-2\,l\,min^{-1}$ and the aortic cannula unclamped and vented. RCP is continued until no more bubbles are seen in the aortic cannula.

The theoretical benefits of intermittent carotid compression (i.e. to reduce antegrade cerebral air delivery and encourage air-flushing from the vertebral arteries during RCP) have to be balanced against the small risk of plaque fissuring and embolization.

The role of pharmacological neuroprotectants remains controversial. Although a number of agents are used in this setting, none have demonstrated unequivocal efficacy and none are licensed for this specific indication (Table 51.4).

Table 51.2 Basic principles of the management of massive air embolism during CPB

Make the diagnosis
Communicate the diagnosis
Identify the source of air embolism
Prevent further air embolism
Limit organ damage
Clear the CPB circuit of air
Re-establish circulation

Table 51.4 Putative neuroprotectants used after cerebral air embolism

Corticosteroids
Antioxidants
Free radical scavengers
General anaesthetic agents
Local anaesthetics

Table 51.3 The roles of surgeon, perfusionist and anaesthetist in the management of massive air embolism during CPB

Perfusionist	Surgeon	Anaesthetist
Stop CPB pump and clamp lines	Clamp arterial cannula Cut arterial line	Carotid compression Steep head-down position Ventilate with 100% oxygen
Add cold fluid to reservoir Re-fill arterial line	Prevent cardiac ejection Connect arterial line to RA Initiate RCP at 20°C Vent air from aortic cannula	Cerebroprotectants?
RCP at $1-2\,l\,min^{-1}$ Stop RCP Restart CPB and cool Slow rewarm	Re-connect arterial line to aorta Complete surgery	Maintain MAP $\sim$80 mmHg Consider hyperbaric oxygen

RCP: Retrograde cerebral perfusion.

Table 51.5 Checklist for inadequate oxygenation during CPB

Gas supply
Gas delivery circuit not compromised
Gas source connected to gas inlet port of oxygenator
Gas flow $>0.5\,l\,min^{-1}$ (visual and by back-pressure in line)
No leak from vaporizer manifold
Ensure adequate F_iO_2 via inline oxygen analyser
Gas scavenging system (if used) not obstructed

Blood flow
Ensure adequate blood flow through oxygenator
Ensure adequate anticoagulation

Patient factors
Ensure depth of anaesthesia is adequate (vaporizer leak)
Check for hyperthermia ($\uparrow CMRO_2$)
Cold agglutinins

CMRO$_2$: Cerebral metabolic rate (for oxygen).

Table 51.6 Causes of inadequate CPB flow

Electrical pump failure
- Impact minimized by
  - uninterruptible power supply
  - backup generators
  - emergency backup batteries incorporated in pump

Mechanical pump failure
- Roller head under occlusion

Venous return
- Air locks, lifting heart

Cannula problem
- Total obstruction: retained clamp
- Partial obstruction: small size, kinking

Aortic dissection
- Increased line pressure and decreased patient arterial pressure

Inadequate oxygenation

Inadequate oxygenation of blood during CPB can occur as a result of failure of the gas delivery system or the oxygenator. The presenting features are darkening of arterial blood and reduced mixed venous oxygen saturation, which may be associated with a rising transmembrane pressure gradient. ABG analysis is used to confirm the clinical diagnosis. As a temporizing measure the pump flow rate can be increased and some of the arterial flow can be diverted (i.e. shunted) back to the venous reservoir, thus increasing SvO_2. The sequence of checks given in Table 51.5 is suggested.

The use of point-of-care anticoagulation monitors means that oxygenator failure due to coagulation is exceedingly rare. Changing an oxygenator *during* CPB requires at least two perfusionists and a period of circulatory arrest. A discussion of the protocols for this unusual procedure is beyond the scope of this chapter.

Inadequate flow

Inadequate flow can result from electrical or mechanical pump failure, a venous 'air lock', cannula obstruction (e.g. kinking, malposition and clamping), covert circulating volume loss and aortic dissection (Table 51.6).

By its nature, electrical power failure during CPB is an unpredictable event. An uninterruptible power supply combined with an on-site backup generator should make total electrical failure in the operating room an extremely rare occurrence. Modern CPB pumps have emergency battery backup, which can be used to drive the pump and critical monitors. Although roller pump heads can be manually cranked during total power loss, this procedure is tiring and requires two individuals if undertaken for more than 5 min. Total power loss causes heater unit failure, which makes rewarming challenging.

As air entrainment interferes with a siphon, venous return to the reservoir may be halted by the presence of a sufficiently large volume of air – an 'air lock'. If elevation of the tubing in sections fails to rectify the problem the venous cannula is clamped and the venous line disconnected and back-filled.

Cannula size determines the flow rate within the venous line. Inappropriately small cannulae or kinks in the lines will lead to decreased venous return and pump flow. Obstruction to flow in the arterial line or oxygenator is confirmed by finding a high CPB flow line pressure and a low patient arterial pressure.

Aortic dissection is generally noticed when CPB is first commenced. CPB arterial line pressure is elevated while patient arterial pressure is low. The aorta may be flaccid on palpation with an obvious mural haematoma. Unrecognized aortic dissection is associated with significant mortality and morbidity. The extent and impact of aortic dissection can be minimized by prompt diagnosis, discontinuation of CPB and repositioning of the aortic cannula. Despite this approach, many surgeons will opt for formal ascending aortic repair (e.g. an interposition graft).

Key points

- Emergencies during CPB are uncommon but potentially catastrophic.
- All staff should be familiar with management protocols for massive air embolism.
- Most management plans include retrograde cerebral perfusion on the grounds that cerebral aeroembolism will have occurred.
- The practice of re-connecting partially used infusion bags should be avoided.

Further reading

Kurusz M, Mills NL. Management of unusual problems encountered in initiating and maintaining CPB In: Gravlee GP, *et al.* (Eds), *CPB: Principles and Practice*, 2nd edition. Philadelphia: Lippincott Williams and Wilkins, 2000; pp. 578–612.

Mills NL, Ochsner JL. Massive air embolus during CPB: causes, prevention and management. *J. Thorac Cardiovasc Surg* 1980; **80(5)**:708–717.

Tovar EA, Del Campo C, Borsari A, Webb RP, Dell JR, Weinstien PB. Postoperative management of cerebral air embolism: gas physiology for surgeons. *Ann Thorac Surg* 1995; **60(4)**:1138–1142.

CARDIAC INTENSIVE CARE

T.W.R. Lee & J.H. Mackay

Haemodynamic instability following CPB is common. The goal of cardiovascular management in the ICU is to maintain adequate oxygen transport to end organs until complete recovery of cardiac function.

Circulation management

Preload optimization

The ventricles compensate for acute changes in venous return and end-diastolic volume (EDV), by varying the force and velocity of myocardial fibre shortening – the Frank–Starling relationship (Figure 4.1). The response to increasing preload can be thought of in three distinct phases (Table 52.1).

Table 52.1 The three phases of the response to increasing preload

1	Intact preload reserve	↑ EDV → ↑ SV and ↑ CO
2	Preload optimization	↑ EDV → unchanged CO
3	Exhausted preload reserve	↑ EDV → ↓ CO and ↓ MAP

In health, preload optimization typically occurs with pulmonary artery wedge pressure (PAWP) 10–15 mmHg. Many cardiac surgical patients have reduced LV compliance, which becomes further reduced by the effects of CPB and catecholamines. In these patients a higher PAWP (i.e. >15 mmHg) is often required to maintain adequate SV.

Rate, rhythm and contractility

HR, rhythm and myocardial contractility are the major determinants of myocardial oxygen consumption (VO_2). Myocardial ischaemia is avoided by homeostatic mechanisms, which balance VO_2 against CO and MAP. Owing to its 30% augmentation of EDV, NSR is desirable whenever possible. Atrial or atrioventricular pacing at 80–100 bpm can improve endocardial perfusion by shortening diastolic filling time and reducing EDV.

VF, and unstable ventricular and supraventricular tachydysrhythmias should be immediately converted by either electrical or chemical means. Maintenance of normal or supranormal $[K^+]$ (i.e. 4.5–$5.5\,mmol\,l^{-1}$) and $[Mg^{2+}]$ reduces ventricular irritability.

Cardiodepressant anti-dysrhythmics should be used with caution in patients with impaired myocardial function. Although amiodarone is the most commonly used anti-dysrhythmic in cardiac surgical patients, other classes of agent may be required for more complex or persistent rhythm abnormalities.

A hypercontractile ventricle, ejecting a maximal SV against a high afterload, does so at the expense of increased VO_2. It is suggested that perioperative β-blockade improves long-term outcome in patients with coronary artery disease. The postoperative use of β-blockers in stable cardiac surgical patients is not uncommon.

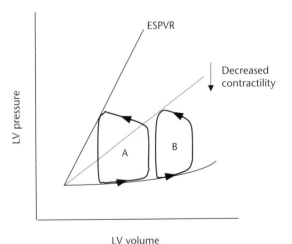

Figure 52.1 LV pressure–volume loops illustrating (A) the normal ventricle, and (B) the decrease in slope of the ESPVR line with decreased contractility. This decrease in contractility can also be accompanied by a decrease in SV, and an increase in LVEDP.

Table 52.2 Correction of hypovolaemia and hypervolaemia

Hypovolaemia

Synthetic colloids (e.g. succinylated gelatin or hydroxyethylstarch) if Hb $> 8.5\,g\,dl^{-1}$

Oxygen delivery (DO_2) maximized at haematocrit 24–30%

Hypervolaemia

Diuretics $\downarrow$ intravascular volume by $\uparrow$ urine output and $\downarrow$ EDV by $\uparrow$ venous capacitance

Direct-acting vasodilators (e.g. nitroglycerine) $\uparrow$ venous capacitance

Enalaprilat, an ACE inhibitor, is also a venodilator; an IV preparation is available for use

Venesection and erect posture

Afterload

Afterload can be viewed as the sum of external forces opposing ventricular ejection, of which SVR is one component. Laplace's law states that wall tension or stress is directly proportional to intracavity pressure and cavity radius, and inversely proportional to wall thickness (see Figure 31.2).

Depending on LV function, increased afterload (Table 52.3) may be associated with either hypertension or hypotension. Both hypertension and hypotension can cause decreased coronary perfusion and systolic dysfunction. Uncontrolled hypertension can cause excessive surgical bleeding.

Table 52.3 Causes of increased afterload in the cardiac surgical patients

- History of preoperative essential or secondary hypertension
- Increased endogenous catecholamines released during CPB
- Hypothermia
- Emergence from anaesthesia
- Response to pain can lead to arteriolar vasoconstriction
- Administration of exogenous vasoconstrictors

Common complications

Left ventricular dysfunction

Ventricular function is commonly decreased for 8–24 h following CPB. The ideal measure of LV performance, the slope of the end-systolic pressure–volume relationship (ESPVR), cannot easily be derived at the bedside. For this reason, surrogate measures of contractility (i.e.

RA pressure, PAWP, MAP, PAP and CO) are used. Although echocardiography can be used to assess ventricular function, the findings are generally load dependent (Figure 52.1).

Decreased contractility can be secondary to metabolic abnormalities, the presence of cardiodepressant agents, reperfusion injury and myocardial ischaemia (coronary vasospasm, thrombosis or occlusion). The incidence of perioperative MI (often clinically silent) is thought to be ~5%. The diagnosis of MI in the post-CABG patient is however a diagnostic challenge (Table 52.4).

Table 52.4 Diagnosis of perioperative MI

ECG	Difficult to interpret in perioperative period, particularly ST- and T-wave alterations. Reliance on Q-wave formation has a low sensitivity in this setting
CK-MB	Traditional enzyme marker used to confirm MI. Found in skeletal muscle and atria. Low specificity following cardiac surgery
TnI	Adenosine triphosphatase inhibitor of actin–myosin complex. Higher sensitivity and specificity than CK-MB. Levels $>60\,\mu mol\,l^{-1}$ correlate with both Q-wave MI and new RWMA

CK-MB, creatinine kinase MB (isoenzyme); TnI, troponin I; RWMA, regional wall motion abnormality.

Before initiating inotropic therapy, all remediable factors (i.e. rate, rhythm, preload and afterload) should be addressed. Myocardial β-receptor desensitization and downregulation make the heart less sensitive to catecholamines. An understanding of the differential effects of inotropes on the heart and circulation, rapid assessment of response and modification of therapy are probably more important than the order in which specific drugs are selected.

Since serum $[Ca^{2+}]$ may be reduced following CPB and the administration of citrated blood products, empirical $CaCl_2$ administration – which causes a transient increase in contractility and vascular tone – may be appropriate.

Mechanical support

In refractory LV failure, where inotrope and vasoactive therapy is maximal, mechanical circulatory support may be necessary. The intra-aortic balloon pump (IABP) decreases systolic ventricular wall tension by providing afterload reduction with balloon deflation, and improves coronary perfusion during diastole by providing diastolic pressure augmentation with inflation (see Chapter 46). Contraindications to the IABP include femoral arterial and abdominal aortic disease, and moderate to severe aortic regurgitation. A mechanical ventricular assist device (VAD) may also be placed intraoperatively in one or both ventricles as a transient strategy to allow for the recovery of contractile function, or as a bridge to cardiac transplantation.

Right ventricular dysfunction

RV failure can be difficult to manage because of the dependence of LV filling on right-sided function. If RV output falls, LV filling and therefore LV output are reduced. The RV is extremely sensitive to increases in afterload (i.e. PVR). Reduced RV contractility or increased RV afterload results in increased wall tension and right heart distension. Isoproterenol or dobutamine are useful first-line agents, as they increase contractility while lowering PVR. More recently, phosphodiesterase (PDE) inhibitors (e.g. enoximone and milrinone), which tend to cause less tachycardia than isoproterenol and dobutamine, have been used to treat RV dysfunction. Although more effective in LV failure, the IABP may reduce RV afterload and improve coronary perfusion. Short-term use of an RV assist device (RVAD) may allow time for RV recovery.

Pericardial tamponade

Pericardial tamponade is characterized by hypotension, tachycardia and elevated CVP. Although it typically occurs acutely within 24 h of cardiac surgery, it can develop chronically over several days. In tamponade, the decrease in the LV filling during inspiration is accentuated. The fall in SV produces a reflex increase in HR and contractility. Diagnostic clues include those described in Table 52.5.

Table 52.5 Clinical signs suggestive of cardiac tamponade

Oliguria
Reduced or no chest tube drainage
Pulsus paradoxus
Equalization of the RAP, PAD and PAWP
Loss of the y-descent in RAP and PAWP
Low-voltage ECG/electrical alternans pattern

In addition to detecting an obvious extracardiac collection, the most common TOE manifestation is collapse of right-sided chambers when their intracavity pressures are at their lowest – the RV in early diastole and the RA in early systole. In the spontaneously breathing patient, transmitral E- and A-wave velocities are

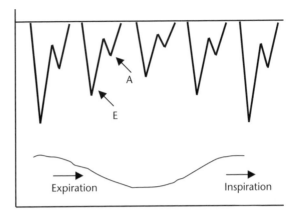

Figure 52.2 Tamponade physiology during positive-pressure ventilation: mitral E-wave velocity increases during the inspiratory phase and decreases during the expiratory phase.

Table 52.6 Resuscitation goals in cardiac tamponade

Preload	Elevated, avoid high PEEP
HR	High, because of reduced SV
Rhythm	Sinus preferable but limited atrial kick
SVR	High
Contractility	Normal or elevated

PEEP, positive end-expiratory pressure.

decreased during inspiration, with reciprocal changes in the right heart. Mechanical ventilation reverses this relationship (Figure 52.2). Management consists of resuscitation (Table 52.6) and prompt surgical drainage.

Postoperative atrial fibrillation

Atrial fibrillation (AF) and atrial flutter are the most common postoperative supraventricular tachy dysrhythmias following cardiac surgery. New onset AF occurs within 24–72 h of surgery in up to 30% patients. Independent predictors of AF include age >65 years, hypertension, male sex, a previous history of AF and valve surgery. Patients undergoing heart transplantation or isolated CABG surgery have the lowest incidence of postoperative AF. Other factors that may contribute to AF include prolonged aortic cross-clamp times, pulmonary vein venting, perioperative pneumonia, chronic obstructive lung disease and prolonged postoperative mechanical ventilation.

Preoperative β-blockade and amiodarone therapy can reduce the incidence of AF following CABG. Other anti-dysrhythmic agents, such as Ca^{2+}-channel blockers and digoxin are less effective as prophylactic regimes. IV magnesium administration and atrial pacing have

Table 52.7 Simplified approach to haemodynamic management in the patient with optimal preload

↑ MAP and ↓ CO	Afterload is likely to be normal or high
	Therapy with an inotrope plus a vasodilator, or with a PDE inhibitor might be considered
↓ MAP and ↑ CO	Afterload is probably low
	Therapy with a vasopressor should be considered
↓ MAP and ↓ CO	Contractility and afterload are reduced
	Therapy with both inotropes and vasopressors should be considered

also been shown to reduce the incidence of AF in some studies. Thoracic epidural anaesthesia may also be of benefit.

In the absence of contraindications, all patients who develop AF should be anticoagulated within 24–48 h. Heparin is an appropriate first-line anticoagulant until therapeutic anticoagulation can be established with oral warfarin. Aspirin therapy may be used as an alternative in patients who cannot be warfarinized. If AF has persisted for more than 48 h and therapeutic anticoagulation has not been maintained, TOE should be performed to exclude the presence of LA thrombus. Electrical or chemical conversion to sinus rhythm is preferred, especially when patients are haemodynamically unstable, symptomatic or unable to receive anticoagulation. Otherwise, pharmacological ventricular rate control alone is acceptable in some cases. IV amiodarone is effective for both conversion to sinus rhythm and ventricular rate control, and can be easily converted to oral therapy. The need for anti-dysrhythmic therapy should be reviewed 6–8 weeks after surgery and discontinued if the patient is in sinus rhythm.

Simplified approach to haemodynamic management

Considering CO, MAP and PAWP in the patient with optimal preload simplifies haemodynamic management (Table 52.7).

Key points

- A PAWP >15 mmHg may be required following CPB.
- Increased afterload may cause hypertension or hypotension.
- Tamponade may be difficult to diagnose clinically and should be considered in all cases of hypotension/low CO following cardiac surgery.
- Intra-aortic balloon counter-pulsation reduces cardiac chamber wall tension by systolic deflation and improves coronary blood flow by diastolic augmentation.
- AF should not be regarded as a benign condition after cardiac surgery.

Further reading

Maisel WH, Rawn JD, Stevenson WG. Atrial fibrillation after cardiac surgery. *Ann Intern Med* 2001; **135(12)**: 1061–1073.

Mangano DT, Layug EL, Wallace A, Tateo I. Effect of atenolol on mortality and cardiovascular morbidity after non-cardiac surgery. Multicenter Study of Perioperative Ischemia Research Group. *N Engl J Med* 1996; **335(23)**: 1713–1720.

Slogoff S, Keats AS. Does perioperative myocardial ischemia lead to postoperative MI? *Anesthesiology* 1985; **62(2)**: 107–114.

Solomon AJ, Greenberg MD, Kilborn MJ, Katz NM. Amiodarone versus a β-blocker to prevent atrial fibrillation after cardiac surgery. *Am Heart J* 2001; **142(5)**: 811–815.

RESUSCITATION AFTER ADULT CARDIAC SURGERY

53

J.H. Mackay & J.E. Arrowsmith

Defibrillation, ventilation, pacing and resuscitation are essential components of cardiac surgical care. Over 3% of cardiac surgical patients require resuscitation for confirmed cardiac arrest during the postoperative period. As patients undergoing cardiac surgery become older and sicker the quality of postoperative care and resuscitation are likely to become increasingly important. Conventional advanced life support (ALS) guidelines provide a useful framework but require modification, particularly in the cardiac surgical ICU setting. This chapter will highlight some of the key differences.

Resuscitation guidelines

Adult basic life support

How should basic life support (BLS) be spelt? According to the current guidelines, the answer is still ABC(D), which means *A*irway, *B*reathing, *C*irculation and *D*efibrillation (rather than cardiac surgical mantra: '*A*ccuse, *B*lame, *C*riticize and *D*eny'). Given the high probability of VF following a witnessed sudden collapse, it has been suggested that a change in order to 'CAB' or 'DCAB' would be more appropriate

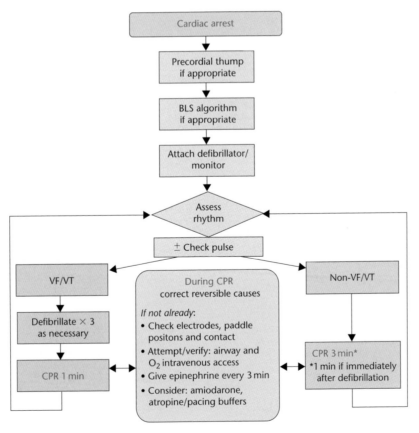

Figure 53.1 ALS algorithm for the management of cardiac arrest in adults. Courtesy of the UK Resuscitation Council and reproduced with permission.

when resuscitating an *adult*. In the setting of the cardiac ICU, when external cardiac massage may be injurious, immediate defibrillation should be the first-line response to a monitored VF arrest (Figure 53.1).

In situations where BLS is undertaken, the recommended ratio of chest compressions to ventilations is now 15 : 2 (per minute) for both one- and two-person CPR. More chest compressions can be given per minute with a ratio of 15 : 2 than with 5 : 1. In the presence of a patent airway, effective chest compressions are considered more important than ventilation in the first few minutes of resuscitation. It should

be borne in mind that coronary perfusion pressure progressively *rises* during chest compressions and rapidly *falls* with each pause for ventilation.

Adult advanced life support

Pulseless VT and VF account for the majority of patients who survive cardiac arrest in a general hospital. For every minute that the dysrhythmia persists, the chances of successful defibrillation decline by 7–10%. Specialist cardiothoracic units should be capable of early detection, rapid defibrillation and superior outcomes (Figure 53.2).

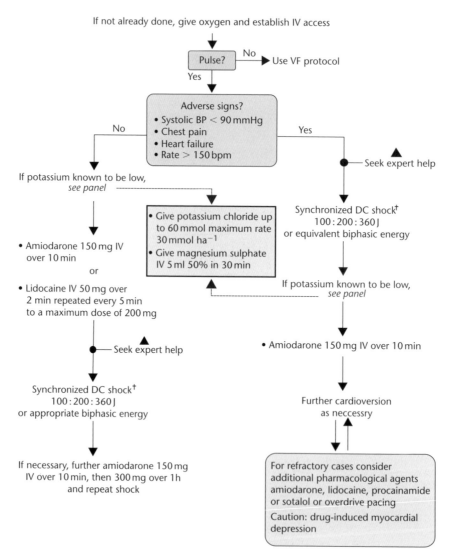

Figure 53.2 ALS algorithm for broad-complex tachycardia. Drug doses are quoted for a 70-kg adult. Paroxysmal torsades may be treated with magnesium or overdrive pacing. [†]The conscious patient should be sedated or anaesthetized before direct current (DC) cardioversion. Courtesy of the UK Resuscitation Council and reproduced with permission.

Table 53.1 An aide memoire to the causes of pulseless electrical activity and asystole

The four 'Hs'	The five 'Ts'
Hypoxia	Tension pneumothorax
Hypovolaemia	Tamponade
Hyperkalaemia	Thromboembolic
Hypothermia	Therapeutic substances in overdose
	Toxic substances

A heterogenous group of conditions may present as non VF/VT cardiac arrest (Table 53.1). Outcome is generally poor unless a reversible cause can be found and treated effectively. The frequent absence of a readily treatable underlying cause means that this type of arrest has a poor prognosis in general hospitals with only 5–10% patients surviving to discharge. In contrast, in the cardiac surgical ICU – where bleeding, hypovolaemia and tamponade are all readily treatable, and where additional therapeutic options are available - outcomes should be considerably better.

When faced with an apparent non VF/VT arrest, it is essential to

- confirm that VF is not being missed and that leads or pads are correctly attached,
- treat bradycardias with epicardial pacing if these are present,
- exclude underlying VF in the presence of fixed-rate pacing,
- consider chest reopening if closed chest CPR is unsuccessful.

Symptomatic bradycardia is extremely common in the cardiac surgical ICU. ALS guidelines recommend atropine as first-line treatment. In the cardiac surgical ICU, where tachycardia is equally undesirable, pacing (when possible) is the preferred option. If pacing is not an option (e.g. no wires *in situ* or failure to capture), isoproterenol or dopamine are often used before atropine is considered.

Drugs

Although the use of vasopressors has become standard practice, the evidence that these drugs are more effective than placebo in humans is weak. Epinephrine 1 mg is recommended every 3 mins to improve coronary and cerebral perfusion. High dose of epinephrine (5 mg every 3 mins) offers no additional benefit. Similar in-hospital resuscitation results are obtained when vasopressin is used as an alternative to epinephrine. A recent out-of-hospital study demonstrated that vasopressin was superior to epinephrine in patients with asystole. However, there was no difference in survival to discharge in patients with VF/VT or pulseless electrical activity.

On the cardiac surgical ICU it may be entirely appropriate to modify the recommended pharmacological management of a monitored cardiac arrest. An α-agonist or smaller initial dosages of epinephrine (0.1–0.5 mg) may be administered to minimize the risk of hypertension and tachycardia following successful resuscitation.

The evidence supporting the use of anti-dysrhythmic drugs in VF/VT was until recently, surprisingly weak. Two recent studies of out-of-hospital VF/VT arrest demonstrated that the administration of amiodarone after three unsuccessful shocks, increased the likelihood of survival to hospital admission. Significantly, neither study demonstrated that amiodarone improved survival to discharge. Despite this latter finding, amiodarone has now been promoted ahead of lidocaine in the VF/pulseless VT algorithm. Pre-filled syringes containing amiodarone (300 mg in 10 ml) are now commercially available. Lidocaine can still be given for VF/VT if the patient has received amiodarone but the evidence supporting its efficacy is weak. Bretylium tosylate no longer appears in the VF/VT algorithm.

Early resuscitation on ICU

Chest opening

Following surgery through a sternotomy, chest reopening is both a diagnostic and therapeutic option in the cardiac surgical ICU. In addition it permits internal cardiac massage, which is considerably more effective than external chest compressions. Bleeding, tamponade, graft occlusion and graft avulsion are conditions likely to be remedied by this approach.

Patients most likely to benefit from chest reopening are:

- those with a surgically remediable lesion,
- those who arrest within 24 h of surgery,
- those in whom the chest is reopened within 10 min of arrest.

Delayed reopening or the finding of a problem that is not amenable to surgery (e.g. global cardiac dysfunction) is associated with a poor prognosis. Chest reopening should not be used as a 'last-ditch' manoeuvre after a prolonged resuscitation sequence.

Cardiopulmonary bypass

The reinstitution of CPB following emergency chest reopening may allow the resuscitation of a patient who would otherwise die. Hypothermic CPB restores organ perfusion, decompresses the heart, and allows the surgeon to consider all possible options in a more controlled setting. Valve replacement, the repair of bleeding cannulation sites, graft revision and additional grafting may be undertaken with often surprisingly successful clinical outcome.

Whenever possible the patient should be transferred to the operating theatre before the emergency reinstitution of CPB.

Late resuscitation on ICU

Patients with greater preoperative surgical risk, adverse intraoperative events and poor physiological state at the time of ICU admission are less likely to survive to hospital discharge. Similarly, refractory multi-system organ failure and recurrent nosocomial infection while on the ICU have been shown to be important determinants of mortality. For some patients, there comes a point when aggressive resuscitation is inappropriate and cardiopulmonary arrest becomes the terminal event in their illness. It is the duty of a doctor to identify these patients and to ensure that they are spared the indignity of futile interventions.

'Do not attempt resuscitation' (DNAR) directives may be instituted in the postoperative period, if it is believed that death is inevitable and that CPR is unlikely to be successful. Sensible guidelines on implementation of DNAR orders can be found on the UK Resuscitation Council's website.

Resuscitation outside ICU

Ward arrests

The management of a cardiac arrest on a cardiac surgical ward differs little from a cardiac arrest on a general surgical or medical ward. Seemingly trivial symptoms and vague 'early warning' signs should be taken seriously as they may herald a more sinister event. The use of a Medical Emergency Team (MET) has been shown to reduce both the incidence and mortality from unexpected ward arrests in the setting of a general hospital (Tables 53.2 and 53.3).

The effectiveness of the MET concept is significantly hampered by incomplete documentation of patient observations. The recording of respiratory rate and hourly urine output are particularly poor.

The relative success of chest reopening following cardiac arrest on the ICU has lead some surgeons to

Table 53.2 Suggested criteria for calling the Medical Emergency Team in a cardiothoracic hospital

Acute change	Physiology
Airway	Threatened
Breathing	All respiratory arrests
	RR <5 or >36
Circulation	All cardiac arrests
	Pulse rate <40 or >140
Neurology	Fall in GCS > 2 points
Renal	Urine output $<0.5\,ml\,kg^{-1}h^{-1}$
	for 2 consecutive hours
Oximetry	SpO_2 $<90\%$ regardless of F_IO_2
Other	Patients giving cause for concern who do not meet above criteria

Oximetry is a widely available and a potentially useful monitor in a cardiothoracic ward. GCS: Glasgow coma sale.

believe that similar results can be obtained from chest reopening on the ward. Unfortunately, as the time out from surgery increases, the proportion of surgically remediable causes of cardiac arrest decreases exponentially. At this time, thromboembolic phenomena and cardiac failure are far more common than bleeding or tamponade. Not surprisingly, therefore, the outcome from chest reopening on the ward is dismal and studies indicate that the practice should be abandoned.

In the event of cardiac arrest on the ward within 72 h of surgery, chest reopening should be considered within the first few minutes of resuscitation. A 'scoop and run' policy is recommended with CPR continuing throughout transfer to the operating theatre.

Catheter laboratory arrests

VF/VT arrests in the catheter laboratory are invariably iatrogenic, are amenable to *very* early defibrillation and are associated with return of spontaneous circulation in $>90\%$ cases, and $>80\%$ chance of survival to discharge. In hospitals with a cardiac catheter laboratory, the inclusion of catheter laboratory arrests in overall hospital statistics can significantly skew the overall hospital survival to discharge rate. In cases of coronary dissection or other surgically amenable conditions early consideration of transfer to the operating theatre and emergency CPB should be considered.

Two recently published, large multi-centre studies, one in Europe and the other in Australia, have demonstrated that mild hypothermia is beneficial in patients successfully resuscitated from out-of-hospital VF cardiac arrest.

Table 53.3 Factors influencing outcome from cardiac arrest and resuscitation on a ward

Geography
- The geographical location and layout of cardiac surgical wards are important.
- Many patients understandably prefer to have their own room while staying in hospital. Given the lack of monitoring in some isolated rooms, cardiac patients may pay a heavy price for their privacy.

Training
- Resuscitation training should place greater emphasis on the identification of the at-risk patient and prevention of cardiac arrests.
- Scenario-based staff training may be of value.

Prevention
- Nowhere is the statement *prevention is better than cure* more true than in the field of resuscitation.
- International studies have shown that many critically ill patients receive sub-optimal care on the general wards. Many terminal arrests on general wards are preceded by unrecognised or inadequately treated deteriorations in their vital signs. Consideration should be given to the pre-emptive transfer of a deteriorating patient to the ICU.
- The appropriate use of DNAR orders significantly reduces the incidence of unexpected cardiac arrest.

Early detection
- Outcomes from witnessed arrests are better than those where the initial arrest is undetected.
- With early detection, the proportion of primary VF/VT arrests is higher and time to defibrillation reduced.

Equipment
- Automated external defibrillators (AEDs) are now increasingly being deployed in public sites. They are now so prevalent that BLS training is being extended to include teaching on the use of these straightforward devices.
- There is a strong argument for putting semi-automated defibrillators on general medical and surgical wards. AEDs for in-hospital use should include an ECG display and a manual override facility for use by the cardiac arrest team.
- Accumulating evidence suggests that biphasic defibrillation waveforms may be superior to monophasic waveforms.

Conclusions

Patients sustaining cardiac arrests in a cardiothoracic surgical unit are twice as likely to survive to hospital discharge as patients who arrest in a general hospital. The essential requirements for a good clinical outcome are early detection of arrests, effective BLS and early defibrillation. Recognition that *prevention is better than cure* will lead to an increasing role for 'the Medical Emergency Team'.

Key points

- ALS algorithms require modification after cardiac surgery.
- Consider the possibility of underlying VF in 'asystolic' arrests and paced patients with apparent electromechanical dissociation.
- Look for epicardial pacing wires in bradycardic arrests before giving atropine and epinephrine!
- Resuscitation after cardiac surgery is associated with better outcomes than resuscitation in general hospitals.

Further reading

Buist M, Moore GE, Bernard SA, Waxman BP, Anderson JN, Nguyen TV. Effects of a medical emergency team on reduction of incidence of and mortality from unexpected cardiac arrests in hospital: preliminary study. *Br Med J* 2002; **324(7334)**: 387–390.

Dorian P, Cass D, Schwartz B, Cooper R, Gelaznikas R, Barr A. Amiodarone as compared with lidocaine for shock resistant VF. *N Engl J Med* 2002; **346(12)**: 884–890.

Gwinnutt CL, Columb M, Harris R. Outcome after cardiac arrest in adults in UK hospitals: effect of the 1997 guidelines. *Resuscitation* 2000; **47(2)**: 125–135.

Mackay JH, Powell SJ, Osgathorp J, Rozario CJ. Six-year prospective audit of chest reopening after cardiac arrest. *Eur J Cardiothorac Surg* 2002; **22(3)**: 421–425.

The Hypothermia After Cardiac Arrest Group. Mild therapeutic hypothermia to improve the neurological outcome after cardiac arrest. *N Engl J Med* 2002; **346(8)**: 549–556.

UK Resuscitation Council: http://www.resus.org.uk

Wenzel V, Krismer AC, Arntz RA, Sitter H, Stadlbauer KH, Lindner KH. A comparison of vasopressin and epinephrine for out-of-hospital cardiopulmonary resuscitation. *N Engl J Med* 2004; **350(2)**: 105–113.

54

M.K. Prasad & F. Falter

Some degree of impairment of respiratory function occurs in all patients undergoing cardiac surgery. This ranges from transient problems, such as retained secretions and atelectasis, to overwhelming acute lung injury (ALI) and the acute respiratory distress syndrome (ARDS). The causes of respiratory complications following cardiac surgery are summarized in Table 54.1. A detailed pathophysiological discussion is beyond the scope of this chapter, which focuses on clinical management.

Respiratory failure

Acute respiratory failure is the inability to perform adequate intrapulmonary gas exchange causing hypoxia *with or without* hypercapnia. The accepted quantitative criteria for the diagnosis are $PaO_2 < 8.0\,kPa$ (60 mmHg) on air and $PaCO_2 > 6.5\,kPa$ (49 mmHg) in the absence of primary metabolic alkalosis. Using this definition many cardiac surgical patients will have postoperative 'respiratory failure' and yet make an uneventful recovery. In this setting the diagnosis of respiratory failure has to be made with reference to the patient's preoperative respiratory function, postoperative cardiac function, the effects of drugs and *trends* in RR, PaO_2 and PCO_2. The major determinant of pulmonary outcome following cardiac surgery is cardiac function.

Atelectasis

Atelectasis, means 'imperfect dilatation' of the lungs. This condition affects dependent areas of lung – particularly the left lower lobe following internal mammary artery harvest. The combined effects of anaesthesia, intermittent positive-pressure ventilation (IPPV) and sternotomy reduce functional residual capacity (FRC), vital capacity and tidal volume (V_T). These effects may be compounded by diaphragmatic dysfunction caused by direct or thermal (cold) injury to the phrenic nerve. Recruitment manoeuvres, such as positive end-expiratory pressure (PEEP) and ensuring that the lungs are fully expanded prior to chest closure, may reverse some of the atelectasis that inevitably occurs during surgery. Postoperative atelectasis is best managed by adequate analgesia, physiotherapy and manoeuvres such as intermittent positive pressure breathing, continuous positive airway pressure (CPAP), incentive spirometry and forced coughing.

The patient with poor gases

As many as 10% of cardiac surgical patients will have impairment of postoperative gas exchange that is sufficient to cause concern, prolong mechanical ventilation and delay discharge from ICU. Before escalating therapy it is essential to examine the patient, review the CXR and consider the problem in the context of the

Table 54.1 Causes of respiratory failure after cardiac surgery. The major determinant of pulmonary outcome following cardiac surgery is cardiac function.

Central neurological	CNS depressant drugs, CVA, pain
Spinal cord	Neuraxial anaesthesia, trauma, ischaemia
Peripheral neurological	Trauma
Neuromuscular	NMBs, severe $\downarrow\downarrow$ K^+, Mg^{2+}, PO_4, myasthenia gravis, starvation
Airway	Retained secretions, asthma
Chest wall	Flail chest, kyphoscoliosis, ankylosis
Pleural	Pneumothorax, pleural effusion
Lung	Smoking-related disease, atelectasis, pneumonia, aspiration, ARDS, PE
Cardiac	LVF, low CO state, valve disease, tamponade, right → left shunt

NMB, neuromuscular blocker; PE, pulmonary embolism; LVF, left ventricular failure.

patient's preoperative respiratory status. As preoperative lung function tests and ABG analysis are not routinely undertaken in most units, preoperative oximetry and the results of the first ABG analysis after induction of anaesthesia ($F_iO_2 \approx 0.6$) can be used as a guide. By definition, the minority of patients who fail to improve with the passage of time, physiotherapy, alveolar recruitment manoevres, satisfy the diagnostic criterion for ALI (Table 54.2). Pre-emptive (i.e. elective) tracheal intubation and mechanical ventilation should be considered in all patients with deteriorating pulmonary function.

Table 54.2 American–European Consensus Conference (AECC) definitions of ALI and the ARDS

ALI	$PaO_2/F_iO_2 < 40$ kPa (300 mmHg)
ARDS	Bilateral pulmonary infiltrates on CXR
	PAWP < 18 mmHg
	$PaO_2/F_iO_2 < 26$ kPa (200 mmHg)

Acute lung injury and acute respiratory distress syndrome

Hypoxia with bilateral pulmonary infiltrates and a relatively low LA pressure following cardiac surgery used to be known as 'pump lung'. The clinical features resemble the so-called 'sepsis syndrome', with increased PVR, increased vascular permeability, and elevated alveolar–arterial O_2 gradient. This ALI usually resolves within 48h or progresses to ARDS (Table 54.2).

The features of ARDS are secondary to inflammatory damage to the pulmonary microvascular endothelium. The natural history of ARDS is classically divided into exudative and infiltrative phases, which progress to either recovery or fibrosis and scarring. The pattern of lung injury is typically heterogeneous, with the process sparing some areas and causing severe alveolar collapse and airway plugging in others.

The incidence of ARDS following CPB is reported to be as high as 2.5% in some series. Predisposing factors include redo cardiac surgery, hypotension, sepsis (both pulmonary and non-pulmonary) and massive transfusion. The aetiology and subsequent complications, rather than respiratory failure itself, dictate mortality from ARDS. Death is usually due to *multiple* organ system failure (MOF). The avoidance of CPB does not eliminate the risk of ALI or ARDS.

Management of ARDS

General measures

The management of ARDS is predominantly supportive. In the acute phase, efforts should be directed towards resuscitation, identification of the cause and prevention of further organ dysfunction and other complications. As a result of capillary leak and subsequent volume resuscitation, most patients are fluid overloaded. Fluid restriction and forced diuresis often improve lung compliance and oxygenation. The potential benefits of this strategy however, have to be balanced against the consequences of vital organ hypoperfusion. In the setting of oliguria and impending renal failure, early institution of renal support therapy should be considered.

Ventilation

Progressive and potentially life-threatening hypoxia is the hallmark of ARDS. Most patients require invasive ventilatory support until lung function improves. The combination of poor pulmonary compliance, ventilation–perfusion mismatch, pulmonary oedema and heterogeneous alveolar infiltration make it impossible to select a ventilatory strategy to suit all lung units. Traditional large V_T (10–15 ml kg^{-1}) IPPV with moderate PEEP (5–10 cmH$_2$O) in ARDS has been shown to be harmful – resulting in ventilator associated lung injury (VALI). The so-called 'baby lung' concept describes the preferential ventilation of less diseased areas of lung resulting in excessive airway pressures (barotrauma) and over-distension (volutrauma). Shear stress at the junctions between collapsed and aerated alveoli may cause alveolar rupture, leading to pneumothorax, pneumomediastinum or subcutaneous emphysema. Modern lung management strategies are based on pressure-controlled, small V_T (5–6 ml kg^{-1}) ventilation, optimal (best) PEEP, manipulation of the inspiratory : expiratory time ratio, permissive hypercapnia and patient posture.

Pressure-controlled ventilation

Pressure-controlled ventilation (PCV) allows time-cycled, pressure-limited breaths to be delivered. Inspiratory V_T is determined by the preset pressure limit and pulmonary compliance, with gas flow being terminated as soon as this pressure is reached. The combination of decelerating flow and maintenance of airway pressure over time means that stiff lung units with low static compliance and long time constants are more likely to be inflated. Although PCV allows spontaneous ventilation, it is not particularly comfortable for the awake patient. Volume alarms require careful setting, as an abrupt fall in compliance will result in hypoventilation.

Pressure-support ventilation

Pressure-support ventilation (PSV), which supplements each spontaneous breath with gas flow until a preset airway is reached, is a much more comfortable mode during weaning.

Positive end-expiratory pressure

PEEP increases FRC and redistributes extravascular lung water, which may in turn improve lung compliance and oxygenation. In the setting of pulmonary oedema, CT has shown that within 30 min of the application of PEEP, there is an increase in lung cross-sectional area and a reduction in dependent lung density. The benefits of PEEP have to be set against impairment of venous return and volutrauma. The optimal level of PEEP can be estimated by reference to the inspiratory part of the pressure–volume curve (Figure 54.1).

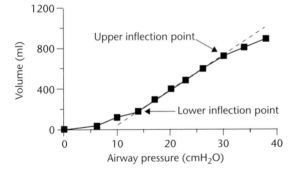

Figure 54.1 Determining the optimal level of PEEP. The lower inflection point represents the start of the part of the curve with the greatest compliance. The use of small tidal volumes prevents the pressure from exceeding the upper inflection point. PEEP should be maintained just *above* the lower inflection point.

Inverse ratio ventilation

Inverse ratio ventilation (IRV) describes any mode of ventilation where the inspiratory time is greater than the expiratory time. The prolongation of inspiration reduces gas flow velocities and induces laminar flow, resulting in a more even distribution of V_T. This theoretically reduces the risk of VALI and increases alveolar recruitment. Unfortunately, concerns about patient comfort, barotrauma (dynamic hyperinflation

and excessive intrinsic PEEP) and haemodynamic instability have reduced the popularity of IRV.

High-frequency oscillatory ventilation (HFOV) is administration of low tidal volumes ($1–3\,\mathrm{ml\,kg^{-1}}$, i.e. smaller than the dead space) at a frequency of $1–50\,\mathrm{Hz}$ ($60–3000\,\mathrm{min^{-1}}$). HFOV is almost exclusively used in neonates. Mixing and diffusion, rather than convection and mass transport, are responsible for oxygenation. Low tidal volumes reduce the potential for barotrauma and the gas flow characteristics may improve ventilation–perfusion mismatch. The adequacy of ventilation has to be assessed clinically and assessment of gas exchange (ABG analysis) as the tidal volume delivered cannot be measured.

Permissive hypercarbia

Permissive hypercarbia is the inevitable consequence of using PEEP and pressure-limited low V_T ventilation (i.e. deliberate alveolar hypoventilation). Although the highest tolerable $PaCO_2$ has not been defined, it has been said that $PaCO_2 > 10\,\mathrm{kPa}$ (75 mmHg) represents *promiscuous* hypercarbia. The adverse effects of respiratory acidosis include hypoxia, myocardial depression, dysrhythmia, intracranial hypertension and the need for patient sedation. Over the course of several days, increased renal bicarbonate reabsorption generates a compensatory metabolic alkalosis. Paralysis and dietary modification may have a marginal impact on metabolic CO_2 production.

Prone position ventilation

Prone position ventilation (PPV) has been shown to improve oxygenation in as many as two-thirds of patients with refractory hypoxia secondary to ARDS. Ventilation–perfusion mismatch in ARDS stems from the fact that pulmonary blood flow is directed by gravity to dependent areas of lung, which are collapsed and underventilated. The preferential ventilation of non-dependent areas of lung further compounds the situation during mechanical ventilation. Dependent areas of lung are, in effect, operating on the part of the pressure–volume curve (Figure 54.1) that lies *below* the lower inflection point. The net effect is an extracardiac shunt. The effects of PPV are

1 to redistribute blood flow from previously dependent areas of lung to previously non-dependent areas of lung
2 to move previously dependent lung units up the pressure–volume curve.

The prone position should be maintained for as long as possible. Failure to respond to PPV should not preclude later attempts. Although studies of PPV have revealed improved oxygenation without haemodynamic compromise, no improvement in outcome has been demonstrated. Most deaths are caused by MOF rather than acute hypoxia.

Adjuvant therapy

Pulmonary hypertension secondary, in part to hypoxic pulmonary vasoconstriction – a constant finding in ARDS – leads to worsening hypoxia. Inhaled pulmonary vasodilators (e.g. nitric oxide (NO) and prostacylin) offer some theoretical benefit. Although, inhaled NO has been shown to improve oxygenation by >20% in two-thirds of patients, the effects are short-lived. Despite improving oxygenation without haemodynamic compromise, no randomized study has demonstrated improved survival in ARDS.

When used as a last resort in adult patients, outcome from extracorporeal gas exchange (e.g. extracorporeal membrane oxygenation (ECMO), extracorporeal CO_2 removal, intravenous oxygenation is invariably poor. In contrast, the outcome from ECMO in children in the setting of congenital heart surgery is considerably better.

Tracheostomy

It is usual for ICU patients requiring long-term ventilation to undergo tracheostomy. There is a wide variation in practice and considerable debate about the optimal timing and operative technique. Improved patient cooperation and comfort, easier pulmonary toilet and reduced dead space are cited as reasons for early (i.e. <10 days) tracheostomy. In contrast, the long list of significant complications – particularly haemorrhage and infection – is often used to justify late (i.e. >14 days) tracheostomy. Institutional and personal preference dictates whether open or percutaneous dilatational tracheostomy is performed.

Cardiovascular management

Both the underlying disease process and its treatment may compromise cardiovascular function. Increased PVR in ARDS leads to an increase in right ventricular end-diastolic pressure and right ventricular stroke work, and displacement of the interventricular septum. Continuous haemodynamic monitoring and assessment of end-organ function is widely used. A disproportionate degree of hypoxia, in the absence of

clinical and radiological signs, should trigger the echocardiographic exclusion of an intracardiac shunt. Despite continuing debate about the use of the PAFC in the general ICU, they are still used in the setting of ARDS following cardiac surgery, where differentiation between ARDS and pulmonary oedema is difficult.

Antimicrobial therapy

Infection may cause or complicate ARDS. As the typical radiological features of ARDS may mask the signs of intrathoracic infection (e.g. lung abscess and empyema) a high index of suspicion is required. CT is routinely used to exclude intrathoracic and intra-abdominal sepsis. Antimicrobial therapy, which initially may be empirical, should be guided by the patient's recent medical and surgical history and advice from local microbiologists.

Key points

- Respiratory failure is common after cardiac surgery.
- Treatment of ARDS is supportive and aims to avoid further organ dysfunction.
- Patients with ARDS tend to die from multiple organ failure.
- Low tidal volume ventilation appears to be associated with significantly lower early mortality.

Further reading

Bernard GR, Artigas A, Brigham KL, Carlet J, Falke K, Hudson L et al. The American-European Consensus Conference on ARDS. Definitions, mechanisms, relevant outcomes, and clinical trial coordination. *Am J Respir Crit Care Med* 1994; **149(3 Pt 1)**: 818–824.

Gattinoni L, Tognoni G, Pesenti A, Taccone P, Mascheroni D, Labarta V et al. Effect of prone positioning on the survival of patients with acute respiratory failure. *N Engl J Med* 2001; **345(8)**: 568–573.

Milot J, Perron J, Lacasse Y, Letourneau L, Cartier PC, Maltais F. Incidence and predictors of ARDS after cardiac surgery. *Chest* 2001; **119(3)**: 884–888.

Petrucci N, Iacovelli W. Ventilation with lower tidal volumes versus traditional tidal volumes in adults for acute lung injury and acute respiratory distress syndrome. (Cochrane Review). In: *The Cochrane Library*, Issue 3, 2003. Oxford: Update Software.

GASTROINTESTINAL COMPLICATIONS 55

A.M. Campbell & M.G. Mythen

Gastrointestinal complications following cardiac surgery are relatively rare (reported incidence <3%) but are associated with significant morbidity. Despite significant improvements in perioperative care, these complications are associated with a high mortality (Table 55.1).

Table 55.1 Common gastrointestinal problems after cardiac surgery

Gastrointestinal haemorrhage
Gastrointestinal perforation
Bowel ischaemia
Acute pancreatitis
Acalculous cholecystitis
Bowel obstruction/ileus

GI complications may develop during surgery and at any time in the postoperative period. Presenting features may include: nausea, vomiting, diarrhoea, constipation, failure to absorb enteral feed, abdominal distension or pain, abnormal liver function tests, and metabolic acidosis. Given the prevalence of minor, transient GI symptoms (e.g. anorexia, nausea, etc.) after cardiac surgery it may be very difficult to determine which patients require further investigation. In high-risk groups a high index of suspicion is required as clinically significant GI tract failure may have an insidious onset, particularly when symptoms and signs are masked by drugs. Delays in diagnosis and management result in excessive mortality.

In many cases the common causal factor is impaired GI tract perfusion and GI mucosal ischaemia. Conditions that result in impaired mucosal oxygen delivery include: low CO states, CPB, vasoconstriction and mesenteric thromboembolism. The presence of an arterial counter-current in the intestinal mucosa renders the distal portions of the villi vulnerable to ischaemia (Figure 55.1). Progressive ischaemia is associated with stress ulceration, mucosal atrophy, increased mucosal permeability and loss of barrier function, which may lead to bacterial translocation, endotoxaemia, sepsis and multi-organ failure (MOF).

The risk of developing GI complications after cardiac surgery is dependent on the presence of pre-existing

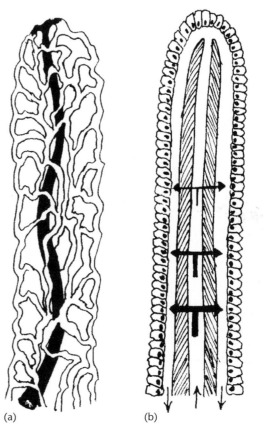

(a)   (b)

Figure 55.1 GI villous blood flow. A central arteriole (a) runs to the tip of the villus before forming a network or palisade of smaller vessels. The arrangement is effectively a counter-current system where diffusion of oxygen from the central arteriole (b) reduces the oxygen content of blood reaching the tip of the villus.

conditions, the type of surgery undertaken and peri-operative events (Table 55.2).

Gastrointestinal bleeding

Bleeding from the upper GI tract is far more common than from the lower GI tract. Haemorrhagic oesophagitis, gastritis or duodenitis accounts for over

Table 55.2 Risk factors for gastrointestinal complications after cardiac surgery

Demographic
Age
Poor nutritional status
History of peptic ulcer disease

Drugs
NSAIDs
Aspirin
Corticosteroids
Warfarin
Splanchnic vasoconstrictors

Types of surgery
Emergency operations (e.g. aortic dissection)
Redo operations
Valve operations
Combined procedures (e.g. valve and CABG)

Preoperative factors
Peripheral vascular disease
Renal insufficiency
Preoperative LVEF <40%
Significant dysrhythmia (e.g. AF)
Cardiogenic shock

Intraoperative
Profound hypotension/hypoperfusion
Prolonged duration of CPB
Inotropic therapy
IABP use

Postoperative
Re-exploration within 24 h
Respiratory failure, prolonged ventilatory support
Renal failure
Sternal/mediastinal infection

LVEF, left ventricular ejection fraction.

Table 55.3 Aetiology of gastrointestinal bleeding during and after cardiac surgery

Upper
Oesophagitis/variceal bleeding
Gastritis/gastric ulceration
Duodenitis/duodenal ulceration

Lower
Mesenteric ischaemia/ischaemic colitis
Antibiotic-associated/pseudo-membranous colitis
Haemorrhoids
Tumours
Diverticulosis
Inflammatory bowel disease
  Crohn's disease, ulcerative colitis
Angiodysplasia
  e.g. Heyde's syndrome (associated with severe aortic stenosis)

a third of all GI complications after cardiac surgery. Rarely, occult GI haemorrhage may occur during CPB and the risk of oesophageal or gastric laceration may be increased by the use of TOE. Lower GI bleeding may be associated with ischaemia, colitis or existing colonic conditions (Table 55.3).

Although the clinical presentation may be dramatic – haematemesis, melaena or rectal bleeding and haemodynamic collapse – anaemia may be the only sign. Opinion varies as to when a patient should be referred for a gastroenterological assessment. Early diagnostic or therapeutic endoscopy is indicated in those patients least able to tolerate the haemodynamic instability associated with repeated episodes of bleeding. Current evidence suggests that rebleeding after therapeutic endoscopy, which occurs in up to 20% of cases, is best treated by further endoscopic intervention rather than

surgery. Surgery for intractable GI haemorrhage following cardiac surgery is associated with significant mortality.

Proctoscopy, sigmoidoscopy or colonoscopy should be performed if upper GI endoscopy is negative or lower GI haemorrhage is suspected. In troublesome cases, mesenteric angiography or a radionuclide scan – performed while the patient is bleeding – allows identification of the bleeding vessel and permits embolization. Vasopressin and the somatostatin analogue, octreotide decrease splanchnic blood flow and may be beneficial in unrelenting haemorrhage. A selective arterial infusion of vasopressin may arrest haemorrhage in up to 90% of patients. The vast majority of patients respond to primary or secondary medical management. Surgical intervention is required in the remainder.

Routine perioperative pharmacological suppression of gastric acid secretion has not been shown to decrease the incidence of GI complications after cardiac surgery. In most cases the aetiology is mucosal ischaemia rather than hyperacidity, as the ischaemic GI tract becomes achlorhydric. Nevertheless, prophylaxis in high-risk cases (e.g. previous gastritis or peptic ulceration, prolonged ventilatory support, coagulopathy, chronic dialysis) is prudent. Although proton pump inhibitors and histamine-H_2 antagonists offer comparable prophylaxis against stress ulceration, the focus of perioperative prevention should be the maintenance of adequate GI perfusion. Only omeprazole has been shown to be effective in reducing further bleeding and the need for surgery in those with bleeding ulcers. Enteral feeding, which stimulates GI tract activity and increases splanchnic blood flow, may also be effective at preventing ulceration. In the presence of critical splanchnic ischaemia, however, enteral feeding may actually *worsen* the situation.

Pancreatitis

Pancreatic cellular injury, indicated by transient pancreatic hyperamylasaemia, is common after cardiac surgery. The aetiology is believed to be pancreatic ischaemia secondary to low CO states and hypoperfusion, although hypothermia, high-dose thiopental and excessive administration of $CaCl_2$ (e.g. $>800 \, mg \, m^{-2}$) may also result in pancreatic injury. In most patients the symptoms of subclinical pancreatitis (e.g. anorexia, nausea, ileus) are mild and resolve within a few days. The incidence of overt pancreatitis in this setting is around 3%. An elevated serum amylase concentration ($>1000 \, i.u. \, l^{-1}$) is diagnostic but has relatively low specificity ($\sim$70%). The simultaneous determination of serum pancreatic lipase increases both the sensitivity and specificity (90–95%). The serum amylase concentration does not appear to correlate with disease severity.

Management is largely supportive. The use of inhibitors of pancreatic autodigestion (e.g. glucagon, somatostatin, octreotide, anticholinergics) does not appear to greatly improve outcome. Anedoctal reports of improved outcome following haemofiltration have not been validated in randomized studies. The routine use of broad-spectrum antibiotics has, however, been shown to reduce the risk of infective complications and abscess formation, and significantly improves outcome from severe acute pancreatitis.

Uncomplicated acute pancreatitis is associated with 5–10% mortality, whereas the mortality from acute necrotizing pancreatitis is up to 50%. If untreated, a pancreatic abscess or infected pseudocyst is invariably fatal. Operative intervention carries a high mortality in acute pancreatitis and CT-guided percutaneous drainage of collections and abscesses is undertaken whenever possible. In aggressive forms of necrotizing pancreatitis, surgery may be the only means of saving the patient.

Cholecystitis

Cholecystitis after cardiac surgery usually occurs in the absence of gallstones (i.e. acalculous). Not infrequently, the symptoms and signs are vague and non-specific. Ultrasound examination should be performed if symptoms persist or the clinical condition of the patient deteriorates. While supportive therapy alone may be adequate, percutaneous drainage should be considered in unstable patients. Delays in diagnosis and treatment

undoubtedly contribute to the high mortality ($\sim$75%) associated with acute cholecystitis in this setting. Cholecystotomy is recommended in the critically ill patient, whereas open or laparoscopic cholecystectomy is preferred in the more stable patient or in the presence of gangrene or perforation of the gall bladder.

Hepatic dysfunction

Mild and transient elevation of the serum concentrations of hepatic enzymes is common after cardiac surgery. While hyperbilirubinaemia occurs in 20% of patients, clinically obvious jaundice is rare and usually indicates other complications of cardiac surgery. Predictors of postoperative hyperbilirubinaemia include RA pressure, preoperative bilirubin level and valve surgery. Significant hepatocellular damage is uncommon and progression to hepatitis and hepatic failure is extremely rare. The presence of hepatic dysfunction usually indicates MOF, which is associated with significantly increased mortality. Patients with severe preoperative liver dysfunction are at significant risk of hepatic failure, bleeding and infective complications after cardiac surgery. Worsening coagulopathy (rising prothrombin time) with persistent hypoglycaemia is an ominous sign. Normal preoperative liver function tests do not preclude the development of significant postoperative hepatic dysfunction. Similarly, abnormal preoperative results do not identify every patient at risk.

Postoperative hepatic dysfunction in the presence of a low CO state carries a poor prognosis. Frank hepatic necrosis is a recognized complication of cardiogenic shock. The only treatment options are supportive – improving cardiac performance and supplying adequate nutritional support. Laboratory tests of liver function (e.g. prothrombin time) are a useful barometer of treatment success.

Mesenteric ischaemia

Mesenteric ischaemia in the setting of cardiac surgery is usually due to low CO or prolonged CPB. Ischaemia secondary to atheroembolism, and arterial or venous thrombosis is less common. Persistent metabolic acidosis may be the only suggestive sign in the sedated and ventilated patient.

Management is, in part, dictated by the severity and rate of progression of symptoms and signs. Angiography may exclude thromboembolism but the absence of vascular occlusion does not rule out ischaemia. Abdominal CT – which may reveal gut dilatation, gut wall thickening, gas in the intestinal wall and peritoneal fluid – is probably the investigation of choice. Diagnostic laparoscopy or laparotomy may be required in some patients.

Ileus and pseudo-obstruction

Paralytic ileus is frequently a benign, self-limited problem, but occasionally it may reflect sepsis or severe intra-abdominal pathology. Simple ileus presents with large nasogastric (NG) aspirates and failure to absorb feed. This will usually improve spontaneously over a few days as the patient's condition improves. A plain abdominal radiograph may reveal distended loops of small or large bowel. Colonic distension (>10 cm in cross section) is associated with an increased risk of colonic rupture.

Contributing factors include gastric distension (possibly related to vagal injury), electrolyte disturbances (decreased K^+), hepatic or splanchnic congestion (systemic venous hypertension), inflammatory processes (e.g. cholecystitis and pancreatitis), retroperitoneal bleeding, pseudo-membranous colitis, mesenteric ischaemia and drugs (e.g. opioids).

Therapy should be directed at any identifiable precipitating process and preventing secondary complications. A NG tube will prevent gastric distension until peristaltic activity returns. Prokinetics such as metoclopramide and erythromycin may be of use. In persistent cases a general surgical opinion should be sought. Failure to diagnose an incarcerated hernia, volvulus or obstruction secondary to adhesion bands has grave implications. Exploratory or diagnostic laparoscopy or laparotomy may be required.

Nutritional management

Most patients undergoing uncomplicated cardiac surgery do not appear to suffer any ill effects from a temporary interruption of their normal diet. Patients requiring prolonged intensive care and those who 'fail to thrive' on the wards require dietetic assessment and nutritional support. Enteral (i.e. oral, NG and nasojejunal) nutrition is preferred as there are few absolute indications for parenteral nutrition (e.g. intestinal obstruction, anatomical disruption and

severe ischaemia). In addition to the benefits of providing energy and protein, enteral nutrition improves splanchnic perfusion, maintains gut integrity (theoretically reducing bacterial translocation) and modulates the immune response. The early introduction of enteral nutrition after surgery is currently encouraged. The small intestine regains motor function within hours of surgery and thus makes jejunal feeding an attractive option.

Randomized controlled trials have demonstrated the benefits of oral feeding in mild to moderate pancreatitis and enteral (nasojejunal) feeding in severe pancreatitis. When compared to total parenteral nutrition, enteral feeding in this setting is associated with less pancreatic and systemic inflammation, a lower incidence of sepsis and MOF, a reduced requirement for operative intervention and significantly lower mortality. Nasojejunal feeding is well tolerated, as it usually does not stimulate pancreatic exocrine function in the same way that oral, gastric or duodenal feeding does.

Key points

- Mucosal ischaemia is responsible for the majority of GI complications after cardiac surgery.
- Upper GI tract bleeding is more common than lower GI tract bleeding.
- Delays in diagnosis and treatment contribute to morbidity and mortality.
- Early postoperative enteral feeding may be of benefit in patients requiring prolonged intensive care.

Further reading

Mythen MG, Webb AR. Perioperative plasma volume expansion reduces the incidence of gut mucosal hypoperfusion during cardiac surgery. *Arch Surg* 1995; **130**(4): 423–429.

van der Voort PH, Zandstra DF. Pathogenesis, risk factors, and incidence of upper gastrointestinal bleeding after cardiac surgery: is specific prophylaxis in routine bypass procedures needed? *J Cardiothorac Vasc Anesth* 2000; **14**(3): 293–299.

Zacharias A, Schwann TA, Parenteau GL, Riordan CJ, Durham SJ, Engoren M *et al.* Predictors of gastrointestinal complications in cardiac surgery. *Tex Heart Inst J* 2000; **27**(2): 93–99.

W.T. McBride & J. Skoyles

At present there is no universally recognized definition of acute renal failure (ARF). Whereas some define ARF as oliguria and an increase (e.g. 50%) in creatinine concentration, others call this combination 'renal insufficiency or dysfunction' and reserve the term ARF for patients requiring renal replacement therapy (RRT) as the definition. The overall incidence of ARF requiring RRT in the adult cardiac surgical population is approximately 5%. The incidence ranges from <1%, for patients with normal preoperative urea and creatinine concentrations to >40% in patients with preoperative creatinine concentration >200 μmol l^{-1} (Figure 56.1). Although rarely the primary cause of death, ARF is associated with 50% mortality. Renal dysfunction after cardiac surgery significantly increases the length of ICU and hospital stay.

Table 56.1 Diagnosis of ARF

Urine output < 0.5 ml kg^{-1} h^{-1}
Complete anuria = obstruction until proved otherwise

$\uparrow$ Plasma urea, creatinine and K$^+$ concentrations
$\downarrow$ Plasma Ca^{2+} and HCO$_3^-$ concentrations

Urine: Plasma creatinine ratio
   >50 suggests pre-renal cause
   <20 suggests renal cause
Urine: Plasma osmolality ratio
   >1.4 suggests pre-renal cause
   ~1.0 suggest renal cause
Urinary [Na$^+$] <20 mmol l^{-1} suggests a pre-renal cause

Concurrent administration of dopamine and diuretics may confuse the interpretation of urinary biochemistry.

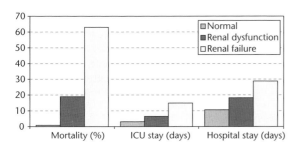

Figure 56.1 The influence of renal function on outcome from cardiac surgery. Data from the 1992–1994 Multicenter Study of Perioperative Ischaemia (McSPI) study – *Ann Intern Med* 1998; **128**: 194–203. Renal dysfunction defined as creatinine >2 mg dl^{-1} (>177 μmol l^{-1}) or rise in creatinine >0.7 mg dl^{-1} (>62 μmol l^{-1}). Renal failure defined as requirement for dialysis.

In clinical practice, renal function is typically assessed using hourly urine output and serum urea and creatinine concentrations. Unfortunately a seemingly adequate urine output (i.e. >0.5 ml kg^{-1}h^{-1}) and normal biochemical indices do not preclude renal dysfunction. Serum creatinine levels tend to remain normal until over 50% of renal tubular function is lost, and doubles with every subsequent halving of function (Table 56.1).

The risk factors for renal dysfunction and renal failure during cardiac surgery is pointed in Table 56.2.

Pathophysiology

Renal blood flow (RBF) accounts for ≈20% of CO. A RBF of *one litre* per minute typically generates *one millilitre* of urine per minute. Renal oxygen delivery is huge (>80 ml 100 g^{-1} min^{-1}) and overall oxygen extraction is low (~10%). Paradoxically, the proximal tubules and medullary loops of Henle function in a hypoxic milieu and have little physiological reserve. The combination of the glomerular portal circulation and a vascular counter-current reduces the PaO$_2$ of blood entering the medulla to 1–2 kPa (Figure 56.2).

Protective control mechanisms

Renal arterial pressure is the major determinant of renal perfusion. In the normotensive patient, RBF is independent of perfusion pressure when MAP is between 90 and 200 mmHg. At MAP < 80 mmHg global RBF and glomerular filtration rate (GFR)

Table 56.2 Risk factors for renal dysfunction and renal failure following cardiac surgery

Patient factors
Increasing age*
Diabetes*
Arterial hypertension/aortic atheroma
Preoperative MI/low CO states*
Preoperative creatinine >130 μmol l^{-1} (>1.4 mg dl^{-1})*
Renal tract obstruction/↑ intra-abdominal pressure
Bladder outflow obstruction

Operative factors
Redo/emergency procedures
Valve/combined surgical procedures
Hyperglycaemia*
Haemorrhage
Infection/sepsis

Pharmacological
Contrast media
Loop diuretics
NSAIDs
Antimicrobials (aminoglycosides, amphotericin)
Ciclosporin

Post-renal causes of renal dysfunction should be excluded before attempting to differentiate between pre-renal and renal aetiologies. *Independent risk factors identified by the Multicenter Study of Perioperative Ischaemia study.

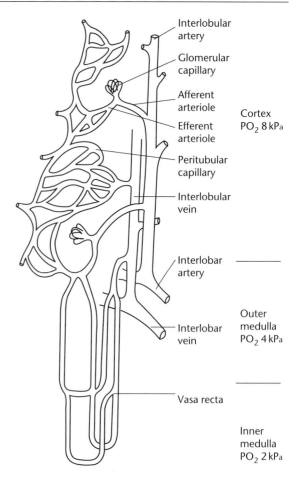

Figure 56.2 Typical partial pressures of oxygen in renal arteriolar blood. Juxtamedullary and intramedullary nephrons are particularly vulnerable to conditions that reduce oxygen delivery.

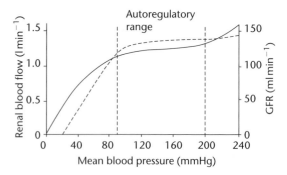

Figure 56.3 Autoregulation of RBF (solid line) and the impact of MAP on GFR (dotted line).

decline. In chronic hypertensives, the autoregulatory curve is shifted to the right (Figure 56.3).

As medullary oxygen delivery falls several protective mechanisms are activated resulting in preservation of outer medullary blood supply at the expense of cortical blood flow and optimization of urinary concentration. The efficiency of these protective mechanisms explains why the normal kidney is better able to tolerate single or short-lived insults (Table 56.3).

Cardiac surgery

During cardiac surgery there is a significant increase in the plasma concentrations of both pro- and anti-inflammatory cytokines. This increase appears to be a response to surgery itself rather than CPB. Nevertheless, the demonstration that experimental CPB can simulate an increase in plasma interleukin 8 (IL-8) and neutrophil adhesiveness, suggests that the interaction between blood and components of the extracorporeal circuit contributes to the perioperative inflammatory response.

Recent evidence suggests that pro-inflammatory cytokines, such as tumour necrosis factor alpha (TNF-α) may cause damage to proximal tubular cell cultures, whereas anti-inflammatory cytokines, such as IL-10 may be renoprotective. These findings suggest that

the balance of cytokines may be an important determinant of renal function. Further support for this hypothesis comes from the demonstration of a correlation between the plasma increases in plasma

Table 56.3 Endogenous renal protective mechanisms

Mechanism	Site/response
Myogenic responses	Stretch-induced Ca^{2+} release. GFR maintained despite falling perfusion pressures by efferent arteriolar constriction.
Glomerulotubular feedback	Macula densa and afferent arteriole (juxtaglomerular apparatus). ↑ Tubular NaCl and water delivery indicates impaired proximal Na^+ reabsorption. Angiotensin II release reduces GFR and nephron oxygen demand.
Autonomic input	Sympathetic stimulation via renal nerves stimulates release of renin, angiotensin and aldosterone. The net effects are ↑ GFR, Na^+ retention and K^+ loss.
Local action of vasodilators	Prostaglandins E_2 and I_2 (prostacyclin), adenosine and nitric oxide produce a fall in net glomerular perfusion pressure, reducing GFR and oxygen demand.

pro-inflammatory cytokines and urinary markers of sub-clinical renal injury in patients undergoing CABG surgery on CPB.

By the same token, normal renal function is required for cytokine balance. Small pro-inflammatory cytokine (e.g. monomeric TNF, IL-1 and IL-8) molecules <20 kD are readily filtered at the glomerulus. In contrast, larger anti-inflammatory cytokines (e.g. IL-10, IL-1ra, TNF-soluble receptors) are less readily filtered. Consequently, the kidneys help to remove pro-inflammatory cytokines while maintaining plasma concentrations of anti-inflammatory cytokines. Although, by inference, glomerular filtrate contains a high concentration of potentially harmful pro-inflammatory cytokine, the normal kidney appears to have mechanisms to ensure their safe disposal. In addition to any direct toxic effect, pro-inflammatory cytokines (e.g. IL-8) may increase neutrophil adhesion causing inflammatory infiltration of small renal vessels. The low incidence of significant renal injury following cardiac surgery is a testament to the powerful intra-renal mechanisms that control the potentially deleterious effects of the pro-inflammatory response. When these mechanisms become overwhelmed (e.g. prolonged CPB, sepsis, etc.) the kidneys are often the first organs to fail.

Prevention of renal dysfunction

It would seem logical that interventions designed to restore and maintain medullary oxygenation should prevent, or at least ameliorate, renal dysfunction after cardiac surgery. Unfortunately, no therapeutic strategy has been shown to be of proven benefit – indicative of the multi-factorial aetiology of renal failure.

In addition to avoiding known nephrotoxic insults, particularly in high-risk patients, a number of (still) controversial strategies can be considered. See Table 56.4.

Table 56.4 Renal protection strategies

Fluid and salt loading
Manipulation of perfusion pressure
Mannitol and loop diuretics
Dopamine and dopamine analogues
Anti-inflammatory strategies

Fluid therapy

The early restoration of renal perfusion in pure pre-renal failure should restore renal function. The maintenance of preload, CO and vital organ perfusion is a fundamental goal of cardiac anaesthesia. The correction of hypovolaemia is key to the prevention and progression of ARF in critically ill patients and should be undertaken *before* instituting any pharmacological intervention.

Perfusion pressure

Renal perfusion pressure is the difference between MAP and IVC pressure. The use of vasopressors such as norepinephrine to increase MAP is controversial. Although norepinephrine undoubtedly raises MAP, a simultaneous increase in renal vascular resistance may actually reduce RBF. While norepinephrine may improve RBF, this is not always translated into an improvement in renal function.

Loop diuretics and mannitol

The use of loop diuretics is driven by the desire to convert oliguric renal failure into non-oliguric renal failure, on the grounds that the latter has a better prognosis. The risks of diuretic therapy include dehydration and direct nephrotoxicity. The logic underlying this approach is that loop diuretics disable the energy-dependent (i.e. Na^+:K^+:Cl^- co-transport) tubular mechanisms that permit urine concentration and reduce renal oxygen demand. Without adequate fluid resuscitation, loop diuretics are ineffective in the prevention of ARF and may worsen tubular function.

Mannitol is an osmotic agent that is freely filterable at the glomerulus and not reabsorbed by the renal tubules. Mannitol has a high diuretic potential and can markedly increase fluid flow rate in all nephron segments, including the proximal tubule. When administered early in the course of ARF, mannitol may flush out cellular debris and prevent tubular cast formation, which in turn may convert oliguric ARF into non-oliguric ARF. Conversion to non-oliguric ARF facilitates the management of fluid and electrolyte imbalance, drug therapy and nutritional needs of the patient. Whether this reduces the requirement for subsequent haemodialysis (HD) or haemofiltration (HF), is uncertain. Combining mannitol with a loop diuretic prevents compensatory increases in ion reabsorption in the loop of Henle. Mannitol is contraindicated in anuric patients.

Dopamine and dopamine analogues

Low-dose infusions of dopamine ($<3\,\mu g\,kg^{-1}\,min^{-1}$) increase CO and RBF. Renal vasodilatation and the inhibition of tubular Na^+–K^+-ATPase result in increased GFR, urine volume and Na^+ excretion in healthy subjects. This diuretic effect has lead to the widespread use of low-dose dopamine to prevent and treat ARF. In the setting of the general ICU, low-dose dopamine had no impact on peak serum creatinine, the requirement for RRT, length of ICU stay or mortality. The authors of a meta-analysis, published in 2001, concluded, *'low-dose dopamine ... should be eliminated from routine ... use'*.

Fenoldopam, a selective dopamine (D_1) agonist is currently under investigation. A small observational study in cardiac surgical patients suggests that low-dose fenoldopam ($0.03\,\mu g\,kg^{-1}\,min^{-1}$ from induction of anaesthesia) may preserve renal function in patients at increased risk of renal dysfunction. Prospective studies are required to validate this finding.

Dopexamine, a potent β_2-adrenergic and dopaminergic agonist, lacks the α-adrenergic effects of dopamine. Any improvement in RBF and GFR is more likely to be the result of increased CO and decreased SVR rather than any direct intrarenal dopaminergic effect. In cardiac surgical practice, dopexamine may cause undesirable hypotension and tachycardia.

Anti-inflammatory strategies

Evidence from animal CPB studies, suggests that methylprednisolone may alter the balance of pro- and anti-inflammatory cytokines (i.e. increased IL-10, decreased IL-8) and reduce sub-clinical renal dysfunction after surgery. Large-scale human studies are awaited.

Pre-existing renal impairment

Pre-existing renal failure significantly increases operative risk – dialysis-dependent renal failure adds 10 points to the Parsonnet score, and a serum creatinine concentration $>200\,\mu mol\,l^{-1}$ adds two points to the EuroSCORE.

A number of issues are of importance to the anaesthetist. It is essential that preoperative RRT does not remove excessive solute and render the patient hypovolaemic. For this reason, haemodialysis is usually discontinued and hypertonic peritoneal dialysis fluids avoided in the 12 h before surgery. Unless the patient is truly anuric, a urethral catheter should be inserted.

The presence of a forearm arteriovenous fistula created for dialysis, interferes with pulse oximetry and reduces the number of sites available for arterial and peripheral venous access. In addition, a fistula may represent a significant shunt, which may be worsened following the administration of vasoconstrictors. Occasionally a large fistula must be excluded from the circulation by ligation or application of proximal tourniquet.

Intraoperative 'neutral balance' HF during CPB may delay the requirement for the reinstitution of RRT in the early postoperative period when anticoagulation may be undesirable. Although peritoneal dialysis avoids many of the potential complications of HF, diaphragmatic splinting may lead to respiratory impairment.

Uraemia-induced platelet dysfunction may lead to excessive perioperative bleeding. Platelet transfusion and desmopressin (1-desamino-8-D-arginine vasopressin; DDAVP) may be of use in this group of patients.

Management of acute renal dysfunction

The treatment of patients with renal dysfunction and renal failure after cardiac surgery is largely supportive. In most centres management is expectant unless there is an indication for intervention or RRT. General measures include those given in Table 56.5.

Table 56.5 Management of renal dysfunction and renal failure after cardiac surgery

Exclude post-renal/obstructive aetiology
Optimize circulation and renal perfusion pressure
Restrict fluid and K^+ intake
Discontinue nephrotoxic drugs
Reduce doses of drugs that accumulate in renal failure
Consider proton pump inhibitor for GI prophylaxis
Exclude and aggressively treat any infection
Treat life-threatening hyperkalaemia, acidosis and dysrhythmias
Slowly correct metabolic acidosis with isotonic bicarbonate
Consider early renal specialist advice.

Key points

- Normal plasma concentrations of creatinine and urea may conceal significantly reduced creatinine clearance.
- Prevention is better than cure. Simple clinical measures – volume resuscitation, and maintenance of adequate CO and perfusion pressure, are essential.
- Any diuresis following loop diuretics and/or dopamine may give false reassurance.
- The benefits of perioperative pharmacological reno-protection and inflammatory response modification remain unproven.

RRT can be considered in three broad categories: peritoneal dialysis, intermittent haemodialysis and continuous venovenous haemofiltration (CVVHF). Most adult patients developing renal failure after cardiac surgery are initially supported with CVVHF, whereas patients with pre-existing renal failure on established peritoneal dialysis may have this therapy reinstituted. Continuous haemodiafiltration, which achieves a greater urea clearance, may be considered in patients who do not respond to simple HF. CVVHF requires insertion of a large-bore, double-lumen cannula specifically designed for CVVHF in a subclavian, internal jugular or femoral vein, and a degree of systemic anticoagulation. A continuous infusion of unfractionated heparin is used to maintain an ACT >200 s. Numerous conditions contribute to the development of thrombocytopaenia during CVVHF. The use of an alternative anticoagulant (e.g. danaparoid) should only be considered if heparin-induced thrombocytopaenia is suspected (Table 56.6).

Further reading

Bellomo R, Chapman M, Finfer S, Hickling K, Myburgh J. Low-dose dopamine in patients with early renal dysfunction: a placebo-controlled randomised trial. Australian and New Zealand Intensive Care Society (ANZICS) Clinical Trials Group. *Lancet* 2000; **356(9248)**: 2139–2143.

Chertow GM, Lazarus JM, Christiansen CL, Cook EF, Hammermeister KE, Grover F *et al.* Preoperative renal risk stratification. *Circulation* 1997; **95(4)**: 878–884.

Garwood S, Swamidoss CP, Davis EA, Samson L, Hines RL. A case series of low-dose fenoldopam in seventy cardiac surgical patients at increased risk of renal dysfunction. *J Cardiothorac Vasc Anesth* 2003; **17(1)**: 17–21.

Kellum JA, M Decker J. Use of dopamine in acute renal failure: a meta-analysis. *Crit Care Med* 2001; **29(8)**:1526–1531.

Mangano CM, Diamondstone LS, Ramsay JG, Aggarwal A, Herskowitz A, Mangano DT. Renal dysfunction after myocardial revascularization: risk factors, adverse outcomes, and hospital resource utilization. The Multicenter Study of Perioperative Ischemia Research Group. *Ann Intern Med* 1998; **128(3)**: 194–203.

Table 56.6 Indications for RRT

Hyperkalaemia
Severe metabolic acidosis
Fluid overload
Severe uraemia – encephalopathy, neuropathy or pericarditis
To facilitate enteral/parenteral feeding
To facilitate blood/blood product administration
Severe hyponatraemia or hypernatraemia
Hyperthermia.

NEUROLOGICAL COMPLICATIONS OF CARDIAC SURGERY

57

J.E. Arrowsmith

Neurological injury following cardiac surgery increases length of ICU and hospital stay, and reduces the likelihood of a return to independent living. Cardiac surgical patients are largely ignorant of this complication.

Clinical spectrum

Brain injury following cardiac surgery ranges in severity from subtle changes in personality, behaviour and cognitive function to fatal brain injury – the 'cerebral catastrophe' (Table 57.1). In most cases, a neurological injury becomes evident as soon as the patient emerges from anaesthesia. In a small number of patients however, significant injury may develop following a 'lucid interval' lasting several hours to several days after surgery.

Pathophysiology

The wide variety of adverse neurological outcomes almost certainly results from a number of distinct pathophysiological processes:

- *Focal* Stroke, reversible ischaemic neurological deficit (RIND) or TIA.
- *Global* Cardiac arrest, prolonged circulatory arrest, profound and prolonged cerebral hypoperfusion, or hypoglycaemia.
- *Diffuse-microfocal* Widespread cerebral microembolism.

Although the mechanisms are imprecisely defined, the so-called 'ischaemic cascade' appears to be the

Table 57.1 Types and initial incidences of neurological complications after cardiac surgery

Complication	Incidence (%)
Fatal brain injury	0.3
Non-fatal diffuse encephalopathy	
Depressed conscious level	3
Behavioural changes	1
Intellectual/cognitive dysfunction	30–79
Seizures	
Choreoathetosis	0.3
Ophthalmological	
Visual field defects	25
Reduced visual acuity	4.5
Focal brain injury (stroke)	2–5
Primitive reflexes	39
Spinal cord injury	0–0.1
Peripheral nerve injury	
Brachial plexopathy	7
Other peripheral neuropathy	6

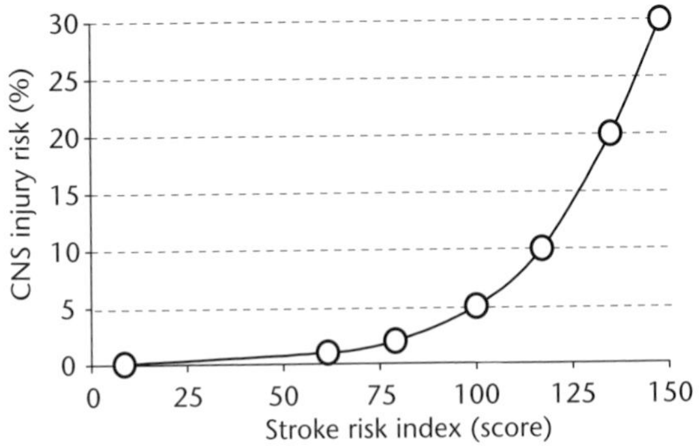

Risk factor	Score
Age	(Age − 25) × 1.43
Unstable angina	14
Diabetes mellitus	17
Neurological disease	18
Prior CABG	15
Vascular disease	18
Pulmonary disease	15

Figure 57.1 Preoperative stroke risk index for patients undergoing CABG (Arrowsmith *et al.*, 2000 adapted from Newman *et al.*, 1996).

final common pathway. The process can be considered in three stages, namely induction, amplification and expression as follows:

- *Induction* Cellular energy failure and receptor-operated ion channel activation leads to an influx of water, Na^+ and Ca^{2+} that cannot be balanced by extrusion and sequestration mechanisms.
- *Amplification* The rise in free cytosolic Ca^{2+} leads to activation of phospholipases and protein kinases, and a cascade of reactions that liberate species with lipolytic, chemotactic, vasoactive and other properties.
- *Expression* Worsening acidosis further inhibits recovery mechanisms. Expression of arachidonic acid metabolites and free radicals results in loss of membrane integrity and irreversible damage to the cytoskeleton. In hypoxia that is not immediately lethal, the rise in intracellular Ca^{2+} may induce certain genes and the expression of neurotrophic and growth factors.

Quantification

The incidence of stroke and cognitive dysfunction are the most commonly used measures of neurological injury after cardiac surgery. Cognitive assessment is labour-intensive and time consuming. Investigational testing schedules are a compromise – short enough to ensure compliance, yet sufficient to assess a meaningful range of cognitive domains.

Biochemical markers of neuronal injury (e.g. astroglial protein S100β and neurone-specific enolase) offer the opportunity to quantify neurological injury without resorting to laborious and expensive clinical testing.

Unfortunately, the magnitude of marker release gives no indication of the anatomical distribution and likely clinical impact. Furthermore, S100β has been an inconsistent measure of neuronal injury in the setting of CPB.

Risk factors

Patient factors, intraoperative factors and post-operative factors all contribute to the risk of perioperative neurological injury (Table 57.2).

A multicentre study of over 2000 patients undergoing CABG identified 13 independent predictors of adverse neurological outcome (Table 57.3). The overall incidence of neurological injury was 6.1%. The incidences of type I (focal) and type II (diffuse) outcomes were 3.1% and 3.0%, respectively.

Using the data obtained in this study, the Duke University group developed a model to predict the likelihood of neurological injury after CABG. Using preoperative patient risk factors, the so-called *stroke index* allows rapid risk assessment (Figure 57.1).

The risk of stroke following combined procedures, such as CABG and MV surgery, has been shown to be 4–6 times greater than that following isolated coronary, aortic or mitral surgery.

Age

Age is probably the most robust predictor of morbidity and mortality after cardiac surgery. The proportion of elderly patients presenting for cardiac surgery is steadily increasing.

Table 57.2 Putative risk factors for adverse neurological outcome after cardiac surgery

Preoperative (patient) factors		Intraoperative factors	Postoperative factors
Demographic	Medical history		
Age	Stroke/TIA	Surgery type	Early hypotension
Gender	Diabetes mellitus	Aortic atheroma	Long ICU stay
Genotype	Cardiac function	Aortic clamp site	Renal dysfunction
Educational level	IABP use	Microemboli	Atrial fibrillation
	Alcohol consumption	Arterial pressure	
	Pulmonary disease	Pump flow	
	Hypertension	Temperature	
	Dysrhythmia	Haematocrit	
	Dyslipidaemia	Use of DHCA	
	Diuretic use		

DHCA, deep hypothermic circulatory arrest; TIA, transient ischaemic attack.

Gender

Women are at greater risk of death and complications following cardiac surgery. Higher-risk profiles, rather than increased gender susceptibility, is the likely cause.

Diabetes mellitus

Diabetes is an independent risk factor for neurological injury following cardiac surgery. Although hyperglycaemia is known to worsen outcome from stroke, the greater incidence of hypertension, vascular disease and renal impairment in diabetics, may partly explain this phenomenon.

Cerebrovascular disease

Patients with a history of symptomatic cerebrovascular disease (CVD) are more likely to sustain neurological injury. In patients with a history of stroke, the risk does not appear to decline over time. Patients undergoing cardiac surgery within 3 months of a focal event are more likely to extend the area of injury whereas patients with a remote stroke (i.e. >6 months) are more likely to have a stroke in a different vascular territory.

Aortic atheromatous disease

The prevalence and severity of aortic atheroma increases with age. There is a strong association between proximal aortic atheroma and stroke following cardiac surgery. Surgical manipulation, cannulation and perfusion of the diseased aorta can liberate atheroemboli. Although TOE assessment of the proximal aorta is superior to digital palpation, the cannulation site is not usually visible. Epiaortic ultrasound represents the gold standard. It is not clear if a change in surgical procedure, prompted by the detection of proximal aortic atheroma, improves neurological outcome.

Genetic predisposition

Apolipoprotein E (APOE) genotype is a risk factor for late-onset and sporadic forms of Alzheimer's disease and as a predictor of adverse outcome following head trauma and subarachnoid haemorrhage. The putative association between APOE-ε4 and worse neuro-psychological outcome after cardiac surgery has not been confirmed. Reduced expression of interleukin-1β receptor antagonist (IL-1ra) during CPB in patients with APOE-ε4 suggests that APOE may play a significant role in modulating the systemic and CNS inflammatory response.

Operative procedure

The risk of neurological injury is, in part, dependent on the type of surgery performed. Intracardiac and major vascular procedures carry the greatest risk, particularly when deep hypothermic circulatory arrest (DHCA), is employed.

Cerebral microemboli, which can be detected (using carotid or transcranial Doppler (TCD) sonography)

Table 57.3 Adjusted odds ratios (95% confidence intervals) for type I (non-fatal stroke, TIA, stupor or coma at discharge, or death caused by stroke or hypoxic encephalopathy) and type II (new deterioration in intellectual function, confusion, agitation, disorientation, memory deficit or seizure without evidence of focal injury) adverse cerebral outcomes after CABG associated with independent risk factors

Risk factors	Type I outcomes	Type II outcomes
Proximal aortic atherosclerosis	4.52 (2.52–8.09)	
History of neurological disease	3.19 (1.65–6.15)	
Use of IABP	2.60 (1.21–5.58)	
Diabetes mellitus	2.59 (1.46–4.60)	
History of hypertension	2.31 (1.20–4.47)	
History of pulmonary disease	2.09 (1.14–3.85)	2.37 (1.34–4.18)
History of unstable angina	1.83 (1.03–3.27)	
Age (per additional decade)	1.75 (1.27–2.43)	2.20 (1.60–3.02)
Admission systolic BP > 180 mmHg		3.47 (1.41–8.55)
History of excessive alcohol intake		2.64 (1.27–5.47)
History of CABG		2.18 (1.14–4.17)
Dysrhythmia on day of surgery		1.97 (1.12–3.46)
Antihypertensive therapy		1.78 (1.02–3.10)

From Roach et al. (1996).

in *all* patients subjected to CPB, have long been considered a significant cause of neurological injury. There is an association between neuropsychological decline and intraoperative cerebral microembolic load. Air may reach the systemic circulation from the bypass circuit and as an unavoidable consequence of intracardiac procedures. Biological particles arise from components of the circulation and the operative site. Non-biological particles arise from the extracorporeal circuit, the cardiotomy reservoir, and from foreign material introduced into the operative site.

Cardiopulmonary bypass

Despite considerable research, the characteristics of 'optimal' CPB perfusion remain to be defined. Profound hypotension combined with prolonged cerebral hypoperfusion is clearly injurious to the brain, particularly the watershed zones. Within the bounds of usual CPB conduct however, pressure, flow rate and flow character appear to have little influence neurological outcome.

Haematocrit

A desire to reduce the use of homologous blood products has resulted in the tolerance of a lower haemocrit during cardiac surgery. In theory reduced oxygen carrying capacity may expose the brain to hypoxia, particularly during rewarming and/or in the presence of significant CVD.

Temperature

Despite considerable research, the cardiovascular benefits and neurological safety of so-called 'normothermic' CPB have yet to be conclusively determined. Methodological shortcomings make it difficult to compare the conflicting conclusions of large studies conducted in this area. Any putative neuroprotection provided by hypothermia has to be weighed against its adverse effects on haemostasis and the requirement for rewarming. Current temperature monitoring methods (i.e. nasopharyngeal and bladder) may grossly underestimate brain temperature during rewarming. Rapid and/or excessive rewarming may cause cerebral metabolism to outstrip substrate delivery and exacerbate excitotoxic neuronal injury. Carefully conducted *and* monitored normothermic CPB reduces the margin for surgical error and probably has little adverse influence on the brain.

Acid–base management strategy

The influence of pH management strategy during hypothermic CPB has been examined in a number of studies. When compared to the pH-stat strategy, the use of the alpha-stat strategy is associated with superior neuropsychological outcome. In patients under-going DHCA, however, the use of the pH-stat strategy during cooling appears to improve neurological outcome.

Dysrhythmia

Postoperative AF is associated with an increased risk of both stroke and cognitive dysfunction.

Improving neurological outcome

With the possible exception of arterial-line filtration, there is a distinct lack of prospective, randomized, controlled studies demonstrating any benefit from physical interventions designed to reduce neurological injury. Potentially neuroprotective strategies include:

- Procedure modification
  - Avoidance of CPB
  - Cancellation of the planned procedure
- Technique modification
  - Single AXC technique for CABG
  - Graft 'top-ends' fashioned before removal of AXC
- Novel techniques/equipment
  - Aortic cannulation 'nets'
  - Proximal aortic anastomotic devices
- Avoidance of known causes of neurological injury
  - Avoidance of prolonged/profound hypotension
  - Avoiding cerebral hyperthermia during rewarming.

Off-pump surgery

Considerable anecdotal evidence suggests that off-pump coronary artery bypass (OPCAB) is associated with fewer cerebral microemboli, reduced S100β release and improved neuropsychological test performance. It is suggested that the greatest benefit of OPCAB will be accrued when all surgical manipulation of the proximal aorta is avoided.

Neuromonitoring

Advanced neurological monitoring remains in the hands of enthusiasts. Neurological monitors may be able to predict clinical outcome and interventional strategies based on multi-modal monitoring may improve outcome (see Chapter 26).

Pharmacological neuroprotection

While each step in the 'ischaemic cascade' offers a potential target for pharmacological intervention,

Table 57.4 Summary of significant studies of putative neuroprotective drugs in cardiac surgery

No.	Drug	Reference	Rx	Ctrl	Result
1	Thiopental	*Anesth Analg* 1982; **61**: 903	110	94	−
2	Thiopental	*Anesthesiol* 1986; **64**: 165	89	93	+ ??
3	Thiopental	*Anesthesiol* 1991; **74**: 406	149	151	−
4	Thiopental	*Can J Anaesth* 1996; **43**: 575	80	174	−
5	Prostacyclin	*J Thorac Cardiovasc Surg* 1987; **93**: 609	50	50	−
6	Nimodipine	*Br J Anaesth* 1990; **65**: 514	18	17	+/−
7	GM1	*Stroke* 1996; **27**: 858	18	11	−
8	Dextromethorphan	*Neuropediatrics* 1997; **28**: 191	6	7	+/−
9	Remacemide	*Stroke* 1998; **29**: 2357	87	84	+
10	Lidocaine	*Ann Thorac Surg* 1999; **67**: 1117	28	27	+
11	Propofol	*Anesthesiol* 1999; **90**: 1255	109		−
12	Chlormethiazole	*Anesthesiol* 2002; **97**: 585	110	109	−

Rx, number in treatment group; Ctrl, number in control group; Results, (−) negative, (+) positive, (+ ??) positive – result challenged, (+/−) equivocal.

it is unlikely that a single drug will prevent brain damage. Nevertheless, considerable effort has been expended in the search for neuroprotective drugs. Studies in cardiac surgery have largely been disappointing (Table 57.4). No drug is currently licensed for the prevention or treatment of neurological injury associated with cardiac surgery.

Key points

- Minor neurological complications are common and often go undiagnosed.
- Neurological complications increase mortality and length of hospital stay.
- Physical interventions, such as arterial-line filtration, cautious rewarming and alpha-stat blood-gas management appear to improve neurological outcome.
- Procedure modification and the use of novel devices and techniques may reduce neurological injury.
- No drug is yet licensed specifically for neuroprotection during cardiac surgery.

Further reading

Arrowsmith JE, Grocott HP, Reves JG, Newman MF. Central nervous system complications of cardiac surgery. *Br J Anaesth* 2000; **84(3)**: 378–393.

Newman MF, Kirchner JL, Phillips-Bute B, Gaver V, Grocott H, Jones RH *et al.* Longitudinal assessment of neurocognitive function after coronary-artery bypass surgery. *N Engl J Med* 2001; **344(6)**: 395–402.

Roach GW, Kanchuger M, Mangano CM, Newman M, Nussmeier N, Wolman R *et al.* Adverse cerebral outcomes after coronary bypass surgery. Multicenter Study of Perioperative Ischemia Research Group and the Ischemia Research and Education Foundation Investigators. *N Engl J Med* 1996; **335(25)**: 1857–1863.

Selnes OA, Goldsborough MA, Borowicz LM Jr., Enger C, Quaskey SA, McKhann GM. Determinants of cognitive change after coronary artery bypass surgery: a multifactorial problem. *Ann Thorac Surg* 1999; **67(6)**: 1669–1676.

van Dijk D, Keizer AM, Diephuis JC, Durand C, Vos LJ, Hijman R. Neurocognitive dysfunction after coronary artery bypass surgery: a systematic review. *J Thorac Cardiovasc Surg* 2000; **120(4)**: 632–639.

MISCELLANEOUS TOPICS

M. Barnard

There are currently approximately 150,000 adults with congenital heart disease in the UK. Over the next decade it is expected that this number will rise by a quarter, and that the number of patients with complex lesions will rise by a half. Although the majority of patients will have undergone previous cardiothoracic surgery, some will have had no intervention or have undiagnosed lesions. Completely normal cardiovascular anatomy and physiology is rarely achieved by corrective surgery during childhood. Problems encountered in patients with grown-up congenital heart (GUCH) disease are listed in Table 58.1.

Table 58.1 Medical problems in GUCH disease

Primary	Secondary
Shunts	Dysrhythmias
Stenotic lesions	Cyanosis
Regurgitant lesions	Infective endocarditis
	Myocardial ischaemia
	Paradoxical emboli
	Polycythaemia
	Pulmonary hypertension
	Ventricular dysfunction

Pathophysiology

Cardiovascular impairment may be due to hypoxaemia, pulmonary vascular disease, myocardial dysfunction or dysrhythmia. Hypoxaemia is associated with either diminished pulmonary blood flow (PBF) and right to left (R–L) shunt, or normal PBF and mixing of pulmonary and systemic venous blood. Polycythaemia is the major adaptive response to hypoxaemia, with blood viscosity increasing exponentially with haematocrit. In addition, microcytosis, secondary to iron deficiency, results in very rigid erythrocytes, which significantly increase viscosity.

When PBF is normal or elevated with venous mixing, SaO_2 is related to the pulmonary:systemic flow ratio ($Q_P:Q_S$). Elevated PBF may excessively increase cardiac work or decrease systemic perfusion although SaO_2 will be higher. In the presence of a systemic to pulmonary (e.g. modified Blalock-Taussig, B-T) shunt PBF is dependent on the size of the shunt, systolic arterial pressure and PVR. Elevated PBF decreases pulmonary compliance, increases airway resistance and work of breathing, and can lead to a maldevelopment of the pulmonary vasculature with characteristic histological features. The estimation of $Q_P:Q_S$ ratio:

$$\frac{Q_P}{Q_S} = \frac{SaO_2 - SsvO_2}{SpvO_2 - SpaO_2}$$

where SaO_2 is the arterial saturation; $SsvO_2$, systemic venous saturation; $SpvO_2$, pulmonary venous saturation and $SpaO_2$, PA saturation. Note that $SpaO_2$ is equal to SaO_2 in patients with PBF supplied through a B–T shunt.

Both systolic and diastolic ventricular dysfunction and abnormalities of ventricular interaction are common. Causes of ventricular impairment include late or inadequate surgical repair, poor intraoperative myocardial protection, pulmonary hypertension and chronic pressure or volume overload. RV dysfunction is seen more commonly than in patients with acquired heart disease. Simple indices of ventricular function (e.g. LV ejection fraction) are often rendered inadequate by complex anatomy and loading conditions. Hypertrophy results in reduced ventricular compliance. Loss of sinus rhythm and dysrhythmias are poorly tolerated.

Chronic cyanosis or hypoxaemia imply the possibility of aorto-pulmonary collateral arteries, haematological abnormalities, renal impairment and myocardial scarring. Collateral arteries may be acquired (e.g. bronchial) or congenital (e.g. complex pulmonary atresia).

Risk assessment

Resternotomy carries a significant risk in patients who have undergone previous surgery for congenital heart disease. This is particularly the case for replacement of retrosternal right heart conduits, when careful assessment of the retrosternal space to determine conduit position is essential. This may be best performed with MRI although a lateral CXR will demonstrate a calcified conduit in many patients.

Higher operative risk is associated with chronic hypox-aemia, $Q_P:Q_S > 2:1$, ventricular outflow tract (VOT) gradient >50 mmHg, elevated PVR, polycythaemia, recent heart failure, syncope or substantial exercise intolerance. With the exception of previous, complete ASD, VSD and patent ductus arteriosus (PDA) clos-ure, infective endocarditis is a risk in most corrected and uncorrected lesions. Conditions that warrant referral to a specialist centre are listed in Table 58.2.

Table 58.2 Abnormalities best treated in specialist congenital heart unit

Valvular atresia
Double inlet/outlet ventricle
Malposition of great arteries
Fontan circulation
Single/common ventricles
Transposition of great arteries
Atrial switch procedure
Rastelli procedure
Eisenmenger reaction
Pulmonary hypertension
Chronic hypoxaemia
$Q_P:Q_S > 2:1$
Ventricular outflow gradient >50 mmHg
↑ PVR
Secondary polycythaemia

Eight questions to consider during preoperative assess-ment are listed in Table 58.3. Whenever possible, records of previous surgical procedures, anaesthesia and investigations should be scrutinized. Echocardiography should be performed in addition to routine investiga-tions (i.e. haematocrit, coagulation studies). Lung func-tion testing should be undertaken in dyspnoeic or scoliotic patients.

Table 58.3 Preoperative assessment of patients with congenital heart disease

What is the anatomy of any previous repair?
Are there any residual structural defects?
Is ventricular function normal?
Are there anatomical or physiological abnormalities of the pulmonary vasculature?
Normal venous anatomy: connections, drainage and monitoring sites?
Are there residual ECG abnormalities?
What antibiotic prophylaxis is necessary?
Is anticoagulation therapy employed and when should it be withdrawn/re-instituted?

Common sequelae of individual lesions are listed in Table 58.4. Previous surgery may have resulted in

recurrent laryngeal or phrenic nerve injury, or Horner's syndrome.

The presence of large collateral arteries (e.g. bronchial) may induce systemic steal (L-L shunt) and ventricu-lar distension during CPB. Selective angiography may be used to assess their anatomy and permits embolization prior to surgery. Although visualization may be difficult, they can be controlled or ligated before instituting CPB. Alternatively, hypothermic arrest or low flow CPB with ventricular venting may be used.

Anaesthetic management

As polycythaemic patients are at risk from dehydration, IV fluids are commenced the night before surgery. Preoperative venesection is performed for very high haematocrits, although usually only when symptomatic hyperviscosity is present. In the presence of dimin-ished PBF, hypoxaemia should be minimized by ensur-ing adequate hydration, maintaining systemic arterial BP, minimizing elevations in PVR and avoiding increases in VO_2. Cardiac medications are typically continued until the time of surgery. Sedative premed-ication is popular, although caution must be exercised in the presence of hypoxaemia.

Vascular access may present difficulties. Interruption of the IVC or thrombosis following previous instru-mentation may preclude femoral vein cannulation. Placement of a PAFC may be technically difficult on account of anatomical abnormalities and might actually be dangerous in the presence of pulmonary reactivity. In the presence of a right subclavian to right PA (modified B-T) shunt, the left arm should be used for arterial pressure monitoring. Patients with cavopul-monary (e.g. Glenn and Fontan) shunts are at risk of venous thrombosis. Although PA pressure monitor-ing with a SVC line is often useful in these patients, a single-lumen line should be used and removed as early as possible to reduce the risk of thromboem-bolism. Meticulous care must be taken to avoid venous air entrainment in patients with shunt lesions as systemic embolization can occur, even when shunt-ing is predominantly L-R.

The selection of induction agent is an individual choice. The choice of drugs is less important than appropriate haemodynamic goals: maintenance of ventricular per-formance and avoidance of large alterations in $Q_P:Q_S$. When a shunt is present, blood leaving the heart may travel in one of two parallel circulations: either to the systemic circulation via the aorta or to the pulmonary circulation via the shunt. The SVR, PVR *and* the

Table 58.4 Common sequelae of surgery for congenital heart disease

ASD	Residual shunt, septal aneurysm, device fracture
Coarctation of aorta	Systolic hypertension, residual gradient, inaccurate left arm BP (subclavian flap repair), aneurysm formation, dissection
PDA	Residual flow, recanalization, laryngeal nerve injury
TGA	
Atrial switch	Dysrhythmias, systemic ventricular dysfunction, baffle leak, venous pathway obstruction
Rastelli	Residual VSD, ventricular dysfunction, LVOTO, conduit failure
Arterial switch	Supravalvar AS/PS, aortic regurgitation, ventricular dysfunction, coronary artery stenosis
Tetralogy of Fallot	Residual VSD, RVOTO, RV dysfunction, PR, RBBB/AV block, ventricular dysrhythmias. B-T shunt, BP inaccurate
Single ventricle	Preload dependence, ventricular dysfunction, cyanosis (fenestration), protein-losing enteropathy, dysrhythmias, diminished functional reserve

TGA: transposition of great arteries; RVOTO, LVOTO: RV and LV outflow tract obstruction.

resistance of the shunt determine the flow through each vascular bed. In the perioperative period the goal is to balance the circulations (i.e. $Q_P : Q_S = 1 : 1$).

IV induction may be slowed if the circulation time is prolonged. R-L shunt theoretically prolongs inhalation induction, but this is rarely of clinical importance. The presence of R-L shunt or common mixing will, however, cause end tidal CO_2 monitoring to underestimate $PaCO_2$. Although vasodilatation during induction tends to increase R-L shunt and reduce SaO_2, this is partially offset by reduced metabolic rate. Narcotic-based anaesthesia may be preferable in the presence of significant ventricular dysfunction. In the presence of maximal sympathetic stimulation ketamine may paradoxically depress cardiac function. The haemodynamic impact of dynamic LVOT obstruction may be reduced by a modest depression of ventricular function.

External defibrillator pads are placed on patients undergoing reoperations, as access for internal paddles is usually impossible during chest opening. VT and VF are common during RV dissection. The femoral vessels are usually exposed *before* resternotomy. If preoperative investigation indicates that a conduit is at risk, femoro-femoral CPB is instituted *before* sternotomy. Induction of hypothermia and circulatory arrest prior to sternotomy is occasionally necessary despite the risk of VF and ventricular distension. Ventricular decompression can be achieved by venting the left heart through the chest wall or by external cardiac massage.

Pulmonary vasodilators (e.g. nitric oxide) are required during ~5% of procedures. TOE is particularly useful in GUCH surgery to confirm preoperative findings and exclude previously undiagnosed lesions. In addition, TOE permits the assessment of ventricular performance, valvular function and blood flow velocity and is essential for confirming adequate anatomical repair.

Post-anaesthesia care

Standard management principles apply to most patients. Experience in the management of PVR, shunt lesions and VOT obstruction is required. Hypovolaemia increases R-L shunting. Cyanotic patients should have their haematocrit measured frequently.

Cardiopulmonary interaction, particularly in the setting of Fontan-like circulations, is very important. Control of ABGs (particularly $PaCO_2$) is fundamental to optimizing PBF. While low airway pressures and early weaning from ventilation are beneficial to PBF, the duration of the inspiratory phase during intermittent positive-pressure ventilation is usually more important than peak inspiratory pressure. Shortening the inspiratory time (with consequent increase in peak inspiratory pressure) may improve PBF. Since the ventilatory response to $PaCO_2$ is normal, adequate analgesia and sedation are required to prevent the patient 'fighting' with the ventilator. This is particularly important in the presence of labile PA pressures.

The hyperbolic relationship between SaO_2 and $Q_P : Q_S$ and the parabolic relationship between $SsvO_2$ and $Q_P : Q_S$ are not often appreciated (Figure 58.1). As a consequence an inappropriately high SaO_2 in a mixing-type circulation may be associated with a very low $SsvO_2$ and should arouse concern. If PBF is too high, SaO_2 will be high and systemic perfusion inadequate leading to hypotension, oliguria, acidosis and increased serum lactate. Treatment is aimed at improving overall CO, reducing PBF by pulmonary vasoconstriction and

Table 58.5 Interpretation of SaO_2 in the presence of different physiological states in patients with shunt

SaO_2	Physiological status	Consequences	$Q_P : Q_S$	Treatment
75%	Balanced Q_P and Q_S	None	~1:1	None
	↓ CO	↑ O_2 extraction, ↓ SvO_2	>1:1	↑ CO, ↑ PVR, ↓ SVR
	Lung disease	↓ $SpvO_2$	>1:1	Optimize ventilation, ↑ PVR, ↓ SVR
>85%	Shunt too big	↑ PBF	>1:1	↑ PVR, revise shunt
<65%	Shunt too small or blocked	↓ PBF	<1:1	Revise shunt
	↑ PVR	↓ PBF	<1:1	↓ PVR, ↑ MAP
	↓ CO	↑ O_2 extraction, ↓ SvO_2	~1:1	↑ CO
	Lung disease	↓ $SpvO_2$	~1:1	Optimize ventilation

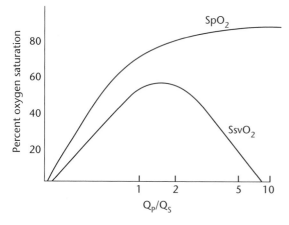

Figure 58.1 Graphical representation of SaO_2 and systemic venous oxygen saturation ($SsvO_2$) as a function of $Q_P : Q_S$. Both curves will move up or down with changes in pulmonary venous oxygen saturation. It is often assumed that $SaO_2 \sim 75\%$ equates to the ideal $Q_P : Q_S$ of ~1:1. This will be the case if there is good systemic perfusion (oxygen extraction resulting in $SvO_2 \sim 50\%$) and normal lung function. It can be misleading to infer $Q_P : Q_S$ from SaO_2 alone as SaO_2 of 75% may also represent a $Q_P : Q_S \gg 1$ in certain situations.

increasing systemic flow by peripheral vasodilatation. In contrast, a low SaO_2 may be due to an undersized shunt, increased PVR, reduced CO or lung disease (Table 58.5).

Key points

- Adults with congenital heart disease present a spectrum ranging from well patients with corrected minor defects to those with extreme deviations from normal physiology.
- Involvement of clinicians with experience of congenital heart disease is essential.
- Thought should be given to the appropriate placement of vascular catheters and avoidance of aeroembolism.
- A detailed understanding of the factors influencing PBF is essential.
- Infective endocarditis guidelines should be followed.

Further reading

Brickner ME, Hillis LD, Lange RA. Congenital heart disease in adults. First of two parts. *N Engl J Med* 2000; **342(4)**: 256–263.

Brickner ME, Hillis LD, Lange RA. Congenital heart disease in adults. Second of two parts. *N Engl J Med* 2000; **342(5)**: 334–342.

Deanfield J, Thaulow E, Warnes C, Webb G, Kolbel F, Hoffman A *et al*. Management of grown up congenital heart disease. *Eur Heart J* 2003; **24(11)**: 1035–1084.

Findlow D, Doyle E. Congenital heart disease in adults. *Br J Anaesth* 1997; **78(4)**: 416–430.

Perloff JK, Warnes CA. Challenges posed by adults with repaired congenital heart disease. *Circulation* 2001; **103(21)**: 2637–2643.

J.E. Arrowsmith & J.H. Mackay

Cardiac disease is the leading indirect cause of maternal mortality and accounted for nearly a third of all maternal deaths in the UK between 1994 and 1996. Although, the prevalence and types of cardiac disease in pregnancy are subject to considerable geographical variation the majority are due to chronic rheumatic heart disease. The various types are:

- *Rheumatic heart disease* MS, AR.
- *Congenital heart disease* Fallot's, ASD, VSD.
- *Other valvular diseases* MV prolpase.
- *Infective endocarditis* IV drug abusers.
- *Aortic dissection* peripartum, Marfan's.
- *Dysrhythmia.*
- *Ischaemic heart disease.*
- *Other* idiopathic hypertrophic subaortic stenosis (IHSS), cardiomyopathy, transplant.

Physiology

The normal physiological changes that accompany pregnancy tend to exacerbate existing cardiovascular disorders (Table 59.1). The rate of physiological change reaches a maximum during the late second and early third trimester therefore the emergence of symptoms (e.g. angina and dyspnoea) in early pregnancy is an omin-ous sign.

The 25–40% increase in CO usually seen during labour may be further increased as a result of postpartum uterine autotransfusion. Cardiac decompensation during labour may therefore occur in patients who have otherwise tolerated pregnancy. The immediate postpartum period is a particularly critical time. A return to normal pre-conception physiology takes 8–12 weeks.

Timing of surgery

Cardiac surgery during pregnancy, whether performed with or without CPB, carries a greater risk than surgery in matched, non-pregnant patients. For this reason surgery is reserved for patients with

---

Table 59.1 Physiology of pregnancy

Circulating volume
- Blood volume ↑ 30%
- Physiological anaemia (plasma ↑ 45%/erythrocytes ↑ 20%)
- ↓↓ Colloid osmotic pressure ⇒ ↑ risk of pulmonary oedema
- Neutrophilia
- Hypercoagulable state

Cardiovascular
- ↑ Sympathetic tone ⇒ SV ↑ 30% + HR ↑ 15% ⇒ CO ↑ 50%
- ↑ Wall stress/contractility ↑ Myocardial O_2 consumption
- CVP and PAWP unchanged (PVR and SVR ↓ 20%)
- Systolic BP – unchanged
- Diastolic BP – initially falls and then returns to normal at term
- Aortocaval compression ⇒ ↓↓ CO
- Increased vascularity of airway – especially nasal passages

Respiratory
- Diaphragmatic splinting
- ↑ Minute ventilation, ↑ RR, ↑ V_T ↓ FRC
- ↓ $PaCO_2$, ↓ HCO_3^-, ↓ buffering capacity
- Total body O_2 consumption ↑ 15–20%

Gastrointestinal
- Delayed gastric emptying
- Increased risk of gastro-oesophageal reflux
- Reduced gut motility – constipation
- Mild hyperbilirubinaemia – pruritis

Genitourinary
- ↑ Renal blood flow and GFR
- Increased risk of vesico-ureteric reflux/infection
- Glycosuria (tubular transport maximum exceeded)
- Uterine enlargement

Metabolic and endocrine
- ↑↑ Prolactin, ACTH, cortisol
- ↓ Growth hormone
- ↑ Thyroid-binding globulin, T_4 and T_3 (free-T_4 near normal)
- ↑ Gastrin

ACTH, adrenocorticotrophic hormone; FRC, functional respiratory capacity; GFR, glomerular filtration rate; PAWP, pulmonary capillary wedge pressure.

life-threatening conditions when the risks to the mother have to be balanced against those to the foetus. Surgery in the first trimester carries a high risk of miscarriage and foetal abnormality. In the second trimester surgery may cause intrauterine death or premature labour. Delivery at or before 26 weeks gestation is associated with very high foetal mortality and morbidity.

In a recent study it was reported that maternal *mortality* was similar whether surgery was performed during pregnancy, immediately after delivery or in the postpartum period. Maternal *morbidity*, however, was considerably greater if surgery was delayed until after delivery. In contrast foetal outcome was improved if surgery was delayed until after delivery.

In the emergency situation, when medical therapy is unlikely to be of help, all efforts are directed to saving the mother. Management in the non-emergency situation depends on the duration of pregnancy. As 80–90% infants will survive an operative delivery at 28 weeks gestation, maximal medical therapy is instituted with the aim of prolonging pregnancy to at least this duration at which time an operative delivery followed by cardiac surgery is performed.

Anaesthetic considerations

The perioperative management of the pregnant cardiac surgical patient combines the basic principles of both obstetric and cardiac anaesthesia. Preoperative invasive monitoring and pharmacological optimization of the circulation should be considered in all cases. The likelihood of haemodynamic instability and the need for anticoagulation are contraindications to the use of neuraxial anaesthetic techniques.

There are no data to suggest that any particular anaesthetic technique or agent is superior in terms of maternal or foetal outcome. Since the risks of nitrous oxide and benzodiazepines remain undetermined, these are probably best avoided.

Tocolytic agents, such as β_2-agonists (e.g. ritodrine), may be poorly tolerated and should not be used prophylactically.

Conduct of bypass

As uteroplacental blood flow is dependent on perfusion pressure and uterine vascular resistance, the foetus is at risk of hypoxia secondary to inadequate placental perfusion. Although off-pump coronary artery bypass

(OPCAB) has been described in the setting of pregnancy, most cases will require CPB. For obvious reasons, there is little experimental data from which the characteristics of optimal CPB in this setting can be determined. The following have been recommended for the preservation of uteroplacental blood flow:

- *CPB onset*   slow (i.e. over 5–10 min).
- *Pump flow*   maintain at $>2.0 \, \text{l min}^{-1} \text{m}^{-2}$.
- *Systemic pressure*   maintain at >60 mmHg.
- *Flow pattern*   pulsatile rather than non-pulsatile.
- *Temperature*   maintain at $>32°C$.
- *Blood gases*   maintain $P_{O_2} >20$ kPa.
- *Acid–base*   alpha-stat, avoid maternal alkalosis.

Continuous foetal heart rate monitoring by an obstetrician should be undertaken during cardiac surgery. Fetal bradycardia, common during hypothermic CPB, may be improved by physical and pharmacological manoeuvres to increase uteroplacental perfusion.

Despite the potential for considerable haemorrhage, particularly when cardiac surgery follows Caesarian section, this complication has not been widely reported. The use of aprotinin has been reported, although this is an unlicensed indication.

Key points

- Cardiac disease remains a leading indirect cause of maternal mortality. The onset of symptoms in early pregnancy is an ominous sign.
- Cardiac decompensation may only occur during or after delivery.
- Whenever possible, cardiac surgery should follow delivery of the foetus.
- The conduct of CPB should take into account the normal physiological changes associated with pregnancy.

Further reading

Department of Health. *Why Mothers Die – Report on Confidential Enquiries into Maternal Deaths in the United Kingdom 1994–6*. The Stationery Office, 1998.

Malhotra M, Sharma JB, Arora P, Batra S, Sharma S, Arora R. Mitral valve surgery and maternal and fetal outcome in valvular heart disease. *Int J Gynaecol Obstet* 2003; 81(2): 151–156.

Weiss BM, von Segesser LK, Alon E, Seifert B, Turina MI. Outcome of cardiovascular surgery and pregnancy: a systematic review of the period 1984–1996. *Am J Obstet Gynecol* 1998; **179(6 Pt 1)**: 1643–1653.

T.W.R. Lee

The so-called 'stress response to surgery' causes a multitude of adverse haemodynamic, metabolic, haematological, endocrine and immunological effects. In the setting of cardiac surgery, attenuation of pain and sympathetic autonomic activity has many theoretical attractions. The introduction of high-dose opioid techniques into cardiac anaesthesia was based, in part, on the belief that they would inhibit the stress response. Failure to block the stress response completely, combined with equivocal evidence of clinical benefit and the need for prolonged postoperative mechanical ventilation made the technique unpopular. The demonstration that thoracic sympathetic blockade improves blood flow in severely diseased coronary arteries, the emergence of less-invasive cardiac surgical procedures and economic pressures have prompted renewed interest in regional anaesthetic techniques.

Thoracic epidural anaesthesia

The first description of the use of thoracic epidural anaesthesia (TEA) for analgesia *after* cardiac surgery appeared in 1976. It was not until 1987 however, that the first report of epidural catheter insertion *before* cardiac surgery was published. In most published series the interspaces between C_7–T_1 and T_3–T_4 have been used for TEA. The higher approaches are technically easier, although it should be borne in mind that the ligamentum flavum in the thoracic region is thinner and more delicate than in the lumbar region. Most practitioners use a midline approach with the conscious patient sitting or lying. The method used to identify the epidural space varies. The avoidance of the 'asleep' epidural in this setting is due to both a function of retaining the ability to assess the efficacy of the block *before* induction of anaesthesia, and to a lesser degree, response to medicolegal implications of neurological injury.

Typical initial doses include 3 ml lidocaine 2% and 5 ml bupivacaine 0.5% with or without fentanyl $\sim$25 μg; repeated after 10 min, as necessary. Regardless of the epidural infusion recipe used, it is imperative that a bilateral T_1–T_5 dermatome block is present before proceeding. A continuous epidural infusion

(e.g. $\sim$0.125% bupivacaine $\pm$ fentanyl 1–5 μg ml^{-1} $\pm$ clonidine $\sim$0.5 μg ml^{-1} at a rate of 4–10 ml h^{-1}) is then started during surgery and usually continued for up to 3 days. The synergy between agents of different classes (i.e. opioids and local anaesthetics) permits the total dose and side effects of each to be reduced. Regular input from an acute pain management team maximizes epidural efficacy and allows early detection of adverse events.

The 'pros' and 'cons' of the potential benefits of TEA and analgesia in cardiac surgery are shown in Table 60.1.

There is little doubt that the uptake of TEA in cardiac anaesthetic practice has been slowed by 'the ill-defined risk of permanent paraplegia in a fully anticoagulated, unconscious patient' and TEA remains in the hands of enthusiasts. Questions commonly asked by anaesthetists include those shown in Table 60.2.

It can be deduced from this list that the risks of bleeding, epidural haematoma and permanent neurological injury are foremost in anaesthetists' minds. The absence of reported complications in relatively small prospective series (i.e. <1000 patients) gives little cause for comfort – the so-called 'zero numerator' problem. While estimates vary from 1 : 1500 to 1 : 150,000, data from neurologists and closed medicolegal claims analyses may provide a more accurate measure of the true incidence of epidural haematoma. In the context of the major risks of cardiac surgery (i.e. death and stroke), the risk of epidural-related paraplegia is very small.

Patient refusal, local or systemic infection, decompensated aortic stenosis and coagulopathy are regarded as absolute contraindications to neuraxial blockade. In practice, coagulopathy means a platelet count $<100 \times 10^9\,l^{-1}$, international normalized ratio (INR) >1.2 or APTT prolonged >45 s. Most patients undergoing elective cardiac surgery will be asked to discontinue taking aspirin and other antiplatelet agents (e.g. NSAIDs and clopidogrel). The magnitude of any additional epidural-related risk, directly attributable to concurrent antiplatelet therapy is unknown. Oral anticoagulation should be stopped 3–4 days before surgery and normalization of the INR confirmed. Patients who cannot have their oral anticoagulation safely withdrawn

Table 60.1 The 'pros' and 'cons' of the potential benefits of TEA and analgesia in cardiac surgery

Cardiac sympathetic blockade

Pro Unmyelinated sympathetic neurones very sensitive to local anaesthetics
Blockade of sympathetic neurones from T_1–T_5
Dilatation of severely diseased coronary arteries
$\downarrow$ Incidence of postoperative dysrhythmias
$\uparrow$ Myocardial contractility – remains unproven

Con Risk of hypotension
May inhibit sympathetic vasodilatation in normal coronary arteries

Attenuation of stress response

Pro Local anaesthetics superior to epidural opioids alone
Attenuation of $\uparrow$ circulating catecholamine levels
BP and HR response to surgery blunted
Less effect on secondary metabolic, immune and haematological responses

Con Unequivocal evidence of stress response attenuation difficult to obtain

Analgesia

Pro Intense intraoperative and postoperative analgesia
Avoids adverse effects of parenteral narcotic analgesics
Early tracheal extubation and mobilization
Improved postoperative pulmonary function
Possible $\downarrow$ incidence of chronic pain syndromes

Con Unilateral block or missed segments render technique ineffective
Motor and proprioception block may limit mobilization

Table 60.2 Questions frequently asked about the use of epidural anaesthesia in cardiac surgery

1 What is the incidence of epidural-associated spinal haematoma?
2 Do normal laboratory coagulation test results give comfort that clotting is normal?
3 Do antiplatelet agents increase the risk of spinal haematoma?
4 How should patients taking oral anticoagulants be managed?
5 What is the safest epidural insertion – heparin administration interval?
6 What is the appropriate response to a 'bloody tap' or 'dural tap'?
7 Is there an 'ideal' intervertebral space for epidural placement?
8 Does TEA make any difference to patient outcome?

before surgery should not have TEA. Opinion regarding the minimum safe interval between epidural catheter insertion and heparin administration varies from 1 to 12 h.

The optimal management of a bloody tap is unknown. Practices vary from the extreme, abandoning TEA and postponing surgery for 24 h to re-siting the epidural and continuing with the surgical procedure. The latter approach is based on the belief that blood clots in 10–12 min and that heparin is not thrombolytic. Due to the theoretical risk of bleeding following removal of the epidural catheter, this is usually performed after normalization of coagulation has been confirmed by laboratory tests. In patients receiving heparin, the epidural catheter is typically removed not less than 4 h *after*

discontinuing an infusion of unfractionated heparin or 1 h *before* any dose of low-molecular-weight heparin. In some centres, the institution of oral anticoagulation is delayed until after the epidural catheter has been removed.

The neurological sequelae that may accompany a spinal haematoma range from vague sensory and motor symptoms to dense paraplegia or even quadriplegia. The presence and extent of any neurological deficit may only be apparent after discontinuation of the block and removal of the epidural catheter. If there is any doubt, CT or MRI must be undertaken urgently and neurosurgical advice sought. Failure to make the diagnosis and institute management will rightly draw criticism.

TEA is almost invariably used as an adjunct to general anaesthetic techniques tailored to early recovery and neurological assessment. Recently some centres have been assessing the feasibility of using TEA as a sole anaesthetic in beating heart surgery. Case reports have demonstrated that it is possible to rise to the challenge and perform heart surgery on awake patients. However, most anaesthetists remain unconvinced that rational and definitive indications exist for awake heart surgery, given the potential risks to patients. Spontaneous respiration with an open pleural cavity is physiologically undesirable, respiratory depression due to paralysis of diaphragmatic or intercostal muscle may occur, and TOE is virtually impossible. The goals of anaesthesia for cardiac surgery should also include the prevention of unanticipated patient movement throughout the operation.

The insertion of an epidural catheter prior to full anticoagulation is less taboo than in the past. Emerging evidence suggests that those most likely to benefit are patients with borderline pulmonary function, opioid addicts and patients likely to be incompletely revascularized by surgery. Recently published prospective studies suggest that TEA is associated with a lower incidence of postoperative respiratory tract infection, supraventricular dysrhythmias and renal failure. No study yet published has had sufficient power to demonstrate any statistically significant improvement in mortality. Double-blind studies of TEA, with placement of a 'non-therapeutic' epidural catheter in the control group patients, have not been undertaken.

Spinal anaesthesia

The first report of spinal anaesthesia in cardiac surgery was published in 1980. In this report, as in the vast majority of subsequent publications, the agent used was morphine sulphate. The potential benefits of spinal anaesthesia in cardiac surgery are the same as those for TEA, although the risk of epidural haematoma is probably less due to the use of small gauge needles and the avoidance of catheter insertion *and* removal. Unlike TEA however, spinal anaesthetic techniques in this setting have tended to be 'single shot' and opioid based. The limited duration of drug action dictates that lumbar puncture has to be performed shortly before heparinization. The major safety concerns therefore are respiratory depression and neuraxial bleeding, although pruritus, nausea, vomiting and urinary retention are usually more troublesome. The low lipid solubility of morphine results in delayed onset of analgesia and unpredictable effects. Although some investigators have demonstrated superior postoperative analgesia, others have reported either no benefit or delayed recovery.

This may explain the failure of intrathecal morphine to attenuate the stress response to surgery.

In contrast, published investigations of intrathecal local anaesthesia in cardiac surgery are scarce. In a retrospective study published in 1994, Kowalewski and colleagues reported that the combination of hyperbaric bupivacaine (30 mg) and morphine (0.5–1.0 mg) produced excellent postoperative analgesia compatible with same-day early extubation. More recently, Lee and colleagues have demonstrated that general anaesthesia combined with high-dose intrathecal bupivacaine (37.5 mg) resulted in significant attenuation of the stress response and improved LV segmental wall motion. When compared to patients who had a 'sham spinal', study patients had significantly lower serum levels of epinephrine, norepinephrine and cortisol, and significantly less atrial β-receptor dysfunction. Infamiliarity with the technique and the perception of haemodynamic instability may limit widespread adoption of high-dose intrathecal bupivacaine by cardiac anaesthetists.

Parasternal and paravertebral blockade

Although used routinely in some centres, parasternal blockade following cardiac surgery is poorly represented in the literature. Prior to skin closure, preservative-free 0.25% isobaric bupivacaine with or without epinephrine (total volume 40–50 ml) is injected along the sternal borders, deep to the posterior intercostal membrane, to block the anterior cutaneous branches of the intercostal nerves for 6–10 h. The technique may be considered in the patient with abnormal coagulation.

Paravertebral blockade is most commonly used to provide analgesia during and after thoracic surgery. Paravertebral blockade for cardiac surgery is used far less frequently. The paravertebral space lies just anterior to the parietal pleural of the lung, and posterior to the intercostal intimus muscle. Small-bore catheters are usually placed percutaneously, by 'walking' a large-bore epidural needle off the superior aspect of the transverse process of the thoracic vertebra (T_3–T_5). As with TEA, a 'loss of resistance' technique is used to identify the paravertebral space. After administration of a bolus of local anaesthetic, an infusion of dilute local anaesthetic (e.g. 0.1% bupivacaine at 6–8 ml h^{-1}) is then commenced. A unilateral approach may be used for minimally invasive cardiac surgery via an anterior short thoracotomy. Although continuous paravertebral blockade provides good analgesia and facilitates early tracheal extubation, difficulty identifying and catheterizing the paravertebral space and a definite failure rate limit its applicability.

Key points

- Cardiac sympathetic blockade, profound postoperative analgesia and attenuation of the stress response *may* improve patient outcome.
- The emergence of less-invasive cardiac surgical procedures has prompted renewed interest in regional techniques.
- Although no longer taboo, the ill-defined risk of paraplegia in unconscious anticoagulated patients has deterred the majority of anaesthetists from using TEA in cardiac surgical patients.
- The optimal management strategy for the 'bloody tap' is unknown.
- Prospective, randomized, multicentre studies are required to demonstrate that TEA or spinal anaesthesia are superior to combined α- and β-adrenergic blockade.

Further reading

Canto M, Sanchez MJ, Casas MA, Bataller ML. Bilateral paravetebral blockade for conventional cardiac surgery. Anaesthesia 2003; 58(4): 365–370.

Chaney MA (Ed.). *Regional Anesthesia for Cardiothoracic Surgery. A Society of Cardiovascular Anesthesiologists Monograph.* Baltimore: Lippincott, Williams & Wilkins, 2002.

Kowalewski RJ, MacAdams CL, Eagle CJ, Archer DP, Bharadwaj B. Anaesthesia for coronary artery bypass surgery supplemented with subarachnoid bupivacaine and morphine: a report of 18 cases. *Can J Anaesth* 1994; 41(12): 1189–1195.

Lee TW, Grocott HP, Schwinn D, Jacobsohn E, *et al.* High spinal anesthesia for cardiac surgery: effects on beta-adrenergic receptor function, stress response, and hemodynamics. *Anesthesiology* 2003; 98(2): 499–510.

Scott NB, Turfrey DJ, Ray DA, Nzewi O, Sutcliffe NP, Lal AB *et al.* A prospective randomized study of the potential benefits of thoracic epidural anesthesia and analgesia in patients undergoing coronary artery bypass grafting. *Anesth Analg* 2001; 93(3): 528–535.

I. Hardy

The prospects of sternotomy and the real possibility of disability or death, give cardiac surgical patients a high expectation of postoperative pain and an understandable degree of apprehension. New procedures and surgical approaches present fresh challenges in acute pain management. The rational application of effective management strategies requires an understanding of pain pathophysiology.

Pathophysiology

Routine cardiac surgery produces a combination of somatic and visceral pain (Table 61.1). Commonly used incisions include cervical, thoracic and lumbar dermatomes (Figure 61.1).

Tissue injury and the associated inflammatory response liberate a 'cocktail' of substances, which act on peripheral nociceptors and nerves. Nociceptive impulses are conducted by unmyelinated C fibres and myelinated Aδ fibres, which synapse in the dorsal horn nuclei of the spinal cord. Under normal conditions C fibres are not stimulated by 'physiological' peripheral stimuli. Their excitation threshold is lowered by noxious stimuli

such as inflammation. In comparison to Aδ fibres, conduction velocity in C fibres is very slow ($\sim 2\,\mathrm{m\,s^{-1}}$ versus $12\text{--}30\,\mathrm{m\,s^{-1}}$). Aδ fibres are responsible for the early detection of tissue injury (the so-called 'first pain') and form the sensory component of the rapid reflex motor response. Synaptic transmission is opioid insensitive. In contrast, C fibres are responsible for the so-called 'second pain' and synaptic transmission is susceptible to opioid blockade.

The *direct* central pathway consists of second-order neurones in the contralateral lateral spinothalamic tract, which synapse in the ventral posterolateral and intralaminar thalamic nuclei and project to the sensory cortex via third-order neurones. In contrast, the *indirect* (multisynaptic) pathway involves the spinoreticular tracts, which transmit pain impulses via the reticular formation to a wide and ill-defined area of cerebral

---

Table 61.1 Types and sources of pain following cardiac surgery

Superficial
- Skin incisions
- Drain and cannulation sites

Musculoskeletal
- Sternal and costal fractures
- Sternoclavicular and acromioclavicular joints
- Costovertebral and cervicothoracic zygoapophyseal joints

Visceral
- Pericardium
- Pleura
- Myocardium (ischaemia)

Neurological
- Peripheral nerve injury
- Nerve entrapment
- Nerve plexus (e.g. brachial) injury

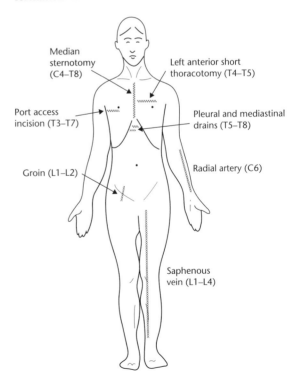

Figure 61.1 Cardiac surgical incisions and corresponding dermatomes.

cortex. Nociceptive signals in the brainstem and thalamus activate descending corticospinal 'antinociceptive' pathways (Figure 61.2), which inhibit or 'gate' afferent nociceptive transmission in the dorsal horn nuclei.

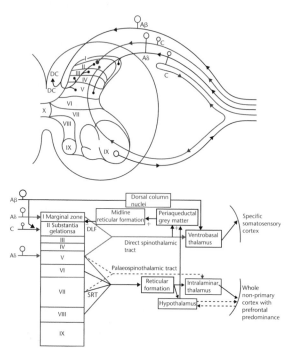

Figure 61.2 Central nociceptive and antinociceptive pathways. DLF, dorsolateral fasciculus; SRT, spinoreticular tract.

If nociceptive input continues, neural pathways undergo both physical and neurochemical changes that make them hypersensitive to nociceptive input and resistant to antinociceptive input. These changes, which are very similar to those involved in memory formation in the brain, can be thought of as 'spinal pain memory'. Reorganization or 'rewiring' of neural pathways in the CNS, a process termed 'plasticity', leads to the abnormal perception of pain in neighbouring anatomical areas.

Acute pain management

The philosophy of acute pain management can be considered under four headings:

1 *Prevention*   Attention to patient positioning and operative technique.
2 *Pre-emptive analgesia*   Prevention of neuronal plasticity (e.g. opioids, N-methyl-D-aspartate (NMDA) receptor antagonists).
3 Depression and reversal of afferent-induced changes in the excitability of central neurones (e.g. opioids).

4 Breaking the vicious cycle of the physiological response to pain.

Some aspects of postoperative pain are preventable. Positioning the arms at the side in internal, rather than external, rotation reduces the incidence of shoulder pain. Similarly, bony fractures and excessive sternal retraction, particularly during internal mammary artery harvesting, should be avoided. The use of endoscopic techniques for saphenous vein and radial artery harvesting may reduce the extent of incisional pain.

In conventional cardiac surgery it is virtually impossible to provide pain relief with local or regional techniques alone (Figure 61.1). For this reason, nurse-controlled intravenous morphine infusions have been the mainstay of postoperative analgesia since the early days. Balanced or 'multimodal' analgesia can be achieved by combining an opioid with regular doses of an NSAID and paracetamol (acetaminophen).

Whenever possible, staff should be conscious of the patient's level of analgesia before embarking on a potentially painful intervention or procedure. The pain associated with chest drain removal, physiotherapy and mobilization may be the only memory a patient has on the 1st postoperative day.

Despite abundant evidence of the safety of NSAIDs in non-cardiac surgery, the routine intraoperative and early postoperative use of NSAIDs in cardiac surgical patients remains controversial. In the absence of any specific contraindication to their use, valid concerns about excessive surgical bleeding, renal dysfunction and GI haemorrhage in an elderly population mean that NSAIDs are usually withheld until at least the 2nd postoperative day. In many centres, NSAIDs are reserved for patients with pleural and pericardial pain. The theoretical advantages of selective cyclo–oxygenase (COX) II inhibitors (e.g. rofecoxib and celecoxib) offer potential benefits in the setting of cardiac surgery.

Occasionally, when severe acute pain does not respond to this traditional multimodal analgesic approach, chronic pain management techniques and early referral to a pain specialist should be considered. Local and regional techniques, transcutaneous electrical nerve stimulation (TENS), acupuncture and adjunctive agents (e.g. α_2-agonists, gamma amino butyric acid (GABA)-agonists, gabapentin, amitriptyline, NMDA antagonists) may be effective.

Chronic pain management

Chronic pain at the operative site that persists for more than 3 months can be defined as chronic (Table 61.2).

Table 61.2 Risk factors for chronic pain after cardiac surgery

Age <60 years
Internal mammary artery harvesting
Body mass index >25 kg m^{-2}
Preoperative angina pectoris
Pre-existing arthritis
Female gender
Poor perioperative analgesia

Using this definition, the incidence of chronic pain after cardiac surgery may be >30% – far more common than most cardiac anaesthetists appreciate. Although mild persistent chest pain is common after sternotomy, it does not usually interfere with daily life. Patients who report chronic post-sternotomy *and* post-saphenectomy pain, however, have a measurably lower quality of life.

The approach to the cardiac surgical patient with chronic pain is no different from that of any patient with chronic pain. The principle aims are to identify the type of pain (i.e. musculoskeletal or neuropathic), exclude the presence of a new diagnosis (e.g. recurrent angina, arthritis, cervical spondylosis or myeloma) and formulate a treatment plan (Table 61.3). A careful history should be taken using the patient's own words

to describe their symptoms and the impact that they have on their quality of life. It is important to document any exacerbating and relieving factors, and to review the effect of previous therapies. It is essential to consider the possibility of co-existing depression and substance abuse.

Examples of drugs that may be used in chronic pain management are shown in Table 61.4. A more detailed description of the application of cognitive-behavioural therapy, temporary nerve blocks, electrical stimulation and neurolysis in chronic pain management is beyond the scope of this chapter.

Role of anaesthetist in chronic refractory angina

As many as 1 in 10 patients undergoing coronary angiography will be found to have coronary anatomy that is amenable to neither percutaneous nor surgical revascularization. When angina occurs in spite of maximal medical therapy the condition is termed chronic refractory angina (CRA), which is a neuropathic pain syndrome. Myocardial ischaemia leads to a chronic elevation of sympathetic tone, which in turn leads to a vicious cycle of myocardial oxygen imbalance and myocardial dystrophy. Patients with CRA rapidly become incapacitated by their symptoms and require

Table 61.3 Patterns of chronic pain and their management

	Musculoskeletal	Neuropathic/neurogenic

Features	Pain related to:
	    Muscle groups
	    Joints
	    Ligamentous insertions
	    Bones
		Dermatomal or band-like
		Related to posture and position
		Stocking/glove distribution

Quality of pain	Heavy Aching Tender Cramping Gnawing	Sharp Shooting Stabbing Hot/burning Nettle rash-like
Treatments	Opioid analgesic 'ladder' NSAIDs – COX-II inhibitors Acupuncture	Combination of tricyclic and anti-epileptic medications

	TENS
	Local anaesthetic joint injection
	Corticosteroid joint injection
		Local anaesthetics/
		    corticosteroids to relevant
		    nerve, plexus or root

	Physiotherapy/hydrotherapy Relaxation techniques Osteopathy Exercise	Antispasmodic agents TENS Acupuncture

Table 61.4 Drug therapy in chronic pain

Antidepressants	Amitriptyline: 25–50 mg at night Nortriptyline: 10–25 mg at night Imipramine: 20–100 mg Paroxetine: 40 mg daily Citalopram: 40 mg daily
Anti-epileptics	Sodium valproate: 100 mg tds increasing to a maximum of 2400 mg daily in divided doses. Maximum effect probably achieved at 200 mg tds Carbamazepine: 200 mg tds increasing to 400 mg tds. Maximum daily dose: 1600 mg Gabapentin: 100 mg tds increasing to a maximum of 3600 mg daily. Maximal effect probably achieved at 400 mg tds
Antispasmodics	Baclofen: 5 mg tds increasing to a maximum of 100 mg daily Dantrolene: 25 mg daily increasing to 100 mg qds Piracetam: 2.4 g tds increasing to 20 g daily
NSAIDs	Ibuprofen: 200 mg tds increasing to 600 mg qds Diclofenac: 150 mg daily as slow-release preparation
COX-II inhibitors	Rofecoxib: 25–50 mg od Celecoxib: 100 mg bd increasing to 200 mg bd
Opioids	Codeine: 100–200 mg qds Dihydrocodeine: 60–120 mg qds Morphine: 1–30 mg bd as slow-release preparation (i.e. MST Continus®) Oxycodone: 10–20 mg bd as modified release preparation Fentanyl: 25–100 µg/h (transcutaneous delivery) Buprenorphine: 35–70 µg/h (transcutaneous delivery)
Others	Tramadol: 50–100 mg bd increasing to 100 mg qds Clonidine: 50 µg bd increasing to 75 µg bd Ketamine: Continuous subcutaneous infusion Capsaicin: Topical 0.075% cream

Table 61.5 Care pathway in chronic retractory angina (CRA)

1	Counselling	Explain management plan Provide advice on diet, smoking, physical activity, etc. Agree a realistic treatment contract
2	Rehabilitation	Exercise Relaxation training
3	Cognitive therapy	Cognitive-behavioural therapy Consider formal psychological assessment
4	TENS	May be used with permanent pacemakers
5	Temporary sympathectomy	Stellate ganglion block T3/4 paravertebral block in stages High thoracic epidural
6	SCS	Alternative to redo surgery in some high-risk patients
7	Opioids	Transdermal, oral, epidural or intrathecal
8	Destructive sympathectomy	Surgical – open or thoracoscopic Phenol – rarely used
9	Laser revascularization	Open (transmyocardial) or percutaneous Efficacy unproven – consider as part of clinical trial
10	Transplantation	If other indications are present (see Chapter 40)

Adapted from the recommendations of The National Refractory Angina Centre, Liverpool, UK. <http://www.angina.org>

frequent hospital admissions. Therapeutic interventions have included transmyocardial and percutaneous laser revascularization, high thoracic epidural analgesia and electrical spinal cord stimulation (SCS).

The care pathway in CRA is shown in Table 61.5.

Electrical stimulation of the spinal cord has been shown to produce a more homogenous pattern of coronary blood flow in patients with myocardial ischaemia. This redistribution of coronary blood flow may explain the subsequent increase in effort tolerance in the face of unchanged total coronary blood flow. Although it has been suggested that SCS alters the balance between sympathetic and parasympathetic tone, patients show no change in HR variability.

Key points

- Cardiac surgical patients worry about death, disability and pain.
- Good preoperative information and counselling can reduce patient apprehension and subsequent pain appreciation.
- An understanding of the pathophysiological of acute and chronic pain allows rational management strategies to be developed.
- Patient monitoring by a dedicated acute pain service may improve patient outcome.
- SCS in CRA *may* reduce the frequency of hospital readmission and improve quality of life.

Further reading

Bruce J, Drury N, Poobalan AS, Jeffrey RR, Smith WC, Chambers WA. The prevalence of chronic chest and leg pain following cardiac surgery: a historical cohort study. *Pain* 2003; **104**(1–2): 265–273.

Meyerson J, Thelin S, Gordh T, Karlsten R. The incidence of chronic post-sternotomy pain after cardiac surgery – a prospective study. *Acta Anaesthesiol Scand* 2001; **45**(8): 940–944.

Svorkdal N. Pro: anesthesiologists' role in treating refractory angina spinal cord stimulators, thoracic epidurals, therapeutic angiogenesis, and other emerging options. *J Cardiothorac Vasc Anesth* 2003; **17**(4): 536–545.

62

J.E. Arrowsmith & J.H. Mackay

Patients with haematological conditions or restrictive religious beliefs may require cardiac surgery. Uncommon problems require advanced warning, a review of current literature and recommendations, formulation of a detailed management plan and specialist haematological advice.

Antiplatelet therapy

Aspirin, clopidogrel and the glycoprotein (GP-IIb/IIIa) antagonists (abciximab, eptifibatide and tirofiban) improve outcome in acute coronary syndromes. The small numbers of patients who subsequently require emergency surgery are at increased risk of major perioperative bleeding as a result of their exposure to these drugs (Table 62.1). It is essential therefore, that the cardiac anaesthetist be aware of the differences between them and the implications of their use.

While the impact of aspirin and clopidogrel on perioperative blood loss and transfusion requirements remains unclear, there is little doubt that the GP-IIb/IIIa antagonists have a much greater potential for causing problems. Where possible, it is recommended that surgery be delayed 12–24 h following abciximab exposure and 4–6 h following eptifibatide or tirofiban. In the Evaluation Prevention of Ischemic Complications (EPIC) study, patients undergoing CABG surgery following abciximab treatment were twice as likely to have major bleeding and three times more likely to die than patients given placebo. Bleeding complications following eptifibatide and tirofiban treatment are far less common. Severe, GP-IIb/IIIa antagonist-induced thrombocytopenia occurs in 0.1–0.5% patients.

The mainstay of treatment for excessive perioperative bleeding is platelet transfusion. Prophylactic platelet transfusion should be considered in abciximab-treated patients. Most anaesthetists give platelets empirically following CPB. Some anaesthetists regard GP-IIb/IIIa antagonist exposure as an indication to reduce the dose of heparin administered before CPB, aiming for a celite-ACT >400 s. The role of off-pump coronary surgery has yet to be evaluated in this setting.

Thrombocytopenia

A low circulating platelet count may be primary (idiopathic) or secondary (fictitious, dilutional, drug induced, paraneoplastic, post-infectious and immuno-deficient). Idiopathic thrombocytopenia (ITP), which is three times more common in women, is a diagnosis of exclusion. Maintenance therapy typically comprises intermittent courses of corticosteroids with or without plasmapheresis, gamma globulin or immunosuppresssion.

Table 62.1 Characteristics of commonly used antiplatelet drugs

Aspirin	Impair ability of platelets to synthesis and release thromboxane
Clopidogrel (Plavix®)	Irreversibly inhibits ADP-induced platelet aggregation Half life of main metabolite 8 h Excreted in urine and faeces Platelet function normalizes ~5 days after discontinuation
Abciximab (Reopro®)	Non-selective monoclonal antibody Duration of platelet inhibition 24–48 h
Eptifibatide (Integrilin®)	Cyclic heptapeptide Duration of platelet inhibition 2–4 h Renal excretion; no active metabolites
Tirofiban (Aggrastat®)	Synthetic non-peptide Duration of platelet inhibition 4–8 h Renal excretion; no active metabolites

While mild degrees of thrombocytopenia are relatively common in patients following cardiac surgery, it is important to identify those with type II heparin-induced thrombocytopenia (HIT) – a paradoxical procoagulant state defined as a platelet count $<100 \times 10^9 \, l^{-1}$ in association with an immunoglobulin (Ig) G or IgM antibodies against the heparin–platelet factor 4 complex. Patient with type II HIT are at significant risk of thromboembolic occlusion of medium and large vessels by platelet aggregates. Further doses of heparin should not be administered and the drug considered an allergen until after the disappearance of circulating anti-heparin–PF4 antibodies.

Patients with known type II HIT present a considerable problem when considering anticoagulation for CPB. Whenever possible, surgery should be postponed until heparin administration is safe. Alternatively, anticoagulation with danaparoid, hirudin, argatroban or prostacyclin may be considered. These agents are discussed in Chapter 12.

Haemoglobin S disease

Patients with sickle cell trait or sickle cell disease are at increased risk of microvascular occlusion during cardiac surgery. All patients in 'at-risk' groups who are unaware of their phenotype should be tested before cardiac surgery. Heterozygotes are unlikely to undergo sickling unless exposed to profound hypoxia (SaO_2 $<40\%$) or hypothermia. In contrast, homozygotes tend to sickle at SaO_2 $<85\%$ and may develop potentially lethal thrombosis during CPB. In addition, auto-splenectomy renders patients susceptible to infection with encapsulated bacteria and renal tubular dysfunction impairs their ability to concentrate urine. Preoperative transfusion and exchange transfusion are used to reduce the level of haemoglobin SS (Hb-SS) to $<30\%$. Hypoxia, acidosis, hypovolaemia and hypothermia should be avoided.

Heparin or protamine allergy

True allergy to these agents is fortunately rare but may cause considerable problems. Some of the alternative therapies are discussed in Chapter 12. Patients with severe fish allergy confirmed by intradermal (skin-prick) testing should probably not receive protamine.

Haemophilia and von Willebrand's disease

Deficiency of either factor VIII (haemophilia A or classic haemophilia) and factor IX (haemophilia B

Table 62.2 Inherited disorders of coagulation

Factor V Leiden
Prothrombin G20210A mutation
Protein S and C deficiency
Antithrombin deficiency
Activated protein C resistance

or Christmas disease) are sex-linked recessive disorders that significantly increase the risk of excessive peri-operative bleeding. Cardiac surgery in haemophiliacs requires considerable planning and close liaison with the local haemophilia service. Perioperative management comprises the administration of exogenous plasma-derived or recombinant anti-haemophilic factors and regular functional assays to assess circulating levels. Patients with factor VIII or factor IX inhibitors may be particularly difficult to manage.

Von Willebrand's disease (vWD) consists of dysfunction or deficiency of von Willebrand factor (vWF) and a variable degree factor VIII deficiency. It may be congenital (autosomal dominant or recessive) or acquired (e.g. rheumatoid arthritis, systemic lupus erythematosus, renal disease and paraneoplastic), and affects females as well as males. Patients with mild forms of the disease respond to desmopressin, which increases circulating levels of vWF–antigen and factor VIII coagulant protein.

Antiphospholipid syndrome

This autoimmune condition, characterized by arterial and venous thrombosis, affects 2% of general population and 7% of hospitalized patients. Paradoxically, antiphospholipid (APL) antibodies act as *in vitro* anticoagulants; interfering with laboratory tests of coagulation (i.e. APTT). The problem for the anaesthetist is that an ACT $>450\,s$ may not represent adequate anticoagulation for CPB. Given that a blood heparin concentration of $3–4\,i.u.\,ml^{-1}$ is adequate for CPB, it has been suggested that the preoperative construction of a heparin–celite-ACT response curve permits known whole-blood heparin concentrations to be correlated with ACTs.

Thrombophilia

The term thrombophilia encompasses a number of inherited hypercoagulable states (Table 62.2). Of these, the factor V Leiden (FVL) polymorphism is the most common, affecting up to 5% of Caucasians.

Table 62.3 Blood conservation strategies in JW patients undergoing cardiac surgery

Preoperative	Anaemia	Consider iron, folate, erythropoietin
	Anticoagulation	Early withdrawal of antiplatelet agents and warfarin
		Switch to unfractionated heparin if necessary
	Patient size	Anticipate haemodilution effect of CPB
Anaesthetic	ANH	10–15 ml kg^{-1} from large-bore central line
	Pharmacological	Consider aprotinin or antifibrinolytic
Bypass	Blood salvage	Needs preoperative discussion with patient
Surgical	Technique	Meticulous attention to haemostasis
Postoperative	Bleeding	Early re-exploration
	Severe anaemia	Increased risk of multi-organ failure and infection
	Renal failure	Consider peritoneal dialysis

JW: Jehovah's witness; ANH: acute normovolaemic haemodilution.

The substitution of glutamine for arginine-506 produces a variant that is resistant to activated protein C (APC). Affected individuals typically present with deep vein thrombosis, pulmonary embolism, stroke and recurrent miscarriage. Homozygotes are at significantly greater risk of these complications than heterozygotes. FVL appears to protect cardiac surgical patients from blood loss and transfusion. Aprotinin, which exacerbates APC resistance, should be used with caution.

Antithrombin (AT) deficiency may be defined as the failure of 500 i.u. kg^{-1} unfractionated heparin to prolong the ACT to >480 s. A reduction in AT activity to 40–70% of normal occurs in congenital AT deficiency (incidence ~1 : 1000). These patients typically present with spontaneous thromboembolic phenomena and recurrent miscarriage. Acquired AT deficiency is a common sequel of heparin administration. Patients with AT levels <70% of normal may be difficult to anticoagulate prior to CPB. Therapeutic options in this situation include: administration of AT concentrate (expensive) or FFP or red cells, which usually contain sufficient AT to prolong the ACT.

Cold agglutinins

IgG or IgM antibodies that induce erythrocyte or platelet aggregation under hypothermic conditions are termed cold agglutinins. The diagnosis is suggested by unexpectedly high arterial-line pressures during hypothermic CPB and massive haemolysis during rewarming. In known cases blood temperature must be maintained above the critical agglutination threshold. For this reason hypothermic CPB and cold cardioplegic solutions are best avoided. Preoperative corticosteroid therapy and plasmapheresis have been used to reduce cold antibody titres.

The Jehovah's Witness

The refusal of Jehovah's Witness (JW) patients to accept allogenic blood products or stored autologous blood increases the risk of cardiac surgery. Preoperative anaemia should be corrected and antiplatelet agents or anticoagulants discontinued at an early stage. Iron and recombinant erythropoietin are often administered if Hb <13 g dl^{-1}.

Most JW patients accept acute normovolaemic haemodilution (ANH) providing the removed blood is maintained in contact throughout surgery (Table 62.3). ANH theoretically reduces the number of RBCs lost during surgery. Platelets and clotting factors in the sequestered blood are protected from damage during CPB.

Key points

- Uncommon haematological problems require specialist advice.
- Heparin induced thrombosis produces a paradoxical procoagulant state.
- Acquired AT deficiency is a common sequel of heparin administration.
- Most Jehovah's witness patients accept acute normovolaemic haemodilution.

Further reading

Boehrer JD, Kereiakes DJ, Navetta FI, Califf RM, Topol EJ. Effects of profound platelet inhibition with c7E3 before coronary angioplasty on complications of coronary bypass surgery. EPIC Investigators. Evaluation Prevention of Ischemic Complications. *Am J Cardiol* 1994; **74(11)**: 1166–1170.

Martlew VJ. Peri-operative management of patients with coagulation disorders. *Br J Anaesth* 2000; **85(3)**: 446–455.

Sreeram GM, Sharma AD, Slaughter TF. Platelet glycoprotein IIb/IIIa antagonists: perioperative implications. *J Cardiothorac Vasc Anesth* 2001; **15(2)**: 237–240.

D.J.R. Duthie

Anaesthetic agents impair thermoregulation. Despite active warming, prolonged exposure of skin and open wounds to ambient temperatures and the IV infusion of unwarmed fluids render cardiac surgical patients mildly hypothermic (34–36°C) during the perioperative period.

Control of temperature

For the purposes of discussion, the human body may be considered to have a central, well-perfused core (head and torso) and a variably perfused periphery. In a normothermic patient, the former comprises two-thirds of body mass and the latter, one-third. Although the temperature within individual organs is not the same, the mean core temperature is normally tightly regulated between 36.4°C and 37.4°C to preserve physiological and metabolic functions. Circadian variation, ovulation and exercise produce small, physiological changes in core temperature. At an ambient temperature of 20–22°C there is typically a 2–4°C core-periphery gradient. In keeping with other homoeostatic mechanisms, thermoregulation relies on sensory (afferent) neural pathways to detect body temperature, central processing within the CNS and effector pathways.

In clinical cardiac surgical practice, core temperature is measured in the nasopharynx, distal oesophagus and PA. Temperature monitoring in the bladder, rectum and tympanic membrane are less frequently used.

The excitation of peripheral thermoreceptors and temperature-sensitive neurones dispersed in the brain stem and spinal cord changes with temperature. Impulses are conveyed via the lateral spinothalamic tracts to the spinal cord, brain stem, midbrain and hypothalamus. Afferent impulses are modulated in regions such as the locus coeruleus and nuclear raphe magnus in the pons before ascending to the principal thermoregulatory centre, the pre-optic anterior hypothalamus.

Vasoconstriction and vasodilatation are the earliest thermoregulatory responses in patients who cannot move, change their clothing or alter their environment. Most anaesthetic techniques cause peripheral vasodilatation by both peripheral and central actions. Lowering of the central threshold for vasoconstriction in a cold environment (i.e. operating theatre) results in the transfer of heat from core-periphery, and mild hypothermia of the core. The rate of heat loss is dependent on the core-periphery gradient. Later responses, such as non-shivering thermogenesis, shivering and sweating, are greatly affected by anaesthesia. Non-shivering thermogenesis is abolished, neuromuscular blockade prevents shivering and anticholinergics impair sweating.

Consequences of hypothermia

The adverse effects of hypothermia are summarised in Table 63.1. Not only is shivering and uncontrollable muscle movement distressing and uncomfortable for patients, it may induce hypertension and myocardial ischaemia. Cold-induced platelet dysfunction, and altered coagulation and fibrinolysis may worsen blood loss and increase transfusion requirements. Decreased skin and subcutaneous blood flow and impaired leucocyte function impairs wound healing and increases the incidence of wound infection. The pharmacology of IV anaesthetics and muscle relaxants may be significantly

Table 63.1 Complications of mild hypothermia	
Shivering	Involuntary movements, ↑ oxygen consumption
Myocardial ischaemia	Effect of hypertension is greater than shivering
Coagulopathy	*In vitro* clotting tests performed at 37°C may be normal
Infection and impaired wound healing	Vasoconstriction reduces subcutaneous PO_2, ↓ T-cell-mediated antibody production and impaired neutrophil function
Delayed recovery	Altered pharmacokinetics and pharmacodynamics

Table 63.2 Mechanisms of heat loss during anaesthesia and surgery and measures that may be used to reduce heat loss

Mechanism	Comments	Countermeasures
Conduction	Cold intravenous and irrigation fluids	Fluid warmer
Convection	Ventilation and laminar airflow (wind-chill)	Surgical drapes and blankets
Radiation	Most significant factor – human skin is an efficient emitter of infrared energy Dependent on surface area : body mass ratio	Reflective (foil) blanket, window blinds/curtains
Evaporation	Vaporization requires considerable energy Skin preparation solutions, surgical site and airway	Heat and moisture exchanger

Table 63.3 Passive and active measures used during anaesthesia and surgery to maintain normothermia

Thermal insulation (e.g. blankets)	Static air, trapped within a blanket, is a poor conductor of heat Limited ability to insulate the legs and torso in cardiac surgery
Forced air warmer	Prevent radiant heat loss by covering the body with a warm outer shell The contact of warm air and skin reduces convective greater than conductive losses Warming proportional to the area of skin covered Considerably more effective than passive measures and heated mattresses
Heated mattress	Modern operating tables are well insulated; therefore most heat is lost through front of body Limited skin contact with mattress minimizes transfer of thermal energy Risk of pressure–heat necrosis (burns) at temperatures >38°C
Radiant heaters	Generate infrared energy Most efficient when placed close to the body and when the direction of radiant energy is perpendicular to the body surface Allows heat transfer without the need for protective coverings Convective losses continue unimpeded Most commonly used in neonatal practice
Fluid warming	The effect of fluid warming is greatest for refrigerated fluids (e.g. blood) and the rapid administration of fluids at room temperature (i.e. 20°C) Warming of maintenance fluids (administered slowly) is of little benefit Packed red cells at 4°C represent a thermal stress of $120\,kJ\,l^{-1}$ ($30\,kcal\,l^{-1}$) 1 unit of red cells at 4°C may reduce adult core temperature by $\sim0.25°C$
Humidification	Respiratory tract heat losses account for $\sim10\%$ of total Passive (i.e. heat and moisture exchangers) measures are less effective but more convenient to use than active humidification systems

altered and the increase in blood solubility of volatile agents at lower temperatures delays recovery.

Maintaining normothermia

Body heat is lost by conduction, convection, radiation and evaporation (Table 63.2). During surgery heat is lost by conduction to adjacent materials and through thin surgical drapes, convection of adjacent air and through open wounds, radiation of heat to enclosing surfaces and evaporation of liquid on the surface of tissues. Radiant losses, which are the most important, are dependent on the fourth power of the temperature difference (in °K) between the skin and enclosing surface. By virtue of their large surface area to volume ratio, neonates are most vulnerable to hypothermia.

Minimizing passive heat loss and active warming measures are required to maintain normothermia (Table 63.3). For patients undergoing anaesthesia of <30 min duration, preoperative vasodilatation and active warming can prevent an intraoperative fall in core temperature. Active peripheral warming abolishes the temperature gradient between the core and peripheries, while vasodilatation increases the mass of tissues at core temperature. This strategy is largely ineffective for longer procedures as initial heat losses are increased by peripheral vasodilatation.

Cardiopulmonary bypass

CPB offers the facility to produce greater and more rapid changes in core temperature than can be achieved in any other type of surgery. Assuming that human tissue has an average specific heat capacity of $\sim 3.5\,\mathrm{kJ\,kg^{-1}\,^\circ C^{-1}}$ ($0.83\,\mathrm{kcal\,kg^{-1}\,^\circ C^{-1}}$), reducing the temperature of a 70-kg adult from $37\,^\circ C$ to $30\,^\circ C$ results in a $>1700\,\mathrm{kJ}$ ($400\,\mathrm{kcal}$) negative energy balance – the same energy required to raise the temperature of 5 l of water from $20\,^\circ C$ to $100\,^\circ C$. While rapid cooling can be achieved with few obvious deleterious effects, rewarming must be undertaken gradually with a smaller gradient between warmed oxygenated blood returning to the aorta and measured core temperature. Even when rewarming is performed slowly, heat is transferred to the core compartment quicker than it can be redistributed to the periphery resulting in substantial core to peripheral gradients. Following the termination of CPB, heat is transferred from core to the inadequately warmed periphery resulting in core temperatures falling below $35\,^\circ C$. This redistribution of heat and subsequent core hypothermia following hypothermic CPB is known as 'after-drop'. Factors influencing the rate and magnitude of after-drop are shown in Table 63.4. In practice, the duration of rewarming after hypothermic CPB is the best measure of the adequacy of rewarming.

The use of vasodilators during the rewarming phase of CPB reduces the core-periphery temperature gradient and slows the rate at which core temperature rises. Although this technique results in a higher peripheral temperature at the end of CPB, the eventual impact that this has on after-drop is small ($\sim 0.3\,^\circ C$) and clinically unimportant. Forced air heating of the legs during rewarming and after CPB is more effective – reducing after-drop by as much as $0.7\,^\circ C$.

Table 63.4 Factors influencing the magnitude of 'after-drop'

Duration of rewarming
Relative masses of core and periphery
Core to peripheral temperature gradient
Core temperature during hypothermic CPB
Heat loss from open chest post-CPB
Use of vaso-active agents
Active warming of peripheries

Traditionally both core and peripheral temperature have been measured on cardiac surgical ICUs, enabling trends in core to peripheral gradient to be observed. Since most clinical decisions (e.g. need for forced air rewarming, timing of tracheal extubation) are based on core temperature measurement, many centres have abandoned peripheral temperature measurement.

Key points

- The most significant cause of intraoperative hypothermia is radiant heat loss.
- Passive measures to prevent intraoperative heat loss are only successful for short procedures.
- Clinical decision-making should be based on core temperature rather than the gradient between core and peripheral temperatures.
- In practice, the duration of rewarming after hypothermic CPB is the best measure of the adequacy of rewarming.

Further reading

Ginsberg S, Solina A, Papp D, Krause T, Pantin E, Scott G et al. A prospective comparison of three heat preservation methods for patients undergoing hypothermic cardiopulmonary bypass. *J Cardiothorac Vasc Anesth* 2000; **14(5)**: 501–505.

Rajek A, Lenhardt R, Sessler DI, Brunner G, Haisjackl M, Kastner J et al. Efficacy of two methods for reducing postbypass afterdrop. *Anesthesiology* 2000; **92(2)**: 447–456.

Sessler DI. Complications and treatment of mild hypothermia. *Anesthesiology* 2001; **95(2)**: 531–543.

MICROBIOLOGY

64

J.E. Foweraker

Anaesthetists need a working knowledge of anti-microbial prophylaxis for routine cardiac surgery, prophylaxis against endocarditis and prevention and treatment of MRSA.

Routine surgical prophylaxis

The primary aim of prophylaxis is to reduce wound infection. Placebo-controlled trials have shown that antibiotics with activity against *Staphylococcus aureus* significantly reduce the rate of infection following cardiac surgery. Antibiotic prophylaxis is also recommended for permanent pacemaker (PPM), implantable cardiodefibrillator (ICD) and ventricular assist device (VAD) insertion. There is less impact on the development of early prosthetic valve endocarditis or infection of other devices. Deep sternal wound infection is mainly caused by *Staphylococcus aureus*; however, there are significant infections with Gram-negative bacilli (coliforms such as *Escherichia coli*, *Klebsiella* spp., *Enterobacter* spp. and occasionally *Pseudomonas aeruginosa*). These are probably introduced via the leg veins contaminated during saphenous vein harvesting.

Table 64.1 Antibiotic regimes and typical adult doses

Antibiotic regime	Typical adult dose
Flucloxacillin +Gentamicin	1 g qds for 24 h 2 mg kg^{-1} as single dose
Cefuroxime	1.5 g for 24 h tds
Vancomycin +Gentamicin	1 g pre-CPB and 1 g post-CPB 2 mg kg^{-1} as single dose

Gentamicin covers a broader range of Gram-negative bacilli than cephalosporins. Furthermore, the combination of gentamicin and flucloxacillin is less likely to cause *Clostridium difficile* diarrhoea. One dose of gentamicin is sufficient to maintain therapeutic levels throughout surgery and is highly unlikely to cause nephro- or oto-toxicity. Patients who carry MRSA or have a significant penicillin allergy should have vancomycin with gentamicin. Erythromycin resistance is too common for it to be recommended.

Antibiotics should be given no earlier than 30 min before induction. There is no evidence that antibiotics given beyond 6 h after completion of surgery have any impact on surgical-site infection. For many general surgical procedures, single-dose prophylaxis is advocated but this is probably not appropriate for cardiac surgery. Blood loss and the haemodilutional effects of CPB may significantly reduce antibiotic levels and a second dose should be given after CPB, if the drug has a short half-life (e.g. flucloxacillin and most cephalosporins). Once CPB is initiated, vancomycin levels drop more than would be anticipated from haemodilution alone. The drug probably binds to the extracorporeal circuit. A second dose of vancomycin should be given when the patient comes off CPB.

Infective endocarditis

The diagnosis of infective endocarditis and treatment of prosthetic endocarditis are discussed in Chapter 22.

The American Heart Association (AHA) and the British Society for Antimicrobial Chemotherapy (BSAC) have published guidelines for the treatment of endocarditis. The general principles are to use a prolonged course of a cidal antibiotic or antibiotic combination. Drugs with a short half-life such as the penicillins are given at high-dose and frequent intervals to optimize the pharmacokinetics of the drug and pharmaco-dynamics of the drug–bacterium interaction. The treatment for infective endocarditis should continue throughout valve surgery, in addition to the antibiotics for surgical prophylaxis (advice should be available from the local microbiologist).

Endocarditis prophylaxis

Most episodes of infective endocarditis cannot be attributed to an invasive procedure. There is still debate around who needs prophylaxis for which procedures because of a lack of controlled trials. The guidance is based on the likelihood of bacteraemia with the organisms that can cause endocarditis during certain

Table 64.2 Endocarditis prophylaxis for commonly encountered procedures in cardiac ICU

Prophylaxis recommended	Prophylaxis not recommended
Rigid bronchoscopy	FOB (±biopsy)
Surgery on the respiratory or gut mucosa	Cardiac catheterization (±PTCA or stent)
Oesophageal dilatation	Endo-tracheal intubation
TOE (high-risk patients)	TOE (moderate-risk patients)
Any surgical procedure in the presence of active bacterial infection	CABG, insertion of PPM, ICO (but give surgical prophylaxis)
Urethral catheterization (no UTI)	GI endoscopy (±biopsy)

UTI, Urinary tract infection; PCTA, Percutaneous transluminal coronary angioplasty.

Table 64.3 Risk of endocarditis and prophylaxis recommendations in common cardiac conditions

Prophylaxis recommended		Prophylaxis not recommended
High risk	**Moderate risk**	**Negligible risk**
Prosthetic heart valve	HOCM	'Innocent' heart murmurs
Previous endocarditis	Acquired valve dysfunction (e.g. rheumatic fever)	PPM, ICD *in situ*
Complex congenital heart disease, constructed shunts or conduits	Uncorrected simple congenital defects (e.g. PDA and VSD)	Surgical repair of ASD, VSD and PDA (after 6 months healing)

Tables modified from: Dajani AS, *et al.* Prevention of bacterial endocarditis. *Circulation* 1997; **96**: 358–366. HOCM, hypertrophic obstructive cardiomyopathy.

procedures, and the risk and potential outcome of endocarditis in individuals with different predispositions. The general principles are that bacteraemia occurs when a mucosal surface is damaged or when an infected site is instrumented. For example, rigid bronchoscopy carries a significant risk but fibre optic bronchoscopy (FOB) or tracheal intubation do not (see Table 64.2).

The risk of acquiring endocarditis can be divided into high, moderate or negligible (see Table 64.3). It should be borne in mind that an individual's risk may be altered as a result of surgery. For example, following prosthetic valve replacement the risk of endocarditis is permanently increased, whereas 6 months after VSD or patent ductus arteriosus (PDA) closure, the risk is that of the general population.

Antibiotics are given to cover the organisms that are likely to cause endocarditis. These are *Streptococcus viridans* (mouth, airway and upper GI tract), *Enterococcus spp.* (GI and genitourinary tracts) and *Staphylococcus aureus* (infected soft tissues, bones and joints). The BSAC has provided relatively simple guidelines which are well summarized in the British National Formulary (BNF). There is also a well-referenced document from the AHA.

Methicillin-resistant *Staphylococcus aureus*

MRSA is resistant to all penicillins and cephalosporins. Many strains are also resistant to aminoglycosides (e.g. gentamicin) and quinolones (e.g. ciprofloxacin). Strains of MRSA appear no more pathogenic than drug-sensitive *Staphylococcus aureus*. Deep infections, such as mediastinitis, osteomyelitis and infective endocarditis, can however be more difficult to treat. The treatment of choice (a glycopeptide such as vancomycin) is not as effective an anti-staphylococcal agent as flucloxacillin is for a sensitive organism. Many of the more recently introduced anti-MRSA antibiotics are bacteriostatic rather than bactericidal. Vancomycin should be used both as treatment in proven MRSA infection and as empirical treatment of infection in MRSA carriers.

When patients are colonized with MRSA it becomes part of their normal flora (living in moist skin sites such as the anterior nares, throat, perineum and axillae). Systemic antibiotics do not achieve effective concentrations on body surfaces and have no effect on MRSA carriage, whereas topical agents (e.g. triclosan, chlorhexidine and mupirocin) may clear colonization.

Spread of MRSA leads to more use of vancomycin and teicoplanin, which can select for vancomycin-resistant bacteria for which there are few therapeutic options. True vancomycin-resistant *Staphylococcus aureus* has recently been described in the USA.

Current laboratory tests can take several days to isolate MRSA, by which time the organism may have already spread. Every patient should be considered a potential MRSA carrier. Known carriers should be isolated and barrier nursed. The risk of spread can be reduced if staff wash hands or use a topical antiseptic after every contact with the patient or their immediate surroundings. To prevent surgical-site infection in a patient who carries MRSA, vancomycin should be included in the operative prophylaxis.

Patients who have been in hospital or institutional care are at increased risk of carrying MRSA and should be screened before or on admission. Some centres screen all patients before cardiothoracic surgery, as many will have been hospitalized in the previous 6 months. MRSA screening samples include swabs from carriage sites (nose, throat and perineum), urine (if catheterized), sputum (if productive) and wound sites (e.g. line or drain insertion sites).

The trend is away from routine screening of staff. MRSA may be carried as part of the normal flora of a health care worker – usually in the nose. If their 'practice' is good, they are unlikely to spread this to a patient unless they have a desquamating skin condition or an infected lesion. Screening of staff can lead to victimization of those who are carriers but not spreading the organism and conversely cause complacency in those who are not carriers but do spread MRSA from patient to patient because they do not wash their hands.

Vancomycin-resistant Enterococci

Enterococcus faecalis and *E. faecium* can become resistant to vancomycin and teicoplanin, leaving very few antibiotics available for treatment. VRE is found as part of the gut flora and on damaged skin sites (e.g.

wounds, drains sites and tracheostomy). It is very hardy and survives well in the environment therefore exemplary infection control practice is needed to stop spread. Fortunately, these organisms are usually of low pathogenicity and rarely cause infection even in the immunocompromised. VRE endocarditis can, however, be very difficult to treat. Measures should be taken to exclude this organism from cardiac wards and ICU. Any patients with VRE should be strictly barrier nursed. Vancomycin and teicoplanin usage should be strictly controlled to discourage the emergence of resistant bacteria.

Key points

- Given at induction of anaesthesia, prophylactic antibiotics reduce the incidence of surgical wound infection.
- Most episodes of infective endocarditis do not follow an invasive procedure.
- Screening, handwashing and barrier nursing prevent the spread of MRSA.
- Deep MRSA infection is difficult to treat.

Further reading

American Heart Association (www.americanheart.org).

Bayer AS, Scheld, WM. Endocarditis and intravascular infections. In: Mandel, Bennett JE, Dolin, R (Eds), *Principles and Practise of Infectious Diseases*, Vol. 1, 5th edition. 2000; pp. 857–902.

British National Formulary (www.bnf.org.uk).

British Society for Antimicrobial Chemotherapy (www.bsac.org.uk).

British Society for Antimicrobial Chemotherapy, Hospital Infection Society and the Infection Control Nurses Association. Revised guidelines for the control of methicillin-resistant Staphylococcus aureus infection in hospitals. *J Hosp Infect* 1998; **39(4)**: 253–290.

Scottish Intercollegiate Guidelines Network. Publication No. 45: *Antibiotic Prophylaxis in Surgery*. July 2000; ISBN 1899893 22 9 (www.sign.ac.uk).

C.R. Rajamohan

Since its introduction into clinical practice in the early 1950s, the indications for CPB have broadened from operations on or within the heart to include non-cardiac thoracic, abdominal and neurological procedures. The indications for CPB for non-cardiac surgery are shown in Table 65.1.

Table 65.1 Non-cardiac surgical applications of CPB	
Thoracic	Surgery of the great vessels
	Pulmonary embolectomy
	Tracheobronchial reconstruction
	Resection of mediastinal tumours
	Lung transplantation
Abdominal	Resection of renal tumours with IVC extension
Neurological	Arteriovenous malformations
	Basilar artery aneurysm
Resuscitation	Accidental hypothermia
	Multiple trauma

Anaesthetic considerations

Similar principles apply to the application of CPB in both cardiac and non-cardiac surgery. In practice however, there are a number of important factors that must be considered. With the exception of thoracic aortic surgery, non-cardiac CPB procedures are performed rarely and frequently involve staff who have little or no experience of CPB. Moreover, non-cardiac surgeons do not routinely operate on anticoagulated patients. Published case series and experience gained in previous cases should form the basis of detailed protocols for future reference.

The use of femoro-femoral CPB, which avoids the need for sternotomy or thoracotomy, is often employed in procedures that do not routinely involve chest opening. In this situation, there is retrograde perfusion of the aorta. Although the size of femoral arterial cannula has minimal impact on CPB flow rates, a small femoral venous cannula may significantly reduce venous return. For this reason the maximal achievable flow

rate may be insufficient at normothermia. To circumvent this problem, partial or incomplete CPB is initated and lung ventilation continued until the degree of hypothermia is compatible with CPB at reduced flow rates. It is essential that hypothermia-induced VF does not occur before reaching this level of hypothermia.

The risk of CPB-related adverse events is the same, regardless of the clinical application. The basic principles of adequate anticoagulation, avoidance of aeroembolism and maintenance of vital organ perfusion are no less important. Femoral cannulation may result in lower limb ischaemia or neurological injury. In difficult cases it should be borne in mind that femoro-femoral CPB can be established under local anaesthesia *prior* to the induction of general anaesthesia.

Thoracic surgery

CPB for surgery on the ascending aorta and aortic arch is discussed in Chapters 34 and 35. Pulmonary embolectomy and thromboendarterectomy, performed for acute and chronic pulmonary thromboembolic disease respectively, requires CPB $\pm$ DHCA.

In the past, resection of tracheal and carinal tumours was routinely performed with CPB. Advances in endoluminal intervention (e.g. stents, cryotherapy, lasers, etc.) have limited the indications for CPB:

- Patients at high risk of airway obstruction following induction of anaesthesia.
- Repair of tracheal dehiscence following heart–lung transplantation.
- Resuscitation of patients suffering massive haemorrhage after pulmonary resection.

Mediastinal surgery

Patients with large anterior mediastinal tumours (e.g. teratoma, lymphoma or seminoma) may develop airway collapse and great vessel compression following induction of anaesthesia. In addition, initiation of intermittent positive-pressure ventilation may cause distal air trapping. Although inhalational induction and maintenance of spontaneous respiration is theoretically attractive, induction even with sevoflurane, may be slow and hazardous. The left lateral position may be preferable as placing the patient in the supine position may lead to cardiac arrest from PA or SVC obstruction. Neither inhalational induction nor awake-intubation, completely avoid the risk of airway obstruction distal to the ETT. If there is any doubt the groin should be prepared for femoral cannulation *prior* to induction.

Transplantation surgery

Although the majority of single- and double-lung transplants can be accomplished using standard thoracic anaesthetic techniques without CPB, a perfusionist should always be immediately available. Induction of anaesthesia and initiation of positive-pressure ventilation in patients with end-stage emphysema commonly results in severe hypotension. Air trapping and breath 'stacking' have been likened to a tourniquet being applied to the right heart. If in doubt, the patient should be deliberately disconnected from the ventilator to let the trapped gas out. The patient with emphysematous lungs will *expire* if given insufficient time to *exhale*!

Intolerance of one-lung anaesthesia, due to haemodynamic instability, severe hypercarbia or hypoxia, is the principal indication for CPB. Severe gas trapping in the dependent lung or, more rarely, a dependent pneumothorax may produce rapid decompensation. The choice of cannulation site is largely dictated by surgical approach (i.e. lateral thoracotomy, sternotomy or 'clam shell') and expediency.

Urological surgery

The principle indication for CPB in this setting is resection of renal tumours (e.g. renal cell carcinoma or hypernephroma, nephroblastoma) with IVC extension. The aim of surgery is radical, curative resection with the operative approach being largely determined by the superior limit of caval extension. In advanced cases tumour may prolapse through the TV and produce haemodynamic compromise. In this situation, sternotomy is required to establish CPB (i.e. SVC to ascending aorta) as IVC obstruction precludes femoro-femoral CPB. A short period of DHCA may be required for removal of tumour from RA.

The anaesthetist should be aware of the potential for massive haemorrhage, tumour fragmentation/embolism and paraneoplastic phenomena (e.g. hyperglycaemia, hypertension, hypercalcaemia and hypokalaemia). Short central venous cannulae and TOE should be used, and PAFCs avoided.

Neurosurgery

First used in the late 1950s, DHCA was widely used for intracranial aneurysm surgery until the late 1960s. Extra-thoracic cannulation techniques largely overcame the need for simultaneous thoracotomy and craniotomy. Subsequent advances in neurosurgery lead to the abandonment of DHCA for all but the most technically demanding cases, for example posterior fossa haemangioblastomas and giant basilar aneurysms.

Resuscitation

In the setting of cardiac surgery, surgical re-exploration and re-institution of CPB is a common means of dealing with cardiovascular collapse in the early postoperative period. CPB may also be of use in major trauma, particularly in the presence of airway disruption. The benefits of heparinization and CPB have to be carefully weighed against the risk of exsanguination or intracranial haemorrhage. Less commonly, CPB has been successfully used to treat accidental hypothermia and drug overdose (e.g. flecainide and bupivacaine). In practise, the logistical difficulties of moving a patient to a centre that offers CPB, the high mortality and low chance of full neurological recovery limit its application.

Key points

- Induction of anaesthesia and initiation of IPPV is hazardous in patients with large anterior mediastinal tumours.
- Maximal achievable flow rates during femoro-femoral bypass may be insufficient at normothermia.

Further reading

Conacher ID. Dynamic hyperinflation – the anaesthetist applying a tourniquet to the right heart. *Br J Anaesth* 1998; 81(2): 116–117.

Gravlee GP, Davis RF, Kurusz M, *et al. Cardiopulmonary bypass: Principles and Practice*, 2nd edition. Philadelphia: Lippincott Williams and Wilkins, 2000.

CARDIOVASCULAR DISEASE AND NON-CARDIAC SURGERY

66

J.E. Arrowsmith & J.H. Mackay

Cardiovascular disease (CVD) is a significant and potentially reversible risk factor for perioperative morbidity and mortality. The risk of perioperative cardiovascular complications is also dependent on patient age and the type of surgery undertaken. Cardiovascular complications may manifest as sudden death, non-fatal MI, heart failure, dysrhythmias and shock. As many as 10% of all patients undergoing non-cardiac surgery have, or are at risk of having, CVD. As many as 30% of patients over 65 years of age and 60% of patients undergoing vascular surgery will have significant CVD. Surgical procedures requiring AXC are associated with a particularly high incidence of perioperative myocardial ischaemia.

General principles

The objectives of preoperative assessment are as follows:

1 Evaluation of the patient with known CVD.
2 Identification of the patient with symptoms and/ or signs of CVD.
3 Identification of the patient who, by virtue of the type of surgery proposed, is at high risk of perioperative cardiovascular morbidity.

In most cases a careful history and thorough physical examination are the best means of identifying the patient with significant cardiac disease (see Chapter 3.15). Risk factors known to contribute to adverse perioperative cardiac outcome (Table 66.1) should be documented; and symptoms such as angina pectoris,

dyspnoea, orthopnoea, palpitation, (pre)syncope and reduced functional capacity (Table 66.2), should be actively sought. The importance of assessing exercise tolerance cannot be overstated. If a patient can walk a mile without becoming short of breath, then the probability of extensive coronary disease is small.

A brief review of other systems should be conducted to elicit any history of renal, hepatic, metabolic, endocrine, neurological or haematological disease. In addition, it is important to document any history or symptoms of upper GI pathology that may contraindicate the use of TOE.

Risk assessment

Having identified the patient at increased risk of adverse cardiac outcome some quantification of risk is required to guide the appropriate use of additional investigations and interventions. Three key questions need to be considered:

1 Are there modifiable operative risk factors?
2 Should the elective operation be modified, delayed or cancelled?
3 Is percutaneous intervention or cardiac surgery indicated?

The assessment of risk requires consideration of the type of surgery planned (Table 66.3), functional status (Table 66.2) and clinical indicators of CVD (Table 66.1). Historically, the Goldman multi-factorial cardiac risk index (CRI) has been used to stratify patients

Table 66.1 Clinical predictors of perioperative cardiovascular risk

Major	Intermediate	Minor
Myocardial infarction within past 30 days	Mild angina pectoris (CCS class I/II)	Advanced age
Unstable coronary syndromes	Prior Myocardial infarction	Abnormal ECG
Decompensated cardiac failure	Compensated or prior heart failure	Rhythm other than sinus
Significant dysrhythmias	Diabetes mellitus	Low functional capacity
Symptomatic dysrhythmias		History of stroke
Severe valvular heart disease		Uncontrolled hypertension

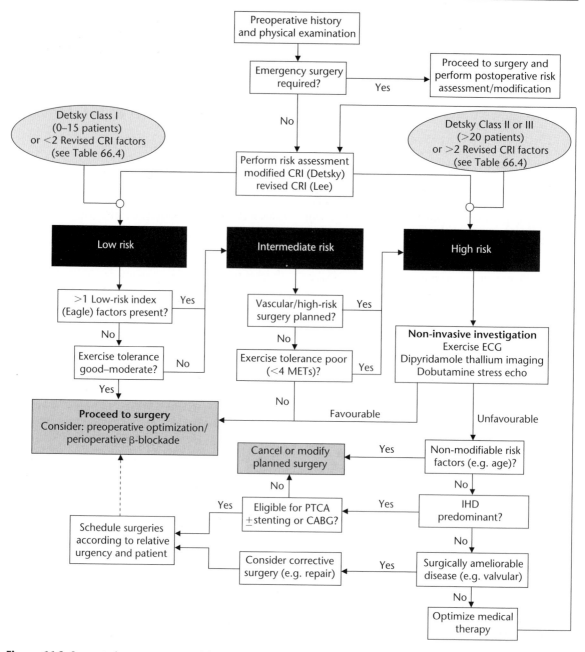

Figure 66.1 Suggested management guidelines for the assessment of risk and management of patients with cardiac disease undergoing non-cardiac surgery. Based on the guidelines published by the American College of Physicians (ACP) and the American College of Cardiology/American Heart Association (ACC/AHA) Task Force. The guidelines are based predominantly on expert opinion and *emerging* clinical evidence rather than being solely evidence based. METs, metabolic equivalents.

according to cardiac risk (Table 66.4). Modifications of the Goldman CRI, that provide better outcome prediction, have been described by Detsky, and more recently by Lee (Table 66.4). A suggested approach to the non-cardiac surgical patient is shown in Figure 66.1.

Patients who require emergency surgery (i.e. within 4 h) should not have their procedure delayed by unnecessary investigations. Cardiac patients undergoing urgent (i.e. 12–24 h) or elective surgery who have had a recent change or recurrence of symptoms

Table 66.2 Assessment of functional capacity

	Activity	Weight	METs
Poor	Walk indoors, such as around your house	1.75	<4
	Do light work around the house – strip and make bed, dusting or washing dishes	2.70	
	Take care of yourself – eating, dressing, bathing and using the toilet	2.75	
Intermediate	Walk one or two blocks on level ground	2.75	4–7
	Do moderate work around the house – vacuuming, sweeping floors, carrying groceries	3.50	
	Do garden work – raking leaves, weeding, pushing a power mower	4.50	
	Have sexual relations	5.25	
	Climb a flight of stairs or walk up a hill	5.50	
	Participate in golf, bowling, dancing, doubles tennis, throwing a baseball or football	6.00	
Good	Participate in swimming, singles tennis, football, basketball, skiing	7.50	>7
	Run a short distance at 5 mph	8.00	
	Do heavy work around the house – scrubbing floors, lifting or moving heavy furniture	8.00	

The Duke Activity Status Index (DASI Hlatky *et al*, 1989) and approximate metabolic equivalents (METs, metabolic equivalents; 1 MET represents an oxygen consumption of $3.5\,ml\,kg^{-1}\,min^{-1}$).

Table 66.3 Risk of cardiac death or non-fatal MI according to type of surgery

High risk (>5%)
- Emergent major operation particularly in elderly
- Aortic or other major vascular
- Peripheral vascular surgery
- Anticipated prolonged surgical procedures associated with large blood loss and/or fluid shifts

Intermediate risk (<5%)
- Carotid endarterectomy
- Head and neck surgery
- Intraperitoneal and intrathoracic
- Orthopaedic surgery
- Prostate surgery

Low risk (<1%)
- Endoscopic procedures
- Superficial procedures
- Cataract surgery
- Breast surgery

or who have new physical signs should undergo further evaluation.

Investigations

'Routine' preoperative investigations have low positive-predictive value in asymptomatic patients without cardiovascular risk factors. The likelihood of obtaining an 'abnormal' result increases with the number of tests performed. Patients <75 years old without risk factors for lung disease do not require a 'routine' CXR. Similarly, the likelihood of detecting an ECG abnormality in an asymptomatic patient <45 years old, is <10%.

Non-invasive investigations, such as exercise ECG, pharmacological stress testing, myocardial perfusion imaging and echocardiography are discussed in more details in Chapters 16, 24 and 25.

Management

A five-step approach is advocated:

- Define the cardiovascular pathology.
- Quantify operative cardiovascular risk.
- Predict the cardiovascular pathophysiology.
- Determine haemodynamic goals.
- Anticipate haemodynamic emergencies.

Cardiac medications should be continued up until the time of surgery. The administration of β-blockers should be considered in every suitable patient as their use before vascular surgery has been shown to significantly reduce both perioperative and late postoperative mortality. Although the use of goal-directed preoperative optimization (i.e. supranormalization of oxygen delivery) has been shown in a number of studies to reduce mortality in vascular surgical patients, access to ICU facilities limit the practicability of this approach. The same principles of management apply

Table 66.4 Calculation of the Goldman multi-factorial CRI, the modified CRI proposed by Detsky *et al.*, the Eagle Low-Risk Index and the Revised CRI proposed by Lee *et al*

	Goldman (1977)	Detsky (1986)	Eagle (1989)	Lee (1999)
Age >70 years	5	5	1	
Emergency surgery	4	10	–	
Intraperitoneal, intrathoracic or aortic surgery	3	–	–	
CCS Class III angina	–	10	–	
CCS Class IV angina	–	20	–	
Unstable angina in previous 6 months	–	10	–	
Any angina	–	–	1	
MI <6 months ago	10	10	–	
MI >6 months ago	–	5	–	
Q-wave on ECG	–	–	1	
S_3 or jugular vein distension	11	–	–	
Pulmonary oedema in previous 7 days	–	10	–	
Any history of pulmonary oedema	–	5	–	
Significant AS (i.e. gradient >50 mmHg)	3	20	–	
ECG rhythm other than sinus with or without APBs	7	5	–	
>5 PVBs min documented on ECG before surgery	7	5	–	
History of ventricular ectopy	–	–	1	
DM	–	–	1	
Poor general medical status*	3	5	–	
High-risk surgery				1
History of IHD				1
History of congestive cardiac failure				1
History of cerebrovascular disease				1
Preoperative treatment with insulin				1
Preoperative serum creatinine >177 μmol$\,$l^{-1}				1
Total possible points	53	120	5	6
Risk Class I	0–5 (1%)	0–15 (0.43)	0 (0–3%)	0 (0.4–0.5%)
Risk Class II	6–12 (6.6%)	20–30 (3.38)	1–2 (6–16%)	1 (0.9–1.3%)
Risk Class III	13–25 (13.8%)	>30 (10.60)	>3 (25–50%)	2 (4–7%)
Risk Class IV	>26 (78%)	–	–	>2 (9–11%)

Observed incidences (Goldman, Eagle and Lee) and likelihood ratios (Detsky) of life-threatening or fatal cardiac complications according to cardiac risk class are shown in parentheses.

*Poor general medical status defined as: $PaO_2 < 8$ kPa, $PaCO_2 > 7$ kPa, $K^+ < 3.0$ mmol$\,$l^{-1}, $HCO_3^- < 20$ mmol$\,$l^{-1}, urea > 18 mmol$\,$l^{-1}, creatinine > 260 μmol$\,$l^{-1}, abnormal serum aspartate aminotransferase, signs of chronic liver disease, bedridden from non-cardiac causes.

APBs, atrial premature beats; IHD, ischaemic heart disease; CCS, Canadian Cardiovascular Society.

in the postoperative phase. Adequate analgesia, supplemental oxygen therapy, cardiorespiratory and fluid balance monitoring all have a part to play in the prevention of cardiovascular decompensation.

Coronary artery disease

It is impractical to define the coronary anatomy and ventricular function of all patients undergoing non-cardiac surgery. It is however, important to identify those who require non-invasive testing and revascularization.

Patients most likely to benefit from revascularization include those with

1 asymptomatic critical left main-stem stenosis;
2 LV dysfunction in the presence of triple-vessel disease;
3 two-vessel disease in the presence of proximal LAD disease;
4 refractory angina despite maximal medical therapy.

The Coronary Artery Surgery Study (CASS) demonstrated that perioperative mortality following non-cardiac surgery was five times greater in patients with angiographic evidence of coronary artery disease who had not undergone revascularization (see Chapter 18). Perioperative MI occurred only in patients with angiographically proven coronary disease.

In patients with a history of MI the overall risk of perioperative re-infarction is around 4–6%. Although a number of studies published in the 1970s suggested that patients operated <3 months after infarction were five to ten times more likely to re-infarct, more recent studies have failed to reproduce this finding. Recent advances in perioperative care are believed to be responsible for this apparent reduction in risk. Nevertheless, truly elective surgery should be postponed for at least 3, and probably 6, months after MI. Patients who have already undergone coronary revascularization within the preceding 5 years usually require no further testing unless they have developed new cardiac symptoms.

Hypertension

The prevalence of arterial hypertension (sustained diastolic pressure >110 mmHg) is as great as 25% of the adult population and increases with age. Untreated or inadequately treated hypertensives exhibit an exaggerated response to surgical stimulation with greater haemodynamic instability. Historically, it has been the practice to defer surgery in uncontrolled hypertensives, although there is little evidence to suggest that this reduces morbidity or mortality. The threshold at which hypertension should give cause for concern should be commensurate with the age of the patient. An elderly patient with diastolic pressure of 110 mmHg who has no symptoms suggestive of end-organ dysfunction (i.e. headache, visual disturbance and congestive cardiac failure) and no other clinical indicators (Table 66.1) is probably at no greater risk of perioperative morbidity. However, a similar BP in a younger patient is more likely to have a renovascular or endocrine cause and should prompt further investigation. Paradoxically, the aggressive management of hypertension in patients >80 years may increase rather than decrease morbidity.

Diabetes mellitus

The cardiovascular, renal and neurological sequelae of diabetes may have a significant impact on a patient's ability to tolerate major surgery. The presence of autonomic neuropathy and the increased incidence of silent myocardial ischaemia should indicate that the long-standing diabetic has significant CVD until proven otherwise.

Heart failure

Heart failure is a major risk factor for adverse outcome in both cardiac and non-cardiac surgical patients (Table 66.4). The symptoms and physical signs of cardiac failure often do not suggest the cause. A CXR, ECG, blood count and serum biochemistry are mandatory. Echocardiography may provide additional information about systolic *and* diastolic ventricular function as well as valvular function. Medical management may include vasodilators, diuretics, digoxin and anticoagulation. The judicious use of β-blockers may have a place but their use remains controversial. A recent study has shown that carvedilol increases LV ejection fraction (LVEF) and reduces mortality. A small number of patients may derive benefit from coronary revascularizaton or valve surgery.

Valvular heart disease

Severe AS (valve area <0.6 cm^2) represents the greatest perioperative risk of all valve lesions – scoring three points on the Goldman CRI and 20 points on the modified CRI. The pathophysiology and haemodynamic anaesthetic goals are discussed in Chapter 31. Untreated hypotension rapidly becomes resistant to inotropes and vasopressors. CPB, which is unlikely to be immediately available, may be the only effective means of salvage. Although valve replacement almost invariably takes precedence over elective surgery, there are exceptions. The timing of surgery for some malignancies remains controversial. In some cases, the non-cardiac procedure should be undertaken *first* in a specialist cardiothoracic centre. The presence of MS may complicate non-cardiac surgery for three reasons: impaired LV filling, AF and anticoagulation. Ventricular rate control, as discussed in Chapter 32, is essential.

Chronic valvular regurgitation is generally better tolerated than stenosis. The principles of anaesthesia for non-cardiac surgery are no different from cardiac surgery (Chapters 31 and 32). In contrast, patients with acute valvular regurgitation (i.e. secondary to infective endocarditis or papillary muscle rupture) are unlikely to be referred for non-cardiac surgery.

Patients with mechanical prosthetic valves will be on warfarin therapy. Some elective surgery (e.g. hip surgery) will necessitate stopping warfarin several days before surgery. The risks of valve thrombosis and embolic problems are greater in the mitral than the aortic position and should be weighed against the risks of haemorrhage and transfusion. For many, the risks of bleeding far outweigh the small risk of stopping warfarin for a few days. Patients at high risk of thrombotic complications can however be switched to continuous heparin therapy the day before surgery with the infusion being discontinued 6 h before surgery. Appropriate antimicrobial prophylaxis should be given in accordance with published national guidelines.

Cardiomyopathy

Hypertrophic, dilated and restrictive cardiomyopathy are discussed in Chapter 39. Hypertrophic obstructive cardiomyopathy poses special problems due to a tendency to LVOT obstruction. Hypotension should generally be treated with volume and β-blockers rather than catecholamines.

Dysrhythmias

Ventricular ectopy is a significant cardiovascular risk factor (Table 66.4) and pharmacological attempts to eliminate them do not appear to improve the outcome. The incidence of AF increases with age and with LA enlargement. The consequent reduction in CO may be poorly tolerated and if the onset is recent, cardioversion should be considered. Patients with long-standing AF should be anticoagulated and have their ventricular rate controlled.

Pacemakers and implantable defibrillators

It is important to establish the indication for implantation and to consider the influence of the device on the surgical procedure as well as the impact of the procedure on the device. The management of patients with implantable devices is discussed in Chapter 37.

Carotid bruit

The presence of a carotid bruit may suggest extracranial vascular disease but gives no indication of location or severity. As the increased risk of perioperative stroke, a history of transient (i.e. dysphasia, amaurosis fugax and tingling) or permanent neurological impairment should be sought in all cases. Symptomatic patient should undergo further non-invasive evaluation to establish cerebrovascular risk and the need for endarterectomy.

Key points

- Considerable effort has been expended in determining the perioperative risks of non-cardiac surgery in patients with CVD.
- The risk of perioperative cardiovascular complications is dependent on cardiovascular risk factors, patient age *and* the type of surgery to be undertaken.
- It is interesting to note that two apparently contradictory regimes, namely β-blockade and supra-normalization of oxygen consumption have each been purported to show impressive improvements.
- With our current level of knowledge the best advice is *keep the diseased heart within its optimal working conditions*.

Further reading

American College of Physicians. Guidelines for assessing and managing the perioperative risk from coronary artery disease associated with major noncardiac surgery. *Ann Intern Med* 1997; **127(4)**: 309–312.

Biccard BM. Peri-operative beta-blockade and haemodynamic optimisation in patients with coronary artery disease and decreasing exercise capacity presenting for major non-cardiac surgery. *Anaesthesia* 2004; **59(1)**: 60–68.

Detsky AS, Abrams HB, McLaughlin JR, Drucker DJ, Sasson Z, Johnston N *et al.* Predicting cardiac complications in patients undergoing non-cardiac surgery. *J Gen Intern Med* 1986; **1(4)**: 211–219.

Eagle KA, Brundage BH, Chaitman BR, Ewy GA, Fleisher LA, Hertzer NR *et al.* Guidelines for perioperative cardiovascular evaluation for noncardiac surgery. Report of the American College of Cardiology/American Heart Association Task Force on Practice Guidelines. Committee on Perioperative Cardiovascular Evaluation for Noncardiac Surgery. *Circulation* 1996; **93(6)**: 1278–1317.

Hlatky MA, Boineau RE, Higginbotham MB, Lee KL, Mark DB, Califf RM *et al.* A brief self-administered questionnaire to determine functional capacity (the Duke Activity Status Index). *Am J Cardiol* 1989; **64(10)**: 651–654.

Palda VA, Detsky AS. Perioperative assessment and management of risk from coronary artery disease. *Ann Intern Med* 1997; **127(4)**: 313–328.

INDEX

Note: page numbers in **bold** denote tables and displayed information.